Graves' Disease

Edited by Robert Gensure

Published in London, United Kingdom

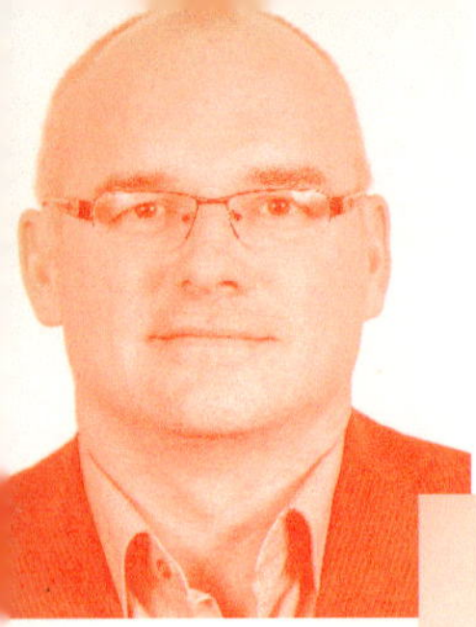
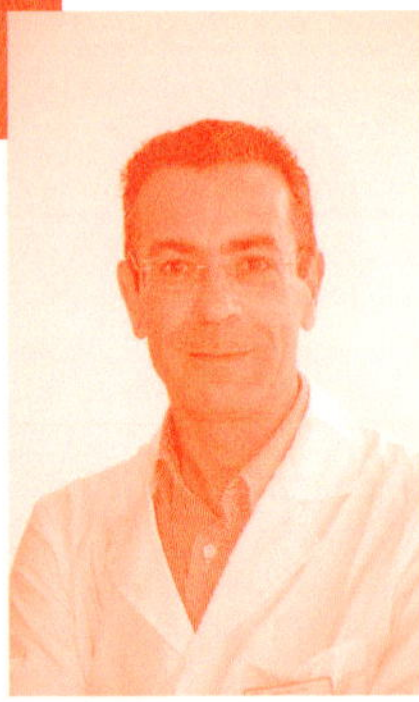
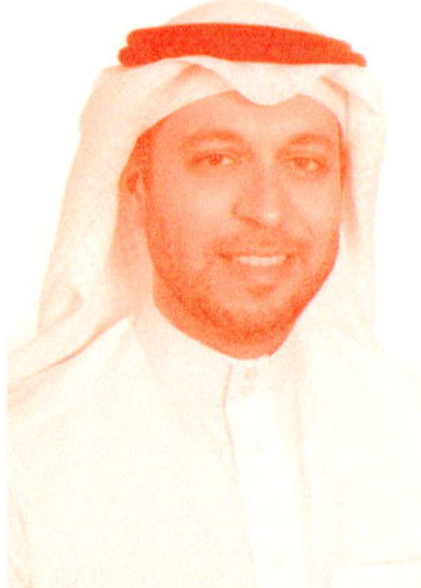
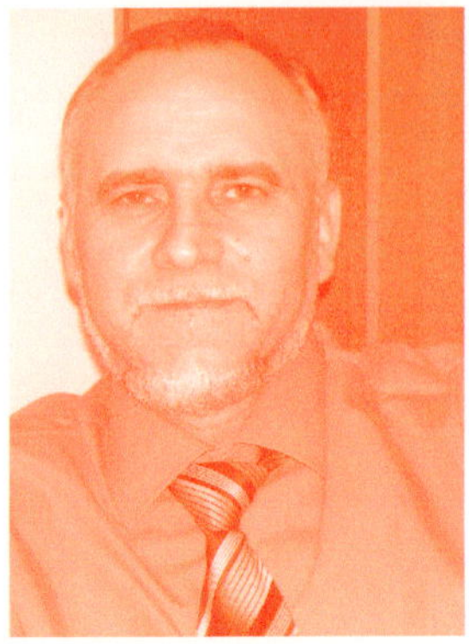
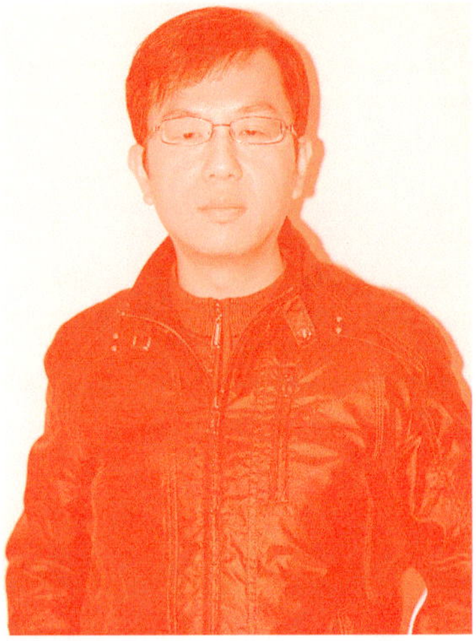
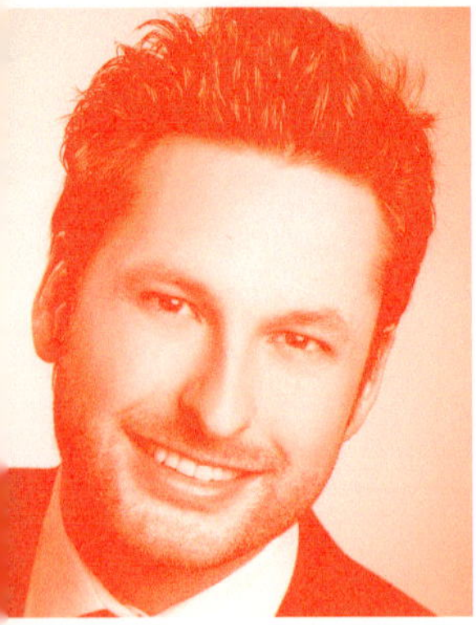
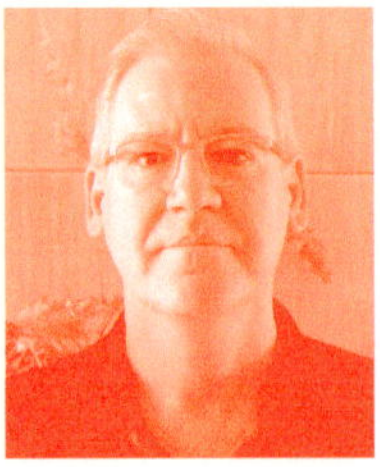

IntechOpen

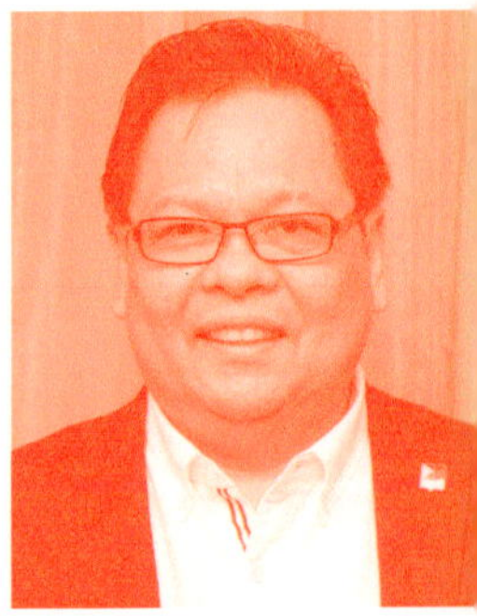
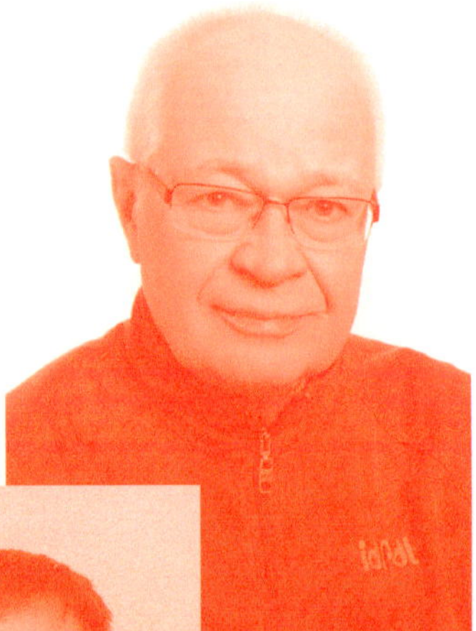
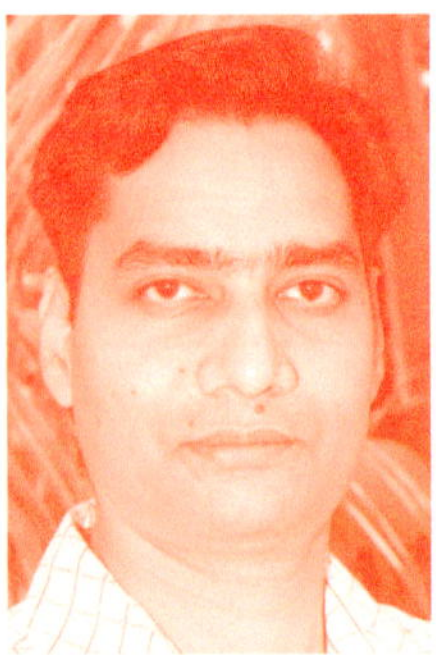
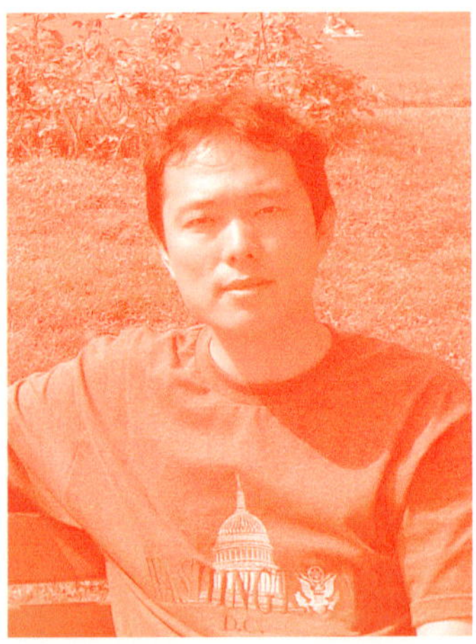
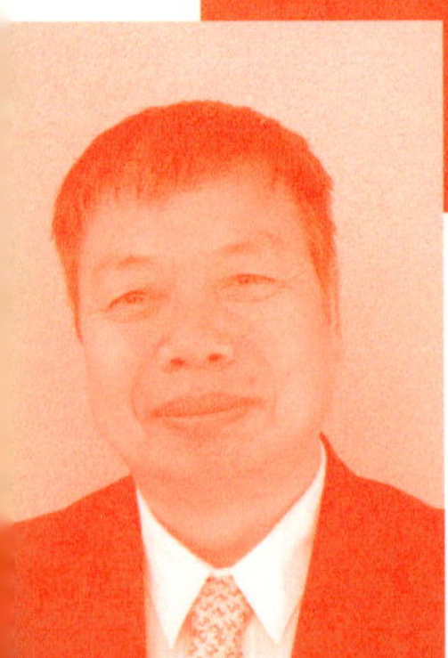
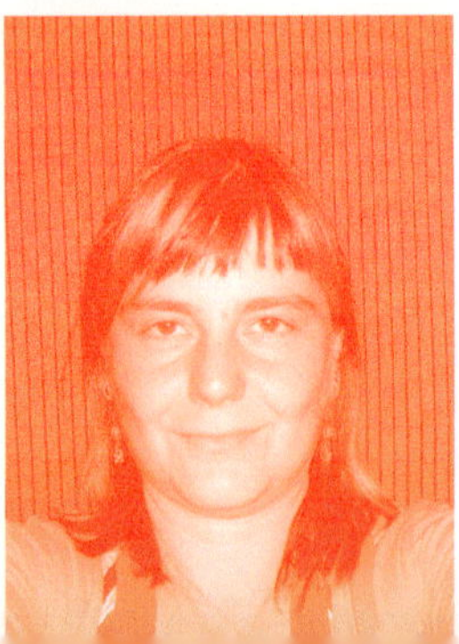

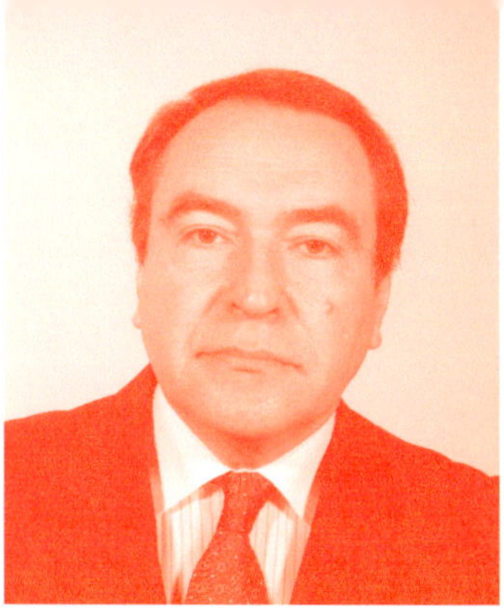
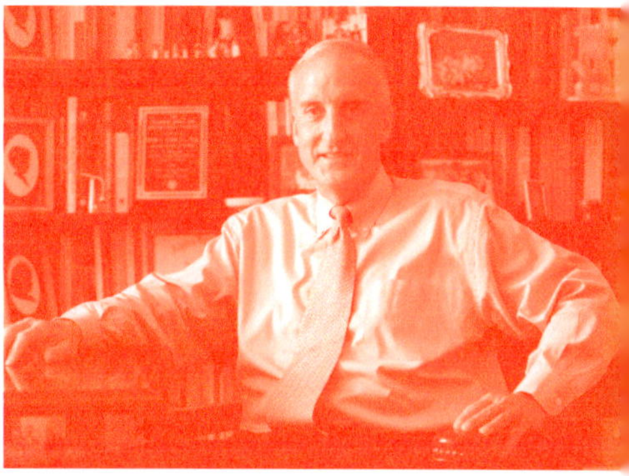
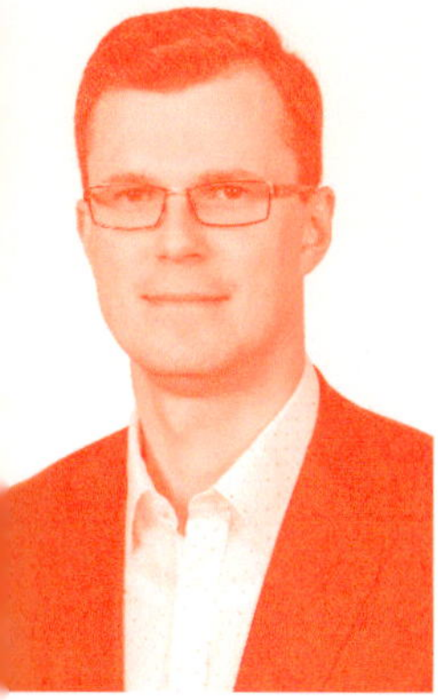
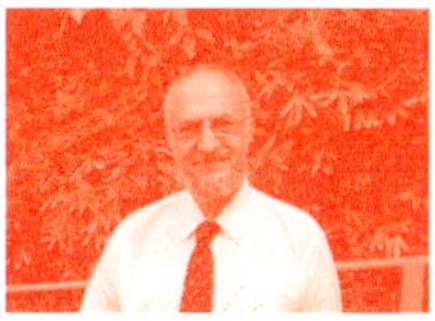
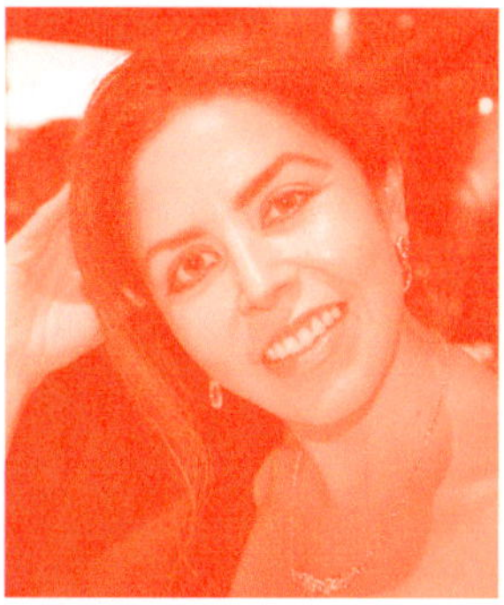

Supporting open minds since 2005

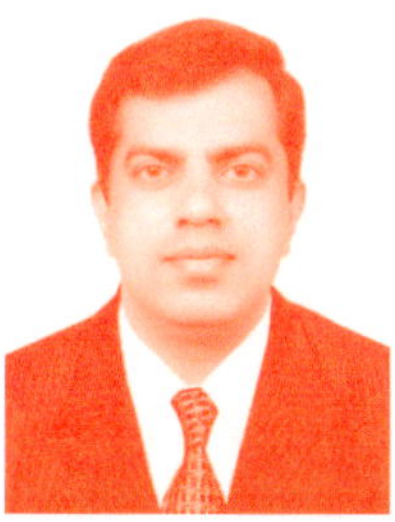
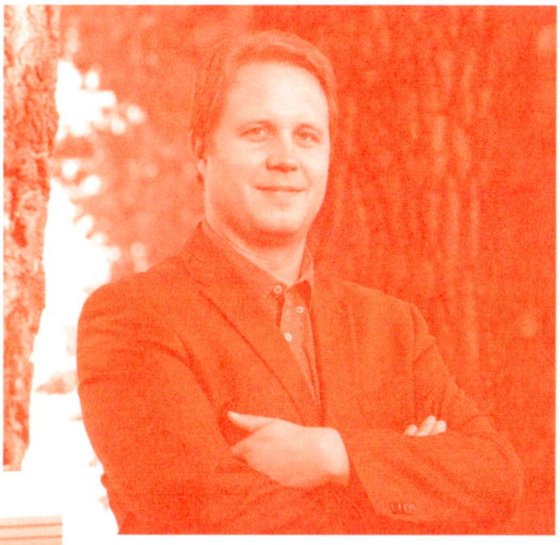
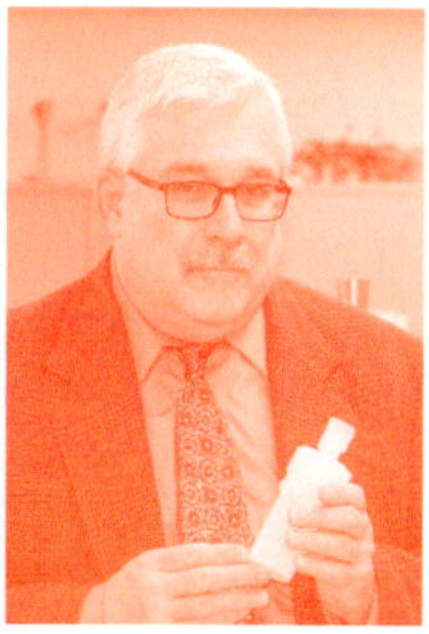
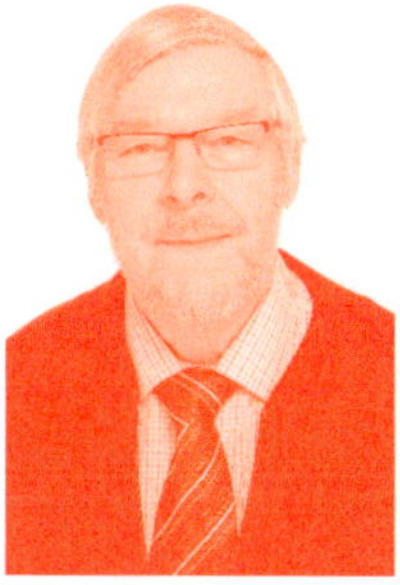
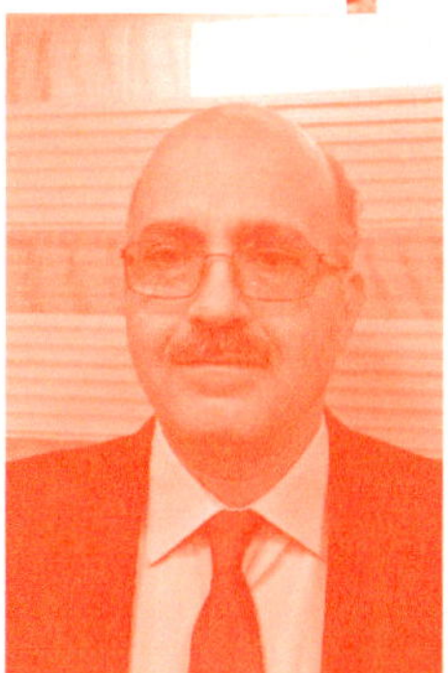
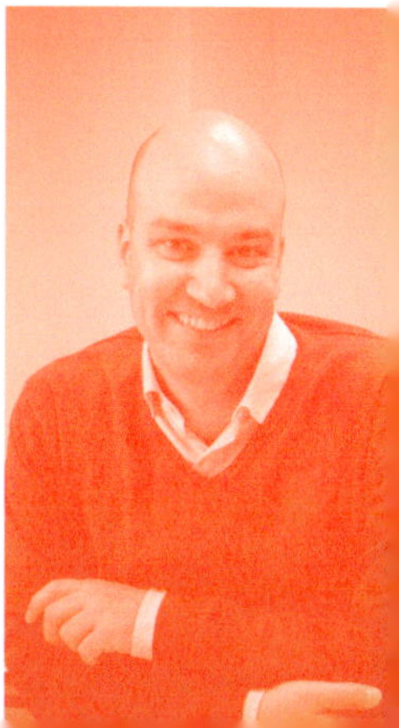
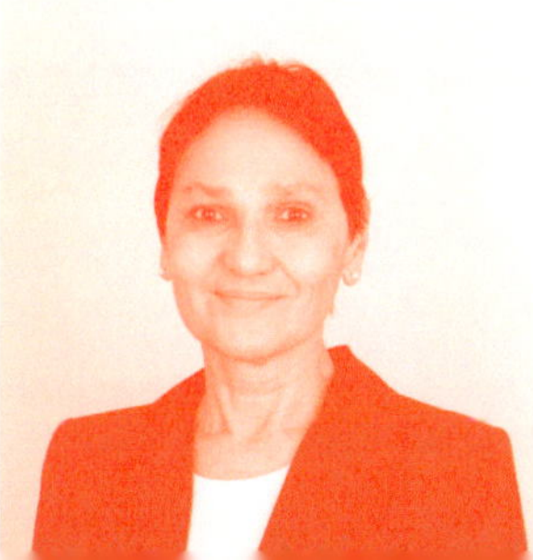

Graves' Disease
http://dx.doi.org/10.5772/intechopen.91498
Edited by Robert Gensure

Contributors
Madhukar Mittal, Vanishri Ganakumar, Sanjay Saran, Ildikó Molnár, Hakan Altay, Abdulla Arslan, Thenmozhi Paluchamy, Aisyah Elliyanti, Anca Panaitescu, Nikolay Botushanov, Aleksandar Botushanov, Albena Botushanova, Mauricio Alvarez Andrade, Lorena Pabón Duarte, Artur Tadeusz Bossowski, Karolina Stożek, Mosin S. Saleem Khan, Suhail S. Lone, Sabhiya Majid, Sunia Shah, Iqra Farooq, Ioannis Iakovou, Evanthia Giannoula, Paraskevi Exadaktylou, Nikitas Papadopoulos, Paula Aragão Prazeres de Oliveira, Eduarda da Silva Souza Paulino, Paula Gabriele Tabosa Lyra, Fernanda Carolinne Marinho de Araujo, Beatriz ONayara Muniz de Oliveira, Anand Kumar Mishra, Kul Ranjan Singh, Ágota Muzsnai, Vasudha Bakshi, Gollapalli Rajeev Kumar, Aulanni'am Aulanniam, Djoko Wahono Wahono Soeatmadji, Zulkarnain Zulkarnain, Dyah Kinasih Wuragil, Yudit Oktanella

First published in London, United Kingdom, 2021 by IntechOpen
IntechOpen is the global imprint of INTECHOPEN LIMITED, registered in England and Wales, registration number: 11086078, 5 Princes Gate Court, London, SW7 2QJ, United Kingdom
Printed in Croatia

British Library Cataloguing-in-Publication Data
A catalogue record for this book is available from the British Library

Additional hard and PDF copies can be obtained from orders@intechopen.com

Graves' Disease
Edited by Robert Gensure
p. cm.
Print ISBN 978-1-83968-773-0
Online ISBN 978-1-83968-774-7
eBook (PDF) ISBN 978-1-83968-775-4

For EU product safety concerns:
IN TECH d.o.o., Prolaz Marije Krucifikse Kozulić 3, 51000 Rijeka, Croatia, info@intechopen.com or visit our website at intechopen.com.

Meet the editor

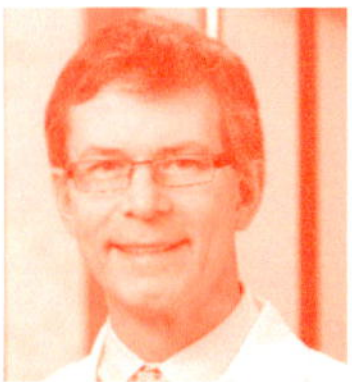

Robert Gensure, MD, Ph.D., is a physician-scientist with significant experience in basic science and clinical research as well as in the clinical practice of pediatric endocrinology. He has authored forty-six publications on topics including parathyroid hormone function, vitamin D supplementation, and inherited disorders of bone and mineral metabolism. He is currently Chief of Pediatric Endocrinology at Tufts Medical Center, Boston, MA.

Contents

Preface

Graves' Disease was first described in 1835, taking its name from the physician who identified it, Dr. Robert Graves. The disorder is caused by autoantibodies to the thyroid gland that mimic thyroid-stimulating hormone (TSH), causing the gland to overproduce thyroid hormone. This speeds up the metabolism of the patient and can lead to dangerous conditions including atrial fibrillation and heart failure. Mainstays of treatment have included antithyroid medication, surgical removal of the thyroid gland, and more recently, radiofrequency ablation of the thyroid gland. Enhancements in diagnostic testing have in turn enhanced our understanding of the natural course of the disease, creating additional therapeutic options. Furthermore, enhanced understanding of the autoimmunity behind the disorder may lead to therapeutic options that address the underlying autoimmunity. This book provides a comprehensive review of these enhancements and how they have resulted in changes in common clinical practice.

Regarding diagnostic testing, there have been improvements in serum assays that allow better characterization of the degree of hyperthyroidism and monitoring of the underlying autoimmune response. The lower limit of detectability of TSH assays has improved and can distinguish between suppression and the low end of the normal range more reliably. Free T4 measurements have effectively replaced the total T4/T3 uptake/TSI combination, allowing direct assessment of bioavailable thyroid hormone and avoiding confounding by variations in thyroglobulin levels. These improvements allow medical therapy to be titrated more effectively to achieve a euthyroid state. TSI assays have improved in accuracy and speed such that the diagnosis of Graves' Disease can often be made without the aid of a thyroid scan.

Remission was thought to be a rare event in adults (more common in children), but this may have been the result of the inability to assess the underlying immune response in a patient receiving medical treatment. Assays for thyroid-stimulating antibodies have improved in accuracy and reliability, and most importantly, the reporting time has decreased from a month to several days. Rather than treating blindly for a fixed amount of time and then initiating a trial of therapy, TSI monitoring allows for withdrawal of treatment when the thyroid-stimulating antibody levels have normalized. This has also improved our understanding of the natural course of the disorder. In particular, the appearance of a second remission after a relapse is now a recognized phenomenon and corresponds to the 'waxing and waning course of other autoimmune disorders.

The mainstays of treatment for Graves' Disease remain medical therapy with thiozonamides and/or iodine to inhibit the thyroid gland, with surgery and radiofrequency ablation providing more definitive therapy. The outcome of more definitive therapy is usually hypothyroidism, which then must be treated with levothyroxine. This is still considered the superior option, as levothyroxine is safe for long-term therapy, but it is still unsatisfying trading one disease for another. Clearly, this is an area where further advances are needed. Likewise, while our understanding of Graves' ophthalmopathy has improved, our capacity to manage it remains limited, typically involving courses of high-dose steroids.

Management of Graves' Disease in children has also benefited from advances in diagnostic and therapeutic tools. TSI monitoring is now an option in neonatal Graves' Disease, although the mix of stimulating and blocking antibodies in this condition still creates challenges to maintain a euthyroid state. Routine use of free T4 measurements (vs total T4) has been especially helpful, as for children, conditions of high or low thyroid-binding globulin may not yet have been discovered. Most importantly, radioactive iodine (RAI) therapy has been extended to ages younger than 18 years. Concerns were raised after the Chernobyl accident regarding increased risk for children of thyroid cancer after exposure to RAI. However, these appear to be the result of tissue damage after low-level radiation exposure and have not been seen after higher doses of RAI in RAI therapy.

As we learn more about the underlying autoimmunity in Graves' Disease, it is intriguing to postulate how future therapies might target this immune response rather than targeting the thyroid gland itself. As it stands now, the definitive therapies for Graves' Disease result in hypothyroidism and the need for lifelong thyroid replacement therapy. This is a superior option to current immune-suppression therapies, which have potentially dangerous side-effect profiles. However, these side effects result not from suppression of TSI production, but rather from suppression of immune function in infection and tumor surveillance. One could imagine a more targeted immune suppressant, which selectively lowers TSI, as a superior option to conventional therapy. While such therapies may seem unrealistic today, we did see similar advancements in targeted radiofrequency ablation of the thyroid gland, which avoids the complications seen with whole-body radiation treatments used for cancer therapy.

Robert Gensure, M.D./Ph.D.
Tufts Medical Center,
Boston, MA, USA

Section 1

Overview of Graves' Disease

Chapter 1

Graves' Disease: Clinical Significance and Management

Thenmozhi Paluchamy

Abstract

Graves' Disease is an autoimmune disease characterized by hyperthyroidism due to circulating autoantibodies. Graves' Disease was originally known as "exophthalmic goiter" but is now named after Sir Robert Graves, an Irish doctor who first described the condition in 1835. A number of conditions can cause hyperthyroidism, but Graves' Disease is the most common, affecting around 1 in 200 people. It most often affects women under the age of 40, but it is also found in men. It affects an estimated 2–3 percent of the world's population. Thyroid-stimulating immunoglobulin (TSIs) binds to and activates thyrotropin receptors, causing the thyroid gland to grow and the thyroid follicles to increase synthesis of thyroid hormone. The overproduction of thyroid hormones can have a variety of effects on the body causes exophthalmic goiter, Graves ophthalmopathy, Graves dermopathy etc.,. Thyroid profile including antithyroid antibodies, radioactive iodine uptake study, and thyroid scan are the main diagnostic investigations to rule out Graves' Disease. The major aim of the treatment is to inhibit the overproduction of thyroid hormones by targeting the thyroid gland, to reduce the symptoms, and prevention of complication is also major challenges.

Keywords: anti-thyroid drug, autoimmune thyroid disease, goiter, Graves' Disease, Graves ophthalmopathy, hyperthyroidism, thyroglobulin, thyroidectomy, thyrotropine receptor antibody, radioactive iodine

1. Introduction

Thyroid diseases are one of the most common endocrinopathies globally [1]. The thyroid gland is a small, butterfly-shaped endocrine gland located in the lower front of the neck synthesizes and secretes mainly two hormones i.e., T4 (Thyroxine) and T3 (Triiodothyronine) [2] into the blood and then carried to every tissues in the body. TSH stands for thyroid stimulating hormone, which is produced by the pituitary gland of the brain. This gland stimulates the thyroid to synthesize and release the thyroid hormones into the blood. Thyroid hormones act on almost all nucleated cells and are essential for normal growth and energy metabolism1. It also controls the body temperature, menstrual cycles, the functioning of the lungs, heart & muscle strength and ancillary vital organs [3]. When thyroid gland secretes either too much or too little of the thyroid hormones T4 and T3, it's called a thyroid disease. There are several different types of thyroid disease, including hyperthyroidism, hypothyroidism, thyroid cancer, thyroiditis, and autoimmune thyroid disease.

Graves' Disease is an autoimmune disorder that leads to overactivity of the entire thyroid gland due to circulating autoantibodies. The synonyms of Graves' Disease are Basedow disease, exophthalmic goiter, Graves' hyperthyroidism, Parry disease and toxic diffuse goiter [4]. Graves' Disease is the commonest cause of hyperthyroidism. Graves' Disease was originally known as exophthalmic goiter but now it is named after Sir Robert Graves, an Irish physician, who described this form of hyperthyroidism in 1830s [5]. Autoimmune thyroid disease ranges from one end of Hashimoto's hypothyroidism (HH) to another end of Graves' hyperthyroidism (GH). Autoimmune diseases are characterized by the activity of autoreactive lymphocytes, which cause tissue or organ damage through the formation of antibodies that react against host tissues, or effector T cells, which are specific for endogenous self-peptides [6]. Thyroid peroxidase (TPO) and thyroglobulin (Tg) are the major autoantigens in Hashimoto's disease whereas in Graves' Disease TPO-Ab and Tg-Ab are also occur in 70% of patients with Graves' Disease [7], but The thyroid-stimulating hormone receptor (TSHR) is the major autoantigen in Graves' Disease. The antibody called thyrotropin receptor antibody (TRAb) and thyroid-stimulating immunoglobulins (TSIs) bind to and activate thyrotropin receptors, causing the thyroid gland to grow and the thyroid follicles to increase synthesis of thyroid hormone.

Graves' Disease is not only affecting the thyroid and often affecting the skin and eyes named as Graves' dermopathy, Graves' orbitopathy and Graves' ophthalmopathy. The overproduction of thyroid hormones can have a variety of effects on the other body systems too. About 3 in every 4 people with an overactive thyroid gland have a condition called Graves' Disease [8]. Graves' Disease is considered to be an autoimmune disorder, but other causes may contribute to its development, including genetic, environmental, and/or other factors. Graves' Disease usually affects people between ages 30 and 50, but can occur at any age [9]. The disease is seven to eight times more common in women than men [10].

2. Epidemiology

Graves' Disease occurs in almost any part of the world. Graves' Disease is the most common causes of spontaneous thyrotoxicosis and it represents 60–90% of all causes of thyrotoxicosis in different regions of the world and it is estimated to affect 2–3 percent of the world's population [4]. Graves' Disease is the most common cause of hyperthyroidism in the United States. The incidence of Graves' Disease in Olmstead County was found to be 30 cases per 100,000 annually [11]. The overall prevalence of hyperthyroidism in the United States is 1.2% with an incidence of 20/100,000 to 50/100,000 in a study conducted in Olmstead County, Minnesota. The incidence of Graves' Disease was 24.8 cases per 100,000 with an adjusted female to male ratio of 3.9:1 [12, 13] but studies specifically on Graves' Disease are rare [14]. In Canada, Graves' Disease is the most common cause of hyperthyroidism affecting one in every 100 people. It appears to becoming even more common. In the Wickham Study in the United Kingdom, the incidence of Graves' Disease was reported to be 100–200 cases per 100,000 population per year which is significantly higher than previous estimates [15] and among women, it has been reported to be 80 cases 100,000 per year [16]. The age adjusted incidence of adult onset Graves' Disease in Sheffield, UK was 24.8 per 100,000 per year. It is more common in women than men and the most common in people with ages 20 to 50 years and the risk for Graves' Disease in women and men are 3% and 0.5%. The 12-year incidence of Graves' Disease among women with 25 to 42 years was as high as 4.6/1000 as per Nurses' Health Study II report. The ratio of 3.9:1 reported in this study is however in keeping with other studies in Iceland and Sweden that reported a gender ratio of 4:1 in hyperthyroidism in general [16]. In Sweden, the reported incidence of Graves' Disease (2003–2005) was 21.4 per 100,000 per year with a Female:Male ratio of 5.6:1 [17].

The prevalence of maternal thyrotoxicosis is approximately 1 case per 500 persons, with maternal Graves' Disease being the most common etiology [10]. Graves' Disease is observed with a rate of 0.1–0.4% in pregnant women [18]. Aside from the infrequent occurrence of postnatal thyrotoxicosis due to maternal antibodies, the incidence of spontaneous Graves' Disease in children before the age of ten is most unusual, but the incidence climbs with each decade until about age 60 [14–15, 19] . Pediatric Graves' Disease accounts for 10–15% of thyroid disorders in patients less than 18 years of age [20]. Graves' Disease is rare under the age of 5 years and has a peak incidence at 10–15 years of age [21]. The incidence of Graves' Disease is believed to be between 0.1 and 3 per 100,000 children [22] with a prevalence of 1 in 10,000 children in the United States [23]. A study found that out of 57 patients with the average age of the 32.8 years, male:female ratio of 1:3.3, 52 (91%) had subacute thyroiditis as the cause of thyrotoxicosis while Graves' Disease was seen in 9% [24]. The Graves' Disease affecting all countries and races equally across the world and it occurs eight times more common in women than men between 30 to 60 years of age group [14, 15].

3. Causes

Graves' Disease is caused by a malfunction in the body's disease-fighting immune system. The immune system usually produces antibodies against the target specific antigens such as bacteria, virus, or other foreign substance. In Graves' Disease, the immune system produces an antibody against the own cell of the thyroid gland. Normally, thyroid gland function is regulated by a hormone thyroid-releasing hormone (TRH) which is secreted from the posterior lobe of the pituitary gland. The immune system produces antibodies called thyrotropin receptor antibody (TRAb) that trigger the TSH receptor, tricking and dominance over the normal function of the thyroid gland and also causing an oversecretion of thyroid hormones. However the exact cause for Graves' Disease is not well understood. Despite there are risk factors like a combination of genetic and environmental factors which triggered the immune system against the thyroid.

4. Risk factors

Although anyone can develop Graves' Disease, many factors (**Table 1**) can increase the risk of disease, including:

Genetic	Environmental Agents
• Genetic background: family history of thyroid disease	• Infectious agents
• Race	• Dietary Iodine
• Age	• Dietary Selenium
• Gender: Women	• Pregnancy and the Postpartum Period
• Other autoimmune disorders	• Medication: (amiodarone,
o Type 1 diabetes	• interferon-a (IFN-a), and CD52 MABs)
o Rheumatoid arthritis	• Smoking
o Pernicious anemia	• Stress
o Lupus erthymatosus	• Radiation Exposure
o Addison's disease	• Toxicants
o Vitiligo	
o Crohn's disease	

Table 1.
Risk factors of Graves' Disease.

4.1 Heredity/genetics

Family history of Graves' Disease is a known risk factor; there is likely a gene or genes that can make a person more susceptible to the disorder. 70%–80% of susceptibility to autoimmune thyroid disease is based on genetics; individuals with a personal history of autoimmune disease or family history of autoimmune thyroid disease are the most susceptible. The specific genes involved include human leukocyte antigen-DR3, cytotoxic T lymphocyte-associated factor 4, CD40, protein tyrosine phosphotase-22 gene, thyroglobulin (Tg), and TSH receptor [25]. Graves' Disease include genes encoding thyroglobulin, thyrotropin receptor, HLA-DRβ-Arg74, the protein tyrosine phosphatase nonreceptor type 22 (PTPN22), and proteins involved in T cell signaling [26–28]. HLA-DRB1 and HLA-DQB1 also appear to be associated with Graves' Disease susceptibility. Cytotoxic T lymphocyte-associated molecule-4 (CTLA4) is a major thyroid autoantibody susceptibility gene, [29, 30] and it is a negative regulator of T-cell activation and may play an important role in the pathogenesis of Graves' Disease. Heredity increases genetic susceptibility to environmental triggers.

4.1.1 Race

The loci associated with autoimmune thyroid diseases are AITD1, CTLA4, GD1, GD2, GD3, HT1, and HT2 among white race and also different loci have been linked in persons of other races. The more susceptible to occur autoimmune thyroid disease is influenced by gene in human leukocyte antigen region on chromosome 6 and in *CTLA4* on band 2q33. It is associated with specific HLA haplotypes and vary with ethnicity [10].

4.1.2 Gender

Women are much more likely to develop Graves' Disease than are men. Women develop it seven to eight times more frequently than men [10] and are due to the production of special proteins (called antibodies) that attack the thyroid gland. The ratio of developing Graves' hyperthyroidism between women and men is 7:1 and is often mediated with either more estrogen or less testosterone and also observed that moderate amounts of estrogen enhance immunologic reactivity [31–33]. However, the X-chromosome is the source of the increased susceptibility rather than sex steroid since the susceptibility continues after the menopause and X-chromosome inactivation has been linked with autoimmune thyroid disease [34].

4.1.3 Age

Typically, Graves' Disease is a disease of young women, but it may occur in persons of any age. Graves' Disease is usually occur in people between ages 30 and 50 years but can occur at any age. The typical age range is 20–40 years and the most affected women are aged 30–60 years [35].

4.1.4 Other autoimmune disorders

People with other autoimmune disorders are more likely to develop Graves' Disease than people without these disorders such as type 1 diabetes, rheumatoid arthritis, pernicious anemia, lupus erthymatosus, addison's disease, vitiligo, or crohn's disease.

4.2 Environmental agents

The remaining 20%–30% contribution to the onset of autoimmune thyroid disease is thought to be due to environmental exposures or triggers. Interfere with thyroid function at multiple sites, including thyroid hormone synthesis, thyroid hormone metabolism and excretion, and thyroid hormone action [36–39]. Most of these agents may influence the pituitary and thyrotropin (TSH) secretion, or even be partial thyroid hormone receptor agonists. There are a number of exposures that have been identified and proposed, both from human and animal studies (11–14) [40–43]. These include infections, life stress, iodine intake, smoking, medications such as amiodarone and interferon, radiation, and environmental toxicants. The environmental parameters commonly reported as contributing factors are infectious agents, iodine, drugs (amiodarone, Interferon-a (IFN-a), and CD52 MABs), tobacco, and stress [44].

4.2.1 Infection

Autoimmune thyroiditis can be induced in experimental animals by certain viral infections. Graves' Disease has been associated with a variety of infectious agents such as Yersinia enterocolitica and Borrelia burgdorferi. Homologies have been shown between proteins of these organisms and thyroid autoantigens [45, 46]. Thyroid autoimmune disease is associated with infections in the thyroid gland itself such as subacute thyroiditis, congenital rubella etc., and could initiate class II molecule expression. When Hepatitis C infection is treated with interferon therapy is a well-recognized precipitator of autoimmune thyroid disease, although less commonly a Graves' Disease develops rather than thyroiditis [47].

4.2.2 Stress

Both physical and emotional stressful life events and illness may act as a trigger for the onset of Graves' Disease among people who have genes that increase their risk. A review of the literature including seven case–control studies has highlighted the preexistence of a 'negative' stressful event in patients with Graves' Disease [48–55]. In general, stress suppresses the immune function, possibly mediated by the actions of cortisol on immune cells. Stress-induced suppression may be followed by rebound immunologic hyperactivity which could precipitate autoimmune thyroid disease in genetically susceptible individuals. The major T helper cells involved in Graves' Disease is Th2 and more recently found that Th17 is favor for the production of the pathogenic antibody directed against the TSH receptor by B lymphocytes both in mice and humans. Stress hormones direct stimulate the Th2, and Th17 or Th1 and also induce IL4, IL6, and IL12 by dentritic cells. Stress causes immature DCs which induce apoptosis in Treg cells leads not to act like regulators of Th2 and Th17 effector cells. It has been found that patients with untreated Graves' Disease have low in Treg cells which is inversely correlated with serum concentration of TSH receptor antibodies [56].

4.2.3 Pregnancy and the postpartum period

Pregnancy or recent childbirth may increase the risk of the disorder, particularly among women who have genes that increase their risk. The immune suppression is associated with the onset of autoimmune diseases especially postpartum thyroiditis. Fetal microchimerism, fetal cells in maternal tissue has maternal immune response is recognized as a trigger for thyroid autoimmunity and development of postpartum autoimmune thyroid disease [57]. During pregnancy severe Graves' Disease is uncommon because hyperthyroidism is associated with increased pregnancy loss pregnancy loss and reduced fertility. Even if pregnancy occurs it can cause complication to mother as well fetus. Both B-cell and T-cell functions are declined during pregnancy, while Tregs increase dampening the disease [44, 58]. After delivery, the slow rebound from immunosuppression results in immune reactivity which contributes to the occurrence of postpartum thyroid disease, including recurrence or the new onset of Graves' Disease [59]. Around 30 percent of young women have a history of pregnancy in the 12 months before the onset of Graves' Disease [60], which shows that postpartum Graves' Disease is a surprisingly common condition and that pregnancy is a major risk factor for susceptible women.

4.2.4 Smoking

Cigarette smoke contains cyanide, which is metabolized to thiocyante, and can interfere with iodine concentration in the thyroid [37]. Cigarette Smoking has been associated with an increased production of T3 and thyroglobulin [61, 62], affect the thyroid hormone action [63], enhanced sympathetic nervous activity, or by affecting thyroid-directed autoimmune responses [49, 62, 64–66]. Cigarette smoking causes complex interactions with the immune system which may increase cytokines in orbit and thyroid causes Graves' Disease and also smokers who have Graves' Disease exacerbating risk of developing Graves' ophthalmopathy [41, 67–68].

4.2.5 Dietary iodine

Iodine is essential for thyroid hormone production, although a number of regulatory factors allow a normal amount of thyroid hormone to be produced across a fairly wide range of iodine intake. Deficient iodine intake is well known to be associated with reduced thyroid hormone production. Excess iodine, however, can also have adverse effects depending on underlying thyroid function, as well as the extent and duration of iodine excess [69]. Patients with multinodular goiter and associated areas of autonomous, TSH-independent, thyroid hormone production can have excess thyroid hormone production in response to iodine, the Jod–Basedow effect. Increased immunogenicity of thyroglobulin, thyroid cell destruction, In response to iodine supplementation in areas of iodine deficiency, there is an increase in thyroid autoantibodies and in some cases autoimmune thyroid disease [42, 43, 70, 71]. The mechanism of stimulation of autoimmune thyroid disease in response to iodine supplementation is not established. Excess iodine intake is associated with highly iodinated Tg, which is thought to be more immunogenic than poorly iodinated Tg [42, 70].

4.2.6 Dietary selenium

Selenium interacts with immune response. Low selenium intake has been associated with an increase in thyroid autoantibodies, and selenium supplementation with a reduction in antibodies [41].

4.2.7 Medications

Medications associated with the onset of autoimmune thyroid disease include lithium, amiodarone, interferon α, interleukin 2, campath-1 h, and highly active anti-retroviral therapy [42]. Some medications, such as lithium, may not trigger autoimmunity, but accelerate the autoimmune process by interfering with thyroid function. It may stimulate the immune response at multiple sites. Medications differ in their mechanisms of stimulating thyroid autoimmunity, as well as the relative effect on promoting hypothyroidism or Graves' Disease [41].

4.2.8 Radiation Exposure

Radiation exposure especially medical radiation is one of the environmental exposures linked to effects on the thyroid which stimulate thyroid autoantibodies, increases thyroid antigens, inflammation. Autoimmune thyroid disease has been linked to therapeutic medical radiation [72–74]. Patients receiving 131I for thyroid disorder develop Graves' Disease later in their life and, sometimes, it can lead Graves' ophthalmopathy [73]. Radiation therapy with 131I causes low level thyroid autoantibody positivity in a sensitive TSH receptor antibody measurement which was associated with the development of Graves' Disease [73].

4.2.9 Toxicants

The main sources of toxicants are industrial chemicals, pesticides and herbicides, toxins in consumer goods, and heavy metals which may impair the thyroid function by recruiting antibodies to attack the thyroid. Most municipal water sources are now closely monitored for a range of toxicants, including those that affect the thyroid and well water also to be tested regularly for contaminants [75, 76].

5. Pathophysiology

Hypothalamic–pituitary-thyroid axis feedback mechanism is controlled the secretion of thyroid hormone by involving the interaction of stimulatory and inhibitory factors. Hypothalamus secretes Thyrotropin-releasing hormone (TRH) which stimulates the anterior lobe of pituitary gland to release Thyroid Stimulating Hormone (TSH). TSH binds with receptors on the thyroid gland leads to the release of thyroid hormones primarily T4 and to a lesser extent T3. Elevated levels of these hormones act on the hypothalamus to decrease TRH secretion and thus the synthesis of TSH and vice versa. Iodine requires for the synthesis of thyroid hormone. Dietary inorganic iodide is carried to the thyroid gland by iodide transporter. In the presence of thyroid peroxidase enzyme inorganic iodide is converted to iodine and bound to thyroglobulin through a process called organification. This causes the formation of Monoiodotyrosine (MIT) and Diiodotyrosine (DIT) and coupled to form triiodothyronine (T3) and thyroxine (T4) and then stored in the thyroid's follicular lumen with thyroglobulin. These preformed hormones which diffuse into the peripheral circulation form thyroid gland. In the peripheral circulation more than 99.9% of T4 and T3 are in inactive form. However, free T3 is 20–100 times more biologically active than free T4. Free T3 acts by binding to DNA-binding proteins in cell nuclei which regulate the transcription of various cellular proteins [77]. Any causes that alter the process leads to an increase in the peripheral circulation of unbound thyroid hormone can cause hyperthyroidism.

Thyroid Stimulating Hormone – Receptor (TSH-R) is a G-protein coupled receptor with seven transmembrane-spanning domains which primarily seen thyroid gland. It is also present in adipocytes, fibroblasts, bone cells and a variety of additional sites [78, 79]. TSHR regulates thyroid growth and thyroid hormone production and secretion and TSH also acting via TSHR. Hyperthyroidism in Graves' Disease manifested by the production of autoantibodies against the TSHR. These autoantibodies mimic the effects of the hormone on thyroid cells thereby stimulating autonomous production of T3 and T4. The derangement of immune function also lead to the production of pathologic autoantibodies complex by involving B and T cells which enhance the several autoantigens in addition to TSH-R. In Graves' Disease, B and T lymphocyte-mediated autoimmunity are known to be directed at 4 well-known thyroid antigens: thyroglobulin (Tg), thyroid peroxidase (TPO), sodium-iodide symporter and the thyrotropin receptor. Thyroid stimulating immunoglobulin binds with thyroid-stimulating hormone (TSH) receptor on the thyroid cell membrane and stimulates the action of the thyroid-stimulating hormone. It stimulates both, thyroid hormone synthesis and thyroid gland growth, causing hyperthyroidism and thyromegaly [3] The stimulating activity of thyrotropin receptor antibodies is found in the immunoglobulin G. Circulating autoantibodies against the thyrotropin receptor continuously stimulate the thyroid gland to increase the secretion of thyroid hormone and thyroglobulin that is mediated by 3,'5'-cyclic adenosine monophosphate which suppresses the secretion of pituitary thyrotropin. These autoanitbodies also stimulate iodine uptake, protein synthesis, and thyroid gland growth [80].

Intrathyroidal lymphocytic infiltration observed in initial histologic examination in autoimmune thyroid disease and can be correlated with thyroid antibodies titer. The thyroid cells express molecules due to being the source of autoantigens that mediate T cell adhesion and complement regulation such as Fas and cytokines which interact the immune system and also the proportion of CD4 lymphocytes is lower in the thyroid than in the peripheral blood. Besides being the source of autoantigens, the thyroid cells express molecules that mediate T cell adhesion and complement regulation (Fas and cytokines) that participate and interact with the immune system. In these patients, the proportion of CD4 lymphocytes is lower in the thyroid than in the peripheral blood. The increased Fas expression in intrathyroidal CD4 T lymphocytes causes CD4 lymphocyte reduction. The autoimmune thyroid disease susceptibility genes are CD40, CTLA-4, thyroglobulin, TSH receptor, and PTPN22 [25, 81] which specific either Graves' Disease or Hashimoto thyroiditis. The two new susceptibility loci are RNASET2-FGFR1OP-CCR6 region at 6q27 and an intergenic region at 4p14 [82]. Positive Graves' Disease is strongly associated with thyroid-stimulating hormone receptor and major histocompatibility complex variants with persistently thyroid stimulating hormone receptor autoantibodies. [83]

5.1 Graves' thyroid gland

The thyroid gland is diffusely enlarged but not always. The pathological change of the thyroid gland is follicular hyperplasia, intracellular colloid droplets, cell scalloping, a reduction in follicular colloid, and a patchy (multifocal) lymphocytic infiltration. The majority of intrathyroidal lymphocytes are T cells but plenty of B cells may be present. In some areas, thyroid epithelial cell size correlates with the intensity of the lymphocytic infiltrate, suggesting thyroid-cell stimulation by local B cells secreting stimulating TSHR-Ab [84].

5.2 Autoantibodies of thyroid

Thyroid autoantibodies, including TSHR-Abs secretes spontaneously from lymphocytes of Graves' thyroid tissue in activated state [85]. It may also secretes activated autoantibodies when decline in serum thyroid autoantibody concentrations after antithyroid drug treatment, after thyroidectomy, and late after radioactive iodine therapy.

5.3 TSH receptor and autoantibodies

Long-acting thyroid stimulator (LATS) was found among patients with Graves' hyperthyroidism [86] and it is proved to be an immunoglobulin which inhibited the binding of radiolabeled thyroid stimulating hormone to thyroid membranes due to the presence of antibodies to the TSH receptor (TSHR-Ab) [87].

5.4 TSHR agonists and antagonists

The characteristics TSHR-Abs are stimulatory or inhibitory or neutral. In case of Hashimoto's thyroiditis, block the binding and action of TSH and, therefore, can cause hypothyroidism. Whereas in Graves' Disease, TSHR-Abs has both stimulating and blocking thereby the clinical presentation may manifest depend upon a balance between these different antibodies. In third category, TSHR-Abs is of the neutral variety which may bind to the receptor but not influencing thyroid stimulating hormone binding. However, these antibodies may not be entirely neutral and can have cell signaling capability of untoward changes [88].

5.5 Similarities with autoimmune thyroiditis

- Lymphocytic infiltration of the thyroid and anti-Tg and anti-TPO antibodies in the serum occur in both Graves' Disease and chronic autoimmune (Hashimoto's) thyroiditis

- The genetic susceptibility of both disorders is HLA

- Areas of cellular apoptosis may be seen even in Graves' thyroid glands [89, 90].

- The presence of antibodies that bind to the TSH receptor in both disorders and differ in biological activities

- Progression from Graves' hyperthyroidism to chronic autoimmune thyroiditis and hypothyroidism is well-recognized [91] and vice versa also occurs [92]. Patients who have hypothyroidism one year, Graves' hyperthyroidism another year, and again hypothyroidism later [93].

- In families of patients, some members may have chronic autoimmune thyroiditis and others may have Graves' Disease [94]

5.6 Immune mechanisms of Graves' Disease

The immune mechanisms involved in the pathogenesis of Graves' hyperthyroidism are molecular mimicry (specificity crossover), thyroid-cell expression of human leukocyte-associated molecules (antigens), and bystander activation [95].

5.7 B cell in Graves' Disease

Monoclonal antibody to the CD 34 antigen on the surface of B cells has demonstrated that changing the B cell repertoire can have profound influences on

Graves' Disease [40]. B cell also plays an important role in TSHR-Ab interaction with retro-orbital TSHRs which expressed on fibroblasts and adipocytes cause Graves Ophthalmology [95].

5.8 T cell in Graves' Disease

T cells are present in the immune repertoire react with appropriate peptides which are derived from thyroid autoantigens in Graves' Disease. Secretion of thyroid-specific autoantibodies from B cells is increase against the activated T cells. The thyroid-specific T cells in Graves' Disease primarily act as helper (CD4+ Th1) cells. However, based on the production of cytokines, subsets of T cells have been distinguished most easily

- CD4+ Th1 cells — Secrete interleukin-2, interferon gamma, and tumor necrosis factor-alpha which in turn activate cytotoxic cells and may induce thyroid cell apoptosis when CD4+ Th1 cells activated
- CD4+ Th2 cells — Secrete interleukin –4 and interleukin –5 and activate antibody production.
- CD4+ Th17 cells — Interleukin –17 is secreted under the influence of interleukin –23 by the CD4+ Th17 cells which is a newly identified pro-inflammatory subset of cells [95].

6. Clinical manifestations

Graves' Disease is a syndrome which consists of hyperthyroidism, goiter, Graves' orbitopathy, and occasionally a Graves' dermopathy referred to as pretibial or localized myxedema (PTM). High amounts of T4, T3, or both can cause an excessively high metabolic rate. Signs and symptoms of Graves' Disease manifested due to the effect of hypermetabolism as well over stimulation of nervous system by T4, T3 or both.

6.1 General

- Muscle weakness
- Fatigue

6.2 Neck

- Enlargement of the thyroid gland (goiter)
- May be palpable thyroid nodules
- Thyroid bruits on auscultation

6.3 Cardiovascular system

- Rapid or irregular heartbeat (palpitations)
- Increased heart rate (Tachycardia)
- High Blood Pressure
- Heart failure

DOI: http://dx.doi.org/10.5772/intechopen.96418

6.4 Respiratory system

- Dyspnea

6.5 Gastro intestinal system

- Diarrhea or increased Frequent bowel movements

6.6 Musculoskeletal

- Proximal muscle weakness
- Easy fatigability
- Back Pain
- Increased risk for fracture

6.7 Neuromuscular system

- A fine tremor of the hands or fingers
- Hyperactive deep tendon reflexes

6.8 Metabolic

- Weight loss, despite normal eating habits
- Worsening diabetes control

6.9 Hematologic

- Easy bruising

6.10 Endocrine/reproductive system

- Change in menstrual cycles
- Erectile dysfunction or reduced libido
- Secondary amenorrhea
- Gynecomastia
- Impotence

6.11 Integumentary

- Heat sensitivity and an increase in perspiration or warm, moist skin,
- Hair loss

- Onycholysis
- Vitiligo
- Thick, red skin usually on the shins or tops of the feet a condition called Graves' dermopathy or Pretibial Myxedema (PTM)

6.12 Extremities

- Edema
- Thyroid Acropachy: is a rare manifestation with characteristic imaging findings. Clinically, it presents as nail clubbing, swelling of digits and toes.
- Onycholysis: Separation of the nail plate starting at the distal free margin and progressing proximally usually starting at the tip and/or sides on the ring finger but can occur on any of the fingernails

6.13 Psychiatric

- Restlessness
- Anxiety
- Irritability
- Insomnia

6.14 Eyes

Bulging eyes (Graves' ophthalmopathy) Graves' ophthalmopathy also called Graves Orbitopathy, Graves Eye Disease, or Thyroid Eye Disease (TED), is an autoimmune inflammatory disorder of the orbit and periorbital tissues, characterized by upper eyelid retraction, lid lag, swelling, redness (erythema), conjunctivitis, and bulging eyes (exophthalmos) It is a problem that develops in people with an overactive thyroid caused by Graves' Disease which increase rate of peripheral blood mononuclear cell conversion into CD34+ fibrocytes. These cells may contribute to the pathophysiology of ophthalmopathy by accumulating in orbital tissues and producing inflammatory cytokines, including TNF-alpha and IL-6. although most cases of thyroid-associated orbitopathy do not result in visual loss, this condition can cause vision-threatening exposure keratopathy, troublesome diplopia, and compressive optic neuropathy.

6.14.1 Early symptom

- Feeling of irritation in the eyes
- Excessive tearing or dry eye
- Forward displacement of the eye
- Sensitivity to light
- Double vision

6.14.2 Late symptoms

- Swelling of the eye
- Inability to move the eye
- Corneal ulceration
- Rarely, loss of vision

7. Complications

7.1 Goiter

An enlarged thyroid gland that has grown big enough to appear as a visible bulge on the neck caused by Graves' Disease is known as a diffuse thyrotoxic goiter. As thyroid enlarges bigger without treatment, goiter gets big enough to make difficulty in swallowing, causes coughing, and sleep disruption.

7.2 Thyroid storm

If Graves' Disease left untreated or treated inadequately, can cause a rare but life-threatening complication called Thyroid Storm also known as thyrotoxic crisis or accelerated hyperthyroidism and requires immediate emergency care. The sudden and drastic raise in thyroid hormones causes fever, sweating, vomiting, diarrhea, delirium, severe weakness, seizures, irregular heartbeat, yellow skin and eyes (jaundice), severe low blood pressure, and coma.

7.3 Heart disorders

Untreated, Graves' Disease can lead to heart rhythm disorders, changes in the structure and function of the heart muscles leads to inability of the heart to pump enough blood to the cells to meet the metabolic demand. Hyper secretion of thyroid hormone causes left ventricular thickening which may lead to heart failure and cardiac-related death. Thyrotoxicosis also has been associated with dilated cardiomyopathy, [96] right sided heart failure with pulmonary hypertension, diastolic dysfunction and atrial fibrillation [97]. An irregular heartbeat that can lead to blood clots, stroke, heart failure, and other heart-related problems such as angina.

7.4 Brittle bones

Untreated hyperthyroidism increase in the rate of bone resorption can lead to weak, brittle bones (osteoporosis). Too much thyroid hormone interferes with body's ability to incorporate calcium into bones. Patients with Graves' Disease have significantly increased in serum calcium and phosphate, plasma FGF-23 compared to healthy individuals and amongst FGF-23 is physiologically related to serum phosphate homeostasis in untreated Graves' Disease [98].

7.5 Maternal/fetal complications

Possible complications of Graves' Disease during pregnancy include miscarriage, preterm birth, fetal thyroid dysfunction, poor fetal growth, maternal heart failure and preeclampsia. Preeclampsia is a maternal condition that results in high blood pressure and other serious signs and symptoms.

8. Assessment and diagnostic investigations

8.1 History collection

Analysis of medical and family history with associated sign and symptoms.

8.2 Physical examination

From head to toe examination and the findings are diffusely enlarged thyroid gland, thyrotoxic signs and symptoms. The unique findings to Graves' Disease such as Graves ophthalmopathy and dermopathy, Myxedematous changes of the skin (usually in the pretibial areas) are described as resembling an orange peel in color and texture, and Onycholysis can be seen usually in the fourth and fifth fingernails.

8.3 Blood investigations including thyroid profile

In case of Graves' Disease, abnormally high levels of T3 and T4, and a very low level of TSH seen as well elevated TSI and positive Thyroid peroxidase antibody

- Thyroid stimulating hormone (TSH)
- Thyroid hormone Triiodothyronine (T3)
- Free T3 or Free triiodothyronine (FT3)
- Thyroid hormone Thyroxine (T4)
- Antithyroid Antibodies: Thyroid peroxidase (TPO) antibody titers provide an evidence for Graves' Disease. More than 95% of patients have positive assays for TPO (thyroperoxidase or microsomal antigen), and about 50% have positive anti-thyroglobulin antibody assays.
- Thyroid-stimulating Immunoglobulin (TSI): It is measured from drawn blood and increase in the level of TSI antibodies reveals that the thyroid gland is more active and release excess amounts of thyroid hormone into the blood (**Table 2**).

Hormone	Normal range
Thyroid stimulating hormone (TSH)	0.40–4.50 mIU/mL
Thyroxine (T4)	5.0–11.0 ug/dL
Free Thyroxine (T4)	0.9–1.7 ng/dL
Triiodothyronine (T3)	100–200 ng/dL
Free triiodothyronine (FT3)	2.3–4.1 pg./mL

Table 2.
Normal range of thyroid profile.

8.4 Radioactive iodine uptake (RAIU) study

A radioactive iodine uptake test and scan will measure the amount of iodine that thyroid gland absorbs and also determines if the entire or only part of the thyroid is overactive. If thyroid absorbs more iodine from blood stream which indicates Graves' Disease.

8.5 Thyroid scan

It shows how and where iodine is distributed in the thyroid. With Graves' Disease, the entire thyroid is involved, so the iodine shows up throughout the gland. It also may confirm hypoechogenicity or intense vascularity of Graves' Disease if a color Doppler flow exam is done.

8.6 Thyroid ultrasound

High-frequency sound waves to produce images of structures inside the thyroid gland. It's most useful when radioactive iodine uptake study is contraindicated such as pregnant women, iodine hypersensitivity.

8.7 Imaging test

computed tomography (CT) scan or magnetic resonance imaging (MRI) scan is indicated for clear picture of thyroid gland when the clinical assessment is not clear. CT scan and MRI of the eye muscles and eye sockets (called orbital imaging) in order to define the exact impact of Graves' Disease on the eyes and to confirm the Graves ophthalmopathy.

8.8 Other investigations to rule out complications

- Electro cardiogram
- ECHO cardiogram
- Blood sugar
- Blood cholesterol
- Serum calcium
- Serum phosphate
- Bone mineral density Test

9. Treatment approaches

The main aims of the management of Graves' Disease are to inhibit the overproduction of thyroid hormones by targeting thyroid gland and to alleviate the effect of an excess hormones on various system of the body thereby correct the thyrotoxic state.

The management includes

- Radioactive iodine therapy
- Anti-thyroid medications
- Beta blockers
- Thyroid Surgery
- Treating Graves' ophthalmopathy
    - Corticosteroids.
    - Teprotumumab (Tepezza)
    - Prisms.
    - Orbital decompression surgery
    - Orbital radiotherapy

9.1 Radioactive iodine therapy

The most commonly used therapy for Graves' Disease is radioactive iodine (radioiodine) since the 1940s. It is still popular because it is non-invasive and highly effective on thyroid gland and has fewer side effects. Graves' Disease with a large thyroid gland, multiple symptoms of thyrotoxicosis, high levels of thyroxine, and high titers of TSI are indicated for radioactive iodine and women who are pregnant or breastfeeding are contraindicated for this therapy. Commonly used radioactive iodine is iodine-131 (I-131) and can be administered orally in the form of capsule or liquid. The dose is calculated based on the age, weight of the thyroid gland and radioiodine uptake and the usual dose ranges from 5–15 mCi. Iodine is essential for thyroid gland to produce hormones, the thyroid absorbs the radioiodine into the thyroid cells and the radiation destroys the hyperactive thyroid cells. This causes the thyroid gland to shrink, hormones to return normal and gradually alleviate the symptoms. It usually takes several weeks to several months. Follow up the patient and monitoring the thyroid profile is very important because it causes hypothyroidism.

9.2 Anti-thyroid medications

Antithyroid medications are one of the prominent methods to treat hyperthyroidism which interfere with the use of iodine by the thyroid to produce hormones. Commonly used antithyroid medicines are thionamides, such as propylthiouracil (PTU), and carbimazole (CBZ). Thionamides are actively transported into the thyroid gland where they inhibit both the organification of iodine to tyrosine residues in thyroglobulin and the coupling of iodotyrosines and hence reduce the synthesis of thyroid hormone [99, 100] and inhibit the function of thyroperoxidase, reducing oxidation and the organification of iodide. Anti-thyroid drugs may be administered before or after radioiodine therapy as a supplemental treatment. Methimazole is considered the first choice of antithyroid medicnes as the risk of liver disease is common in Propylthiouracil. However, propylthiouracil is the preferred anti-thyroid drug during the first trimester of pregnancy, as methimazole has a slight risk of birth defects and can continue the methimazole after the first trimester. Side effects of anti-thyroid drugs are allergic reactions such as skin rash, itching, lower resistance to infection due to decrease in white blood cells and rarely liver disease.

9.3 Beta blockers

Beta blockers do not have the direct effect on thyroid gland to reduce the hormone secretion but can minimize the symptoms until the effect other treatments occur. Beta-blockers, such as propranolol and metoprolol, are often the first line of treatment. The action of beta blockers in hyperthyroidism is to antagonize beta-receptor-mediated effects of catecholamines thereby reduce the heart rate, blood pressure, tremors, anxiety or irritability, heat intolerance, sweating, diarrhea, and muscle weakness. Beta blockers may trigger an asthma attack so aren't often prescribed for people with asthma and also complicate management of diabetes.

9.4 Thyroid surgery

Removal of part or total tissue of thyroid gland namely subtotal or total thyroidectomy is another option for the management of Graves' Disease. Surgery is less common and it is indicated when other treatment fails to manage. Pre-operatively, reduce the size of thyroid gland and bring to the euthyroidal state to reduce the risk of complications post-operatively. The complications of thyroidectomy include hypothyroidism, hypoparathyroidism, recurrent laryngeal nerve, hemorrhage. Patient undergone thyroidectomy has to receive the thyroid replacement hormone medication such as levothyroxine in remaining life.

9.5 Treating Graves' ophthalmopathy

9.5.1 Over-the-counter artificial tears

Mild symptoms of Graves' ophthalmopathy may be managed by using over-the-counter artificial tears during the day and lubricating paraffin-based gels can be applied at night.

If symptoms are more severe:

9.5.2 Corticosteroids

Corticosteroids, such as prednisone, may lessen swelling behind eyeballs. Side effects may include fluid retention, weight gain, elevated blood sugar levels, increased blood pressure and mood swings.

9.5.3 Teprotumumab (Tepezza)

It's given through an IV in the arm every three weeks and is given eight times. TEPEZZA targets and blocks IGF-1R and inhibits fibroblast activation via the IGF-1R/TSHR signaling complex at the source of the disease [101, 102] and decreases proptosis by [103–105] by reducing inflammation, preventing muscle and fat tissue remodeling, and preventing tissue expansion behind the eye. It can cause side effects such as nausea, diarrhea, muscle spasms and elevated blood sugar levels.

9.5.4 Prisms

Prisms in eye glasses may correct the double vision as double vision is one of the effects of Graves' Disease.

9.5.5 Orbital decompression surgery

Removal of bone between eye socket (orbit) and sinuses, the air spaces next to the orbit. This decompression moves the eye back to their original position to release pressure on the optic nerve. This treatment is indicated if pressure on the optic nerve threatens the vision and treats the possible complication of double vision.

9.5.6 Orbital radiotherapy

It is common method of treatment using targeted X-rays to destroy the tissue behind the eyes but the underlying mechanism and benefits are not clear. It can be administered over the course of several days and is recommended if the Graves' ophthalmopathy is worsening and not respond to corticosteroids or not tolerated well.

10. Patient education

10.1 Diet

National Institute of Diabetes and Digestive and Kidney Diseases (NIDDK) stated that Graves' Disease can cause sensitivity to iodine. The symptoms of Graves' Disease may be worsening when consuming foods rich in iodine such as kelp and dulse or iodine supplements. The NIDDK warns to consult the physician before taking a multivitamin supplement or cough medicine, as these can contain iodine.

10.2 Exercise

Exercising can enhance the improvement in some symptoms during treatment. It controls the metabolism as there is a tendency to gain weight when the hyperthyroidism is corrected. Brittle bones also can occur with Graves' Disease, and weight-bearing exercises can help maintain bone density.

10.3 Stress reduction

It may be helpful, as stress may trigger or worsen Graves' Disease. Yoga, meditation, relaxation technique such as Listening to music, taking a warm bath or walking can help to reduce the stress and plan to follow in daily routine.

10.4 Optimal levels of iodine and selenium

Optimal iodine and selenium intake has been found to attenuate the toxic effects that heavy metals and perchlorate can have on the thyroid.

10.5 Avoid stimulants

Avoid consuming coffee, tea and quit the habit of smoking and alcohol as it worsens the symptoms of Graves' Disease.

10.6 Wear sunglasses

Eyes are more vulnerable to ultraviolet rays and more sensitive to bright light when eyes protrude. Wearing sunglasses that wrap around the sides of head will also lessen the irritation of eyes from the wind.

10.7 Elevate the head end

Keep the head higher than the body lessens fluid accumulation in the head and may relieve the pressure on the eyes.

10.8 Cold compresses

Apply cold compress to the eyes to keep the eyes moisture which may soothe eyes.

11. Prognosis

Many patients with Graves' Disease remain well after the course of treatment with anti-thyroid drugs, radioactive iodine or surgery, but recurrence can happen at any time. Treatment approaches are very effective, but often results in abnormally low levels of thyroid hormones cause hypothyroidism. The Graves' ophthalmology also tends to improve slowly with anti-thyroid drug treatment over years. However, some element of the staring appearance often remains.

12. Conclusion

This chapter briefed on epidemiology, causes and risk factors, pathophysiology, clinical manifestations, diagnostic investigations, management and complications of Graves' Disease. Graves' Disease is the autoimmune disorders of thyroid gland and the common cause of hyperthyroidism. It often poses complex challenges in diagnosing and managing the clients with Graves' Disease. Graves' Disease in some patients is curable within a limited time period with modern treatment but in some patients it is a chronic and relapsing. However untreated Graves' Disease causes the complications of thyroid storm, cardiac and ophthalmic complications and over treated Graves' Disease leads to hypothyroidism. Patient education is also plays an vital role in managing and preventing complications.

Acknowledgements

The author would like to thank the IntechOpen publishers for offering me an opportunity to write the chapter on Graves' Disease.

Conflict of interest

The author declared that no competing interests exist.

Author details

Thenmozhi Paluchamy
Saveetha College of Nursing, Saveetha Institute of Medical and Technical Sciences, Saveetha University, Chennai, Tamilnadu, India

*Address all correspondence to: thenmozhi.sethu@gmail.com

References

[1] Kalra S, Unnikrishnan AG, Sahay R. The global burden of thyroid disease. Thyroid Research and Practice. 2013;10:89-90

[2] Marieb E, Hoehn K. Regulation and integration of the body. The endocrine system. Human Anatomy and Physiology. 7th edition. San Francisco, CA: Pearson Education Inc. 2007: 620-625.

[3] Jameson J, Weetman A, Fauci A, Braunwald E, Kasper D, Hauser S, et al. Disorders of the thyroid gland. Harrison's Principles of Internal Medicine. 17th edition. USA: The McGraw Hill Companies Inc. 2008: 2224-2247.

[4] https://rarediseases.org/rare-diseases/graves-disease/

[5] Ellis H. Robert. Graves: 1796-1852. British Journal of Hospital Medicine. 2006;67(6):313.

[6] Sinha A A., et al. Autoimmune diseases: the failure of self-tolerance. Science 1990;248.4961: 1380-1388.

[7] G Effraimidis, WM Wiersinga. Mechanisms in endocrinology: autoimmune thyroid disease: old and new players. European Journal of Endocrinology. 2014; 170(6): R241-R252.

[8] https://www.nhs.uk/conditions/overactive-thyroid-hyperthyroidism/causes

[9] Smith TJ, Hededüs L. Graves' disease. The New England Journal of Medicine. 2016;375(16):1552-1565.

[10] Yeung SJ, Habra MA, Chiu AC. Graves' disease. Medscape emedicine website. http://emedicine.medscape.com/article/120619-overview#a6 External link. Updated March 2017. Accessed December 14, 2020.

[11] Furszyfer J, Kurland LT, McConahey WM, Elveback LR. Graves' disease in Olmsted County, Minnestoa, 1935 through 1967. Mayo Clinic Proceeding. 1970; 45:636.

[12] McGrogan A, Seaman HE, Wright JW, de Vries CS. The incidence of autoimmune thyroid disease: a systematic review of the literature. Clinical Endocrinology. 2008;69(5):687-696.

[13] Cooper GS, Stroehla BC. The epidemiology of autoimmune diseases. Autoimmunity Reviews. 2003;2(3):119-125.

[14] Tunbridge WM, Evered DC, Hall R, et al. The spectrum of thyroid disease in a community the Whickham survey. Clinical Endocrinology. 1977; 7(6):481-493.

[15] Vanderpump MP, Tunbridge WM, French JM, et al. The incidence of thyroid disorders in the community: a twenty-year follow-up of the Whickham Survey. Clinical Endocrinology. 1995;43(1):55-68.

[16] Y S Hussain, J C Hookham, A Allahabadia, S P Balasubramanian. Epidemiology, management and outcomes of Graves' disease-real life data. Endocrine. 2017;56(3):568-578.

[17] Nystrom HF, Jansson S, Berg G. Incidence rate and clinical features of hyperthyroidism in a long-term iodine sufficient area of Sweden (Gothenburg) 2003-2005. Clinical Endocrinology. 2013;78(5):768-776.

[18] Glinoer D. Management of hypo- and hyperthyroidism during pregnancy. Growth Hormone IGF Research. 2003;13:S45–S54.

[19] Hollowell JG, Staehling NW, Flanders WD, Hannon WH,

Gunter EW, Spencer CA, Braverman LE. Serum TSH, T(4), and thyroid antibodies in the United States population (1988 to 1994): National Health and Nutrition Examination Survey (NHANES III). Journal Clinical Endocrinology and Metabolism. 2002 ;87(2):489-499.

[20] Zimmerman D, Lteif AN. Thyrotoxicosis in children. Endocrinology&Metabolism Clinics of North America. 1998;27:109-126.

[21] Kaguelidou F, Alberti C, Castanet M, Guitteny MA, Czernichow P, Le'ger J. Predictors of autoimmune hyperthyroidism relapse in children after discontinuation of antithyroid drug treatment. Journal Clinical Endocrinology and Metabolism. 2008;93:3817-3826.

[22] Lavard L, Ranløv I, Perrild H, Andersen O, Jacobsen BB. Incidence of juvenile thyrotoxicosis in Denmark, 1982-1988. A nationwide study. European Journal of Endocrinology. 1994;130:565-568.

[23] Rivkees SA,Mattison DR. Propylthiouracil (PTU) hepatoxicity in children and recommendations for discontinuation of use. International Journal of Pediatric Endocrinology. 2009:132041.

[24] Philip R, Sivaraman Nair SA, Kuruvilla V, John SM, Amal D, Sankaran KC. Incidentally detected thyrotoxicosis-etiology and natural course: A study from Central Kerala. CHRISMED Journal of Health and Research. 2016;3:203-206.

[25] Jacobson EM, Tomer Y. The CD40, CTLA-4, thyroglobulin, TSH receptor, and PTPN22 gene quintet and its contribution to thyroid autoimmunity: back to the future. Journal of Autoimmunity. 2007;28(2-3):85-98.

[26] Tomer Y. Mechanisms of autoimmune thyroid diseases: from genetics to epigenetics. Annual Review of Pathology. 2014;9:147-156.

[27] Brix TH, Kyvik KO, Christensen K, Hegedüs L. Evidence for a major role of heredity in Graves' disease: a population-based study of two Danish twin cohorts. Journal of Clinical Endocrinology and Metabolism. 2001;86:930-934.

[28] Limbach M, Saare M, Tserel L, Kisand K, Eglit T, Sauer S, et al. Epigenetic profiling in CD4+ and CD8+ T cells from Graves' disease patients reveals changes in genes associated with T cell receptor signaling. Journal of Autoimmunity. 2016;67:46-56.

[29] Zaletel K, Krhin B, Gaberscek S, Pirnat E, Hojker S. The influence of the exon 1 polymorphism of the cytotoxic T lymphocyte antigen 4 gene on thyroid antibody production in patients with newly diagnosed Graves' disease. Thyroid. 2002; 12(5):373-376.

[30] Zaletel K, Krhin B, Gaberscek S, Hojker S. Thyroid autoantibody production is influenced by exon 1 and promoter CTLA-4 polymorphisms in patients with Hashimoto's thyroiditis. International Journal of Immunogenetics. 2006;33(2):87-91.

[31] Kincade PW, Medina KL, Smithson G, Scott DC. Pregnancy: a clue to normal regulation of B lymphopoiesis. Immunology Today. 1994; 15:539.

[32] Paavonen T. Hormonal regulation of immune responses. Ann Med 1994; 26:255.

[33] Da Silva JA. Sex hormones, glucocorticoids and autoimmunity: facts and hypotheses. Annals of Rheumatic Disease. 1995; 54:6.

[34] Yin X, Latif R, Tomer Y, Davies TF. Thyroid epigenetics: X chromosome inactivation in patients with

autoimmune thyroid disease. Annals of the New York Academy of Science. 2007; 1110:193.

[35] Smith TJ, Hededüs L. Graves' disease. The New England Journal of Medicine. 2016;375(16):1552-1565.

[36] Brucker-Davis F. Effects of environmental synthetic chemicals on thyroid function. Thyroid. 1998;8:827-856.

[37] Pearce EN. Braverman LE. Environmental pollutants and the thyroid. Best Practice & Research Clinical Endocrinology & Metabolism. 2009;23:801-813.

[38] Brent GA. Braverman LE. Zoeller RT. Thyroid health and the environment. Thyroid. 2007;17:807-809.

[39] Zoeller RT. Dowling ALS. Herzig CTA. Iannacone EA. Gauger KJ. Bansal R. Thyroid hormone, brain development, and the environment. Environmental Health Perspectives. 2002;110(Suppl 3):355-361.

[40] Strieder TGA. Tijssen JGP. Wenzel BE. Endert E. Wiersinga WM. Prediction of progression to overt hypothyroidism or hyperthyroidism in female relatives of patients with autoimmune thyroid disease using the thyroid events Amsterdam (THEA) score. Achieves of Internal Medicine. 2008;168:1657-1663.

[41] Prummel MF. Streider T. Wiersinga WM. The environment and autoimmune thyroid diseases. European Journal of Endocrinology. 2004;150:605-618.

[42] Burek CL. Talor MV. Environmental triggers of autoimmune thyroiditis. Journal of Autoimmunity. 2009;33:183-189.

[43] Tanda ML. Piantanida E. Lai A. Lombardi V. Dalle Mule I. Liparulo L. Pariani N. Bartalena L. Thyroid autoimmunity and environment. Hormone and Metabolic Research. 2009;41:436-442.

[44] Weetman AP. Autoimmune thyroid disease: propagation and progression. European Journal of Endocrinology. 2003;148 1-9.

[45] Benvenga S, Guarneri F, Vaccaro M, et al. Homologies between proteins of Borrelia burgdorferi and thyroid autoantigens. Thyroid. 2004;14:964-966.

[46] Gangi E, Kapatral V, El-Azami El-Idrissi M, et al. Characterization of a recombinant Yersinia enterocolitica lipoprotein; implications for its role in autoimmune response against thyrotropin receptor. Autoimmunity. 2004;37(6-7):515-520.

[47] Menconi F, Hasham A, Tomer Y. Environmental triggers of thyroiditis: hepatitis C and interferon-α. Journal of Endocrinological Investigation. 2011; 34:78.

[48] Bagnasco M, Bossert I & Pesce G. Stress and autoimmune thyroid diseases. Neuroimmunomodulation. 2006;13:309-317.

[49] Winsa B, Karlsson A, Bergstrom R, Adami HO, Gamstedt A, Jansson R, Adamson U & Dahlberg PA. Stressful life events and Graves' disease. Lancet. 1991;338: 1475-1479.

[50] Sonino N, Girelli ME, Boscaro M, Fallo F, Busnardo B & Fava GA. Life events in the pathogenesis of Graves' disease, A controlled study. Acta Endocrinologica. 1993;128:293-296.

[51] Kung AW. Life events, daily stresses and coping in patients with Graves' disease. Clinical Endocrinology. 1995;42:303-308.

[52] Radosavljevic´ VR, Jankovic´ SM & Marinkovic´ JM. Stressful life events

in the pathogenesis of Graves' disease. European Journal of Endocrinology. 1996;134: 699-701.

[53] Yoshiuchi K, Kumano H, Nomura S, Yoshimura H, Ito K, Kanaji Y, Ohashi Y, Kuboki T & Suematsu H. Stressful life events and smoking were associated with Graves' disease in women, but not in men. Psychosomatic Medicine. 1998; 60: 182-185.

[54] Martin-du Pan RC. Triggering role of emotional stress and childbirth. Unexpected occurrence of Graves' disease compared to 96 cases of Hashimoto thyroiditis and 97 cases of thyroid nodules. Annales d'Endocrinologie. 1998;59:107-112.

[55] Matos-Santos A, Nobre EL, Costa JGE, Nogueira PJ, Macedo A, Galva˜o-Teles A & De Castro JJ. Relationship between the number and impact of stressful life events and the onset of Graves' disease and toxic nodular goitre. Clinical Endocrinology. 2001;55:15-19.

[56] Ge'raldine Falgarone, Hassan M Heshmati, Re'gis Cohen, and Ge'rard Reach. Role of emotional stress in the pathophysiology of Graves' disease. European Journal of Endocrinology. 2013;168:R13–R18.

[57] Ando T, Davies TF. Clinical Review 160: Postpartum autoimmune thyroid disease: the potential role of fetal microchimerism. Journal Clinical Endocrinology & Metabolism. 2003;88:2965.

[58] Fainboim L, Arruvito L. Mechanisms involved in the expansion of Tregs during pregnancy: role of IL-2/STAT5 signalling. Journal of Reproductive Immunology. 2011; 88:93.

[59] Stagnaro-Green A. Postpartum thyroiditis. Best Practice & Research Clin Endocrinology & Metabolism. 2004;18:303.

[60] Jansson R, Dahlberg PA, Winsa B, et al. The postpartum period constitutes an important risk for the development of clinical Graves' disease in young women. Acta Endocrinologica. 1987;116:321.

[61] Bartalena L. Bogazzi F. Tanda ML. Manetti L. Dell'Unto E. Martino E. Cigarette smoking and the thyroid. European Journal of Endocrinology. 1995;133:507-512.

[62] Bertelsen JB. Hegedus L. Cigarette smoking and the thyroid. Thyroid. 1994;4:327-331.

[63] P.N. Taylor, D. Albrecht, A. Scholz, G. Gutierrez-Buey, J.H. Lazarus, C.M. Dayan, O.E. Okosieme, Global epidemiology of hyperthyroidism and hypothyroidism. Nature Reviews Endocrinology. 2018;14:301-316.

[64] Muller B. Zulewski H. Huber P. Ratcliffe JG. Staub JJ. Impaired action of thyroid hormone associated with smoking in women with hypothyroidism. New England Journal of Medicine. 1995;333:964-969.

[65] Wiersinga W M. Smoking and thyroid. Clinical Endocrinology. 2013;79:145-151.

[66] Shine B, Fells P, Edwards OM, Weetman AP 1990 Association between Graves' ophthalmopathy and smoking. Lancet 335:1261-1263.

[67] Bartalena L, Martino E, Marcocci C, Bogazzi F, Panicucci M, Velluzzi F, Loviselli A, Pinchera A. More on smoking habits and Graves' ophthalmopathy. Journal of Endocrinological Investigations. 1989;12:733-737.

[68] Hegedius L, Brix TH, Vestergaard P. Relationship between cigarette smoking and Graves' ophthalmopathy. Journal of Endocrinological Investigations. 2004;27:265-271.

[69] Zimmerman MB. Iodine deficiency. Endocrine Reviews. 2009;30:376-408.

[70] Papanastasiou L, Vatalas IA. Koutras DA. Mastorakos G. Thyroid autoimmunity in the current iodine environment. Thyroid. 2007;17:729-739.

[71] Laurberg P, Jorgensen T, Perrild H, Ovesen L, Knudsen N, Pedersen IB. Rasmussen LB, Carle A. Vejbjerg P. The Danish investigation on iodine intake and thyroid disease, DanThyr: status and perspectives. European Journal of Endocrinology. 2008, 71(3):440-445.

[72] Skla C, Whitton J, Mertens A, Stovall M, Green D, Marina N, Greffe B, Wolden S, Robison L. Abnormalities of the thyroid in survivors of Hodgkin's disease: data from the childhood cancer survivor study. Journal of Clinical Endocrinology and Metabolism. 2000;85:3227-3232.

[73] Dunkelmann S, Wolf R, Koch A, Kittner C, Groth P, Schuemichen C. Incidence of radiation-induced Graves' disease in patients treated with radioiodine for thyroid autonomy before and after introduction of a high-sensitivity TSH receptor antibody assay. European Journal of Nuclear Medicine and Molecular Imaging. 2004;31:1428-1434.

[74] Simon Z, Ress Z, Toldi J, Trauninger A, Miltenyi Z, Illes A. Rare association of Hodgkins lymphoma, Graves' disease and myasthemia gravis complicated by post-radiation neurofibrosarcoma: coincidence or genetic susceptibility?. International Journal of Hematology. 2009;89:523-528.

[75] National Academy of Sciences 2005 Health Implications of Perchlorate Ingestion. National Research Council, National Academy Press; Washington, DC:

[76] Howdeshell KL. A model of development of the brain as a construct of the thyroid system. Environmental Health Perspectives. 2002;110(Suppl 3):337-348.

[77] Stephanie L Lee, Hyperthyroidism and Thyrotoxicosis. Updated: Oct 19, 2020, https://emedicine.medscape.com/article/121865-overview#a4

[78] Davies TF, Ando T, Lin RY, et al. Thyrotropin receptor-associated diseases: from adenomata to Graves' disease. Journal of Clinical Investigations. 2005; 115:1972.

[79] Latif R, Morshed SA, Zaidi M, Davies TF. The thyroid-stimulating hormone receptor: impact of thyroid-stimulating hormone and thyroid-stimulating hormone receptor antibodies on multimerization, cleavage, and signaling. Endocrinology and Metabolism Clinics of North America. 2009; 38:319.

[80] Sai-Ching Jim Yeung, Graves Disease, Updated: Apr 17, 2020. https://emedicine.medscape.com/article/120619-overview#a5.

[81] Iwama S, Ikezaki A, Kikuoka N, et al. Association of HLA-DR, -DQ genotype and CTLA-4 gene polymorphism with Graves' disease in Japanese children. Hormone Research. 2005;63(2):55-60.

[82] Chu X, Pan CM, Zhao SX, et al. A genome-wide association study identifies two new risk loci for Graves' disease. Nature Genetics. 2011;43(9):897-901.

[83] Bell L, Hunter AL, Kyriacou A, Mukherjee A, Syed AA. Clinical diagnosis of Graves' or non-Graves' hyperthyroidism compared to TSH receptor antibody test. Endocrine Connections. 2018;12:7354673.

[84] Paschke R, Brückner N, Eck T, et al. Regional stimulation of thyroid epithelial cells in Graves' disease by

lymphocytic aggregates and plasma cells. Acta Endocrinologica. 1991; 125:459.

[85] McLachlan SM, Pegg CA, Atherton MC, et al. TSH receptor antibody synthesis by thyroid lymphocytes. Clinical Endocrinology.1986;24:223.

[86] Adams, DD, Purves, HD. Abnormal responses in the assay of thyrotropin. Proceedings of the University of Otago Medical School. 1956; 34:11.

[87] Smith BR, Hall R. Thyroid-stimulating immunoglobulins in Graves' disease. Lancet. 1974;2:427.

[88] Morshed SA, Latif R, Davies TF. Characterization of thyrotropin receptor antibody-induced signaling cascades. Endocrinology. 2009; 150:519.

[89] Feig C, Peter ME. How apoptosis got the immune system in shape. European Journal of Immunology. 2007;37 Suppl 1:S61.

[90] Bossowski A, Czarnocka B, Bardadin K, et al. Identification of apoptotic proteins in thyroid gland from patients with Graves' disease and Hashimoto's thyroiditis. Autoimmunity. 2008; 41:163.

[91] Tamai H, Kasagi K, Takaichi Y, et al. Development of spontaneous hypothyroidism in patients with Graves' disease treated with antithyroidal drugs: clinical, immunological, and histological findings in 26 patients. Journal of Clinical Endocrinology & Metabolism. 1989;69:49.

[92] Takasu N, Yamada T, Sato A, et al. Graves' disease following hypothyroidism due to Hashimoto's disease: studies of eight cases. Clinical Endocrinology. 1990; 33:687.

[93] Kraiem Z, Baron E, Kahana L, et al. Changes in stimulating and blocking TSH receptor antibodies in a patient undergoing three cycles of transition from hypo to hyper-thyroidism and back to hypothyroidism. Clinical Endocrinology. 1992; 36:211.

[94] Tamai H, Ohsako N, Takeno K, et al. Changes in thyroid function in euthyroid subjects with a family history of Graves' disease: a follow-up study of 69 patients. Journal of Clinical Endocrinology & Metabolism. 1980; 51:1123.

[95] Terry F Davies, Douglas S Ross, Jean E Mullder. Pathogenesis of Graves' disease, Uptodate.

[96] White A, Bozso SJ, Moon MC. Thyrotoxicosis induced cardiomyopathy requiring support with extracorporeal membrane oxygenation. Journal of Critical Care. 2018;3.45:140-143.

[97] Dahl P, Danzi S, Klein I. Thyrotoxic cardiac disease. Current Heart Failure Reports. 2008;5(3):170-176.

[98] Park SE, Cho MA, Kim SH, Rhee Y, Kang ES, Ahn CW. The adaptation and relationship of FGF-23 to changes in mineral metabolism in Graves' disease. Clinical Endocrinology. 2007;66(6):854-858.

[99] Cooper DS: Antithyroid drugs in the management of patients with Graves' disease: an evidence-based approach to therapeutic controversies. Journal of Clinical Endocrinology & Metabolism. 2003; 88: 3474-3481.

[100] Cooper DS: Antithyroid drugs. New England Journal of Medicine. 2005; 352: 905-917.

[101] Douglas RS. Teprotumumab, an insulin-like growth factor-1 receptor antagonist antibody, in the treatment of active thyroid eye disease: a focus on proptosis. Eye (Lond). 2019;33(2):183-190.

[102] Patel A, Yang H, Douglas RS. A new era in the treatment of thyroid eye disease. American Journal of Ophthalmology. 2019;208:281-288.

[103] TEPEZZA (teprotumumab-trbw) [prescribing information] Horizon.

[104] Bahn RS. Graves' ophthalmopathy. New England Journal of Medicine. 2010;362(8):726-738.

[105] Dik WA, Virakul S, van Steensel L. Current perspectives on the role of orbital fibroblasts in the pathogenesis of Graves' ophthalmopathy. Experimental Eye Research. 2016;142:83-91.

Chapter 2

Graves' Disease: A Review

Sanjay Saran

Abstract

Graves' Disease (GD) is an autoimmune disorder characterized by presence of TSH receptor autoantibody. It is most common cause of hyperthyroidism worldwide. Though GD can occur any age but peak incidence is seen during adulthood in between 20 to 50 years of age. GD is more commonly seen in female. GD is primarily disease of thyroid gland but affects multi organ system i.e. heart, liver, muscle, eye and skin. Symptoms and signs are result from hyperthyroidism or a consequence of underlying autoimmunity. Weight loss, fatigue, heat intolerance, tremor, and palpitations are the most common symptoms. Diffuse goiter presents in most of younger patients with thyrotoxicosis but less common in older patients. Graves' ophthalmopathy and pretibial myxedema are extrathyroidal manifestations of GD which results from action of TSHR autoantibodies on TSHR present onfibroblast, adipocyte and T cells in extrathyroidal tissue. Treatment of GD remains in between antithyroid drugs, radioiodine or surgery. In this review we discuss the diagnosis and management of GD.

Keywords: autoimmune thyroid disease, Graves' Disease, hyperthyroidism, radioactive iodine

1. Introduction

Graves' Disease (GD) is the most common cause of hyperthyroidism worldwide [1, 2]. It was first described by German physician Carl Adolf Von Basdow. It is an autoimmune disorder characterized by presence of TSH receptor autoantibody [3]. These autoantibodies stimulate TSH receptors on thyroid cells and cause hypertrophy and hyperplasia resulting thyroid gland enlargement. TSHR autoantibodies also cause increased synthesis and secretion of thyroid hormones. GD is primarily disease of thyroid gland but affects multi organ system i.e. heart, liver, muscle, eye and skin. Graves' ophthalmopathy and pretibial myxedema are extrathyroidal manifestations of GD which results from action of TSHR autoantibodies on TSHR present onfibroblast, adipocyte and T cells in extrathyroidal tissue.

2. Epidemiology

Graves' Disease accounts for 70–80% cases of hyperthyroidism in iodine sufficient population, where as it accounts for 50% cases of hyperthyroidism in iodine deficient areas of world [4, 5].

Annual incidence for GD is 20–50 person per 100,000 population and life time risk for developing GD is 3% for women and 0.5% for men [6, 7]. Though GD can occur any age but peak incidence is seen during adulthood in between 20 to 50 years

IntechOpen

of age [8]. GD is more common in Caucasians as compare to Asian and least common among black African [9, 10]. The annual incidence of thyroid associated orbitopathy is 16 cases per 100000 in women and 3 cases per 100000 in men and is more in smokers [11]. Pretibial myxedema is a very rare complication of GD, is seen in 1.5 cases per 100000 case of GO [12]. Studies have shown that GD with nodule formation have higher incidence of thyroid carcinoma perticularly tall Cell Variant of papillary thyroid cancer (a more aggressive form of cancer) was significantly more common [13, 14].

3. Risk factors

3.1 Genetic factors

Genetic component is considered a major risk factor for development of GD. Twin studies show concordance rate of GD in monozygotic twins in between 0.29 to 0.36, and in dizygotic twins between 0.00 and 0.04 [15]. GD predisposition appears to be polygenic [16]. Recently, bioinformatics and next-generation sequencing (NGS) based pangenomic analyses have identified many predisposing genes which are implicated in autoimmune disease, autoimmune thyroid disease and Graves' Disease [16]. These are various genes which take part into the pathogenesis of GD: cytotoxic T lymphocyte-associated antigen 4 (CTLA-4), TSH-R, Tg, CD40, protein tyrosine phosphatase-22 (PTPN 22), HLA, and CD25 [17]. Association with various HLA region is also seen, DR3 haplotype (i.e. DQB1*02, DQA1*0501, DRB1*03) predisposes to GD, whereas the DR7 haplotype (i.e., DQA1*0201, DQB1*0302, DRB1*07 or DQA1*0201, DQB1*02, DRB1*07) appears to be protective [18].

3.2 Sex

GD is more commonly seen in female, and estrogen receptor ESR2 polymorphisms are frequently seen in GD. Association of disease fluctuation and estrogen level variations which are seen during pregnancy, the menstrual cycle, and menopause further clarify its role in pathophysiology of the disease [19]. Estrogen receptor expression is present on orbital fibroblasts, and glucocorticoids can modulate it [20].

3.3 Environmental factors

Smoking adversely affects immune system and thyroid gland health. Current smoking doubles the risk of Graves' hyperthyroidism and triples the risk of developing Graves' ophthalmopathy (GO) the effect was found to be dose dependent and more pronounced in women [21–23]. Conversely four large studies confirm that smoking decreases the risk of hypothyroidism and autoimmune thyroid diseases (AITD) by decreasing Anti-TPO antibodies [24–27]. Three large studies have shown that smoking lowers the serum TSH level accompanied by slight increase in serum level of FT3 and FT4 and this effect is dose dependent [23, 28, 29].

Pestisides and halogenated organochlorides have thyroid disrupting properties that can alter the thyroid functions by binding to thyroid hormone transport proteins [30].

3.4 Stress

Relationship in between stressful life events and onset of GD was documented in 1825. Major stress is positively associated with increased risk of GD. By modulating the cortisol pathway stress can alter the course of many other autoimmune diseases also [31].

3.5 Pregnancy

Pregnancy is associated with major changes in thyroid anatomy and physiology. Hyperthyroidism of GD is increased in early pregnancy and during postpartum. As pregnancy advances GD tends to improve which may be due to better maternal immune tolerance or altered B cell and T cell functions [32]. Decrease immune tolerance after delivery may cause increase in autoimmune thyroid diseases in postpartum [33].

3.6 Viruses

Many viruses affect the thyroid gland some of which associated with presence of thyroid autoantibodies i.e. congenital rubella, hepatitis C virus, subacute thyroiditis. But these are not appearing to be associated with development or progression of GD [34]. However, the potential influence of various common infections (such as Epstein–Barr virus and influenza virus) on the epigenetic characteristics of a variety of susceptibility genes remains a major hypothesis for the etiology of GD.

3.7 Iodine and related drugs

Iodine and iodine-containing drugs, such as amiodaroneand iodine-containing contrast media, precipitate GD or its recurrence in a genetically susceptible individual which may be due to presence of some cryptic epitope on Thyroglobulin antibodies [35, 36]. Amiodarone is an iodinated derivative of benzofuran used in tachyarrhythmias. Each molecule of amiodarone contains two iodine atoms, which constitute 37.5% of its mass and its metabolism results in the daily release of approximately 6 mg of free iodine into the circulation which is 20–40 times higher than the daily iodine intake. Amiodarone can cause hypothyroidism or thyrotoxicosis by various mechanisms depending on duration of therapy, autoimmunity and other characteristics [36].

3.8 Drugs

Various drugs can cause supression of TSH by their direct cytotoxic effect on thyroid follicular cells. Interferon and ribaverin used in the treatment of HCV disease can aggravate hyperthyroidism associated with GD. Highly active antiretroviral therapy (HAART) for human immunodeficiency virus (HIV) infection Alemtuzumab humanized anti-CD52 monoclonal antibody, Ipilimumab is a monoclonal antibody against CTLA4, Nivolumab and pembrolizumab antibodies against programmed death protein 1 (PD1) can also precipitate hyperthyroidism by immune mechanisms [37–41].

4. Clinical features

Clinical manifestations of Graves' Disease related to age of onset, severity and the duration of hyperthyroidism. Symptoms and signs (**Table 1**) are result from hyperthyroidism or a consequence of underlying autoimmunity. Weight loss, fatigue, heat intolerance, tremor, and palpitations are the most common symptoms, occurring in more than 50% of patients. Elderly person more commonly presents with Weight loss, decreased appetite, and cardiac manifestations. Atrial fibrillation is seen in more than 10% of elderly but rare in younger patients. Goiter presents in most of younger patients with thyrotoxicosis but less common in older patients. Goiter is

Symptoms
Weight loss (weight gain in 10% of patients)
Palpitations
Dyspnea
Tremor
Tiredness, fatigue, muscle weakness
Heat intolerance, increased sweating
Increased stool frequency
Anxiety, altered mood, insomnia
Nervousness, hyperactivity
Pruritus
Thirst and polyuria
Menstrual disturbances in women (oligomenorrhea or amenorrhea)
Loss of libido
Neck fullness
Eye symptoms (swelling, pain, redness, double vision)
Physical signs of hyperthyroidism
Tachycardia, atrial fibrillation
Systolic hypertension, increased pulse pressure
Cardiac failure
Weight loss
Fine tremor, hyperkinesis, hyperreflexia
Warm, moist skin
Palmar erythema and onycholysis
Muscle weakness
Hair loss
Diffuse, palpable goiter and thyroid bruit
Mental-status and mood changes (e.g., mania or depression)
Extrathyroidal physical signs
Ophthalmopathy
Eyelid lag, retraction, or both
Proptosis (exophthalmos)
Double vision (extraocular-muscle dysfunction)
Periorbital edema, chemosis, scleral injection
Exposure keratitis
Optic neuropathy
Localized dermopathy
Acropachy
Developed from: Ref. [7].

Table 1.
Major symptoms and physical signs in Graves' Disease.

present most commonly as diffuse thyroid enlargement but nodular goiter can also be present perticularly in those who reside in iodine deficient areas (**Figure 1**).

Varying degree of orbital involvement can be seen in GD which is a consequence of thyroid autoimmunity which occur parallel to the thyroid involvement. It usually present with tearing, congestion, redness and irritation in eyes. In severe cases proptosis may occur due to inflammation and edema of extraoccular muscle and retrobulbar tissue expension owing to fluid accumulation as a result of accumulation of glycolsaminoglycan. Double vision and sight threatening complications i.e. corneal ulceration, dysthyroid optic neuropathy can occur as a consequence of damage to extraoccular muscles. For selecting appropriate patient for treatment EUGOGO classified GO in mild, moderate to severe and sight threatening. Activity of GO can be easily assessed by clinical activity score (CAS) (**Table 2**). A CAS ≥3/7 is indicative of active GO (**Figure 2**).

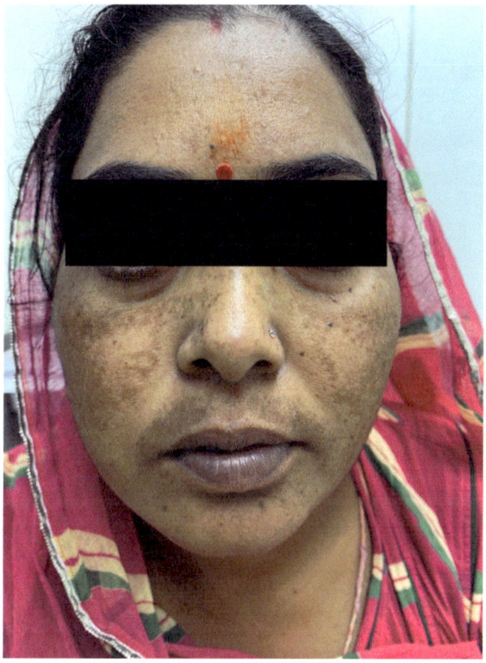

Figure 1.
Graves' orbitopathy.

Spontaneous retrobulbar pain
Pain on attempted up- or down gaze
Redness of the eyelids
Redness of the conjunctiva
Swelling of the eyelids
Inflammation of the caruncle and = or plica
Conjunctival oedema

A CAS ≥3/7 indicates active GO.
Developed from: Ref. [42].

Table 2.
Measures of clinical activity score (CAS).

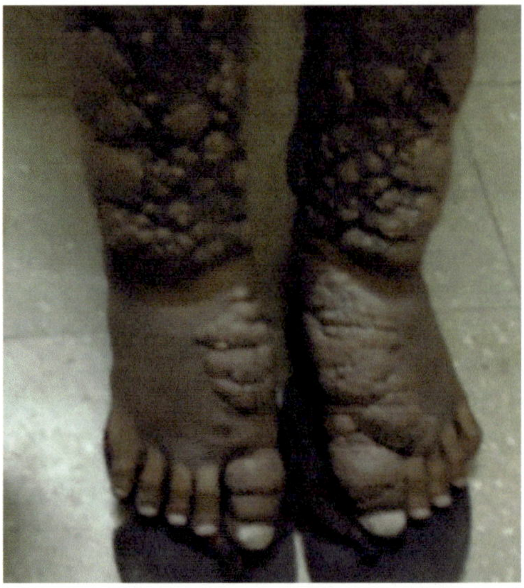

Figure 2.
Graves' dermopathy.

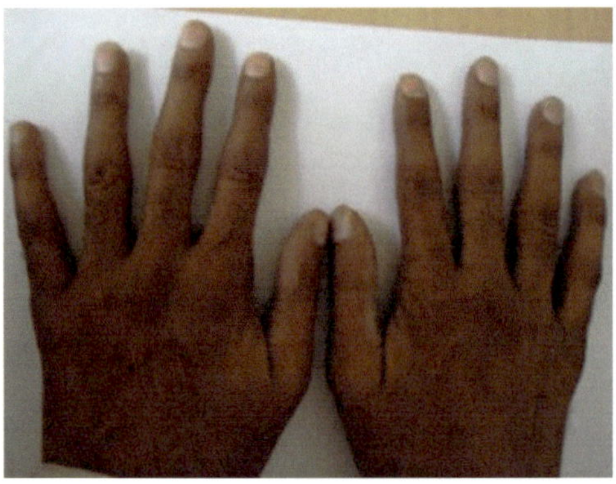

Figure 3.
Thyroid acropachy.

Graves' dermopathy is seen in 1–4% case of GD. It frequently localize to pretibial region but it may be seen on elbow, feet, toe and areas of trauma. Lesion can be described as erythematous, non-pitting thickening of dermis in pretibial region. In mild cases it gives "orange Peel" appearance. Graves' dermopathy is almost always associated with GO (**Figure 3**).

Acropachy is very rare extrathyroidal manifestation of GD. Acropachy is defined as skin tightness, digital clubbing, small-joint pain, and soft tissue edema progressing over months or years with gradual curving and enlargement of the fingers [43]. The pathogenesis of acropachy is not known. In most of cases acropachy remain asymptomatic.

5. Diagnosis

5.1 Graves' hyperthyroidism

Diagnosis of GD is based on clinical manifestations of thyrotoxicosis and biochemical abnormalities. If orbitopathy is present than diagnosis of GD is certain but in the absence of orbitopathy serum TSH Receptor Antibody (TRAb) and imaging may be required to for the diagnosis.

5.2 Biochemical evaluation

5.2.1 Thyroid hormones

Serum TSH measurement has the highest sensitivity and specificity of any single blood test used in the evaluation of suspected thyrotoxicosis [44]. Diagnostic accuracy improves when a serum TSH, free T4, and total T3 are assessed at the initial evaluation. In overt hyperthyroidism, serum free T4, T3, or both are elevated, and serum TSH is subnormal (usually <0.01 mU/L in a third-generation assay). In mild hyperthyroidism, serum T4 and free T4 can be normal, only serum T3 may be elevated, and serum TSH will be low or undetectable. These laboratory findings have been called "T3-toxicosis" and may represent the earliest stages of hyperthyroidism caused by GD [45]. Ratio of total T3 to T4 may also be useful in differentiating GD from thyroiditis. In one study the ratio of total T3 to total T4 (ng/lg) was >20 in GD and toxic nodular goiter, and <20 in painless or postpartum thyroiditis [46].

5.2.2 TSH receptor antibodies (TRAb)

In a hyperthyroid patient with a diffuse goiter and recent history of orbitopathy, the diagnosis of GD is likely so no further testing is required but hyperthyroid patient with a diffuse goiter and no definite orbitopathy, TRAb measurement can be of useful in distinguish GD from other etiologies.

5.3 Imaging

5.3.1 Thyroid ultrasound

Currently ultrasonography has become an important and practical tool for the thyroidologist; beside its role in thyroid nodule it can easily distinguish toxic multinodular goiter from GD. Increased blood flow in Doppler ultrasonography can distinguish GD from thyroiditis where blood flow is decreased.

5.3.2 Radioiodine uptake (RAIU) and thyroid scan

RAIU measures the percentage of administered RAI that is concentrated into thyroid tissue after a fixed interval, usually 24 hours. Technetium uptake measurements utilize pertechnetate that is trapped by the thyroid, but not organified. A technetium (TcO4) uptake measures the percentage of administered technetium that is trapped by the thyroid after a fixed interval, usually 20 minutes. Uptake study is not indicated routinely. It is recommended only when diagnosis is difficult. Uptake is increased in GD, toxic multinodular goiter and toxic adenoma. Uptake is decreased in subacute, postpartum, painless thyroiditis.

6. Management

After establishing the diagnosis of GD treatment options include antithyroid drugs, radioiodine, and surgery. Although RAI is preferred in United States and ATDs in Europe but long term quality of life was found to be same in all three treatment group [47]. Selection of treatment depends on local availability, cost of treatment, presence of active GO and physician preference. The main goal of management is to normalize thyroid hormones level and make the patient asymptomatic.

6.1 Pharmacological therapy

6.1.1 Antithyroid drugs

Thionamides are class of ATDs which inhibit thyroid peroxidase thereby inhibit thyroid hormone synthesis. Methimazole (MMI) and propylthiourecil (PTU) are used in United States where as Carbimazole (converted to methimazole in liver) is used in other part of world. MMI is preferred over PTU as initial therapy because of long duration of action and reduced risk of major side effect, except during first trimester of pregnancy where PTU is preferred because of lesser teratogenic effects [48]. Starting dose of MMI is 10 to 30 mg daily and of PTU is 50 to 10 mg three times daily. Dose of ATDs should be kept lowest to maintain T4 in normal range because higher doses are associated with high risk of adverse effect. Adverse effect of ATDs can be divided in minor allergic reaction and serious allergic/toxic effects agranulocytosis, liver injury and vacuities [48–52]. Hepatotoxicity and agranulocytosis are seen more commonly with propylthiouracil. Initial complete blood cell count and liver function test required before starting these drugs and patient should be instructed to report if he develops high grade fever with sore throat. American Thyroid Association recommends ATDs should be continued for 12–18 months if chosen as primary therapy then can be discontinued if TSH and TRAb levels are normal. Remission rate with ADTs treatment is 40–60% and is not associated with duration and dose of ATDs. If patient becomes hyperthyroid after completion of treatment, RAI or thyroid surgery should be considered.

6.1.2 Beta-adrenergic blocker

Beta-adrenergic blocker should be given to all symptomatic thyrotoxic patients, especially elderly. Goal of beta blocker treatment is to decrease heart rate less than 90 per minute. Propranolol is preferred non-selective beta blocker which decreases deiodinationof T4 to T3 [53]. In patient with asthma, obstructive airway disease and Raynaud's phenomenon selective β_1 blocker can be used with cautions. Calcium channel blockers verapamil and diltiazem can be used when β blockers are contraindicated [45].

6.1.3 Lithium

Lithium carbonate inhibits secretion of thyroid hormones. It does not decrease the efficacy of RAI so it can be used to control hyperthyroidism during RAI therapy or in patient who are allergic to ATDs.

6.1.4 Cholestyramine

It interfarewith enterohepatic circulation thereby decrease thyroid hormone leves rapidly. It can be used as adjunctive therapy in resistant thyrotoxicosis.

6.2 Radioactive iodine

RAI is one of definitive treatment for GD. It has been used for more than seven decade in the management of GD. Effect of ionizing radiation leads to cellular death and consequently reduction in functioning thyroid tissue and thyroid size. The goal of RAI is to render the patient hypothyroid for that 10–15 mci dose is sufficient in most of the patients. RAI can be used as primary therapy in mild cases but in severe thyrotoxic patient β blockers and ATDs are used first to render the patient euthyroid to avoid radiation induced thyroiditis. ATDs should be discontinued 2–3 days prior and till 3–7 day of RAI treatment to enhance the efficacy of treatment. Regular follow up should be at 4–6 weeks interval with biochemical testing include TSH, FT4 and T3 till 6 months or till patient become hypothyroid. Around 40% of patient treated with RAI become hypothyroid by 8 weeks and 80% by 16 weeks [54]. Levothyroxine replacement therapy should be started once patient become hypothyroid. Most of studies found no increase in prevalence of thyroid cancer or secondary malignancy in RAI treated patients. RAI is associated with development and worsening of orbitopathy as compare to ATDs and thyroid surgery [55, 56]. So presence of orbitopathy may influence the treatment option.

6.3 Thyroid surgery

Thyroid surgery is least preferred treatment option for GD. It's preferred when large nodular goiter is present. Total or Near-total thyroidectomy is procedure of choice if surgery is chosen as treatment option. Patient should be rendered euthyroid before surgery by ATDs and β blockers to minimize risk of thyroid storm [57]. Saturated solution of potassium iodide (SSKI) may be used preoperatively to normalize thyroid functions and to decrease the vascularity of thyroid gland [58]. ATA recommends measurement of calcium and 25-hydroxy vitamin D before surgery and if abnormal then should be normalized. Surgery should be performed by experienced surgeon at high volumeCentre to minimize postoperative complications [59].

6.4 Treatment of Graves' orbitopathy in patients with Graves' Disease

The optimal treatment of GO require restoration of euthyroidism and management of orbitopathy. Smoking should be discouraged as smoking increases progression and severity of GO and worsens the outcome [60]. Management of orbitopathy depends on its severity and activity. Mild inactive disease can be managed conservatively by artificial tear films only. In severe and active disease intravenous pulse steroid therapy may be required to decrease inflammation. External beam radiotherapy has also been used in severe cases. In patient with sight threatening and dysthyroid optic neuropathy (DON) orbital decompressive surgery is the only option proven to be effective. Rituximab, a anti CD20+ monoclonal antibody that causes B Cell depletion shown to be very effective in decreasing severity and activity od orbitopathy [61].

6.5 Treatment of Graves' Disease during pregnancy

Pregnancy is a hyper vascular state so, clinical signs of thyrotoxicosis and normal pregnancy remarkably overlap. Moreover, estrogen induces high serum levels of thyroid hormones make the diagnosis difficult. Graves' Disease affects 0.1–0.2% of pregnancy and carries a considerable risk to mother and new born if not controlled adequately [62]. All ATDs are teratogenic and having risk of birth defects in new born [63]. During pregnancy ATDs should be used in lowest dose to main thyroid hormone levels in upper normal range and monitoring of thyroid function should be done monthly. As pregnancy is a state of immune tolerance so in about 50% of patients ATDs can be discontinued after first trimester [62]. Breast feeding is considered safe during ATDs treatment. ATA recommends measurement of TRAb at diagnosis, then at 18–20 weeks of pregnancy, if elevated then repeat at 30–34 weeks to guide decision regarding fetal monitoring.

6.6 Treatment of dermopathy and acropachy

Treatment of dermopathy and acropachy remain ineffective. Topical and intralesional injection of steroid have been used without substantial success [64]. Trials using systemic steroid, rituximab and immunosuppressive drugs are underway with mixed results.

7. Emerging therapy

For last many years treatment of Graves' Disease has not been substantially changed. In future we can see some great change in management of GD as many newer drugs are under trials. These newer therapies are mainly directed to TSH-receptor. A human anti-TSHR monoclonal antibody (K1–70) is in a phase I trial of development [65]. A novel highly selective inhibitor for the TSHR is has promising potential for further development for the treatment of GO [66].

Author details

Sanjay Saran
Department of Endocrinology and Diabetes, SMS Medical College and Associated Group of Hospitals, Jaipur, Rajasthan, India

*Address all correspondence to: drsanjaysaran@gmail.com

References

[1] Peter N Taylor, Diana Albrecht, Anna Scholz, Gala Gutierrez-Buey, John H Lazarus, Colin M Dayan. Global epidemiology of hyperthyroidism and hypothyroidism. Nat. Rev. Endocrinol. 14, 301-316 (2018).

[2] McLeod, D. S. and Cooper, D. S. The incidence and prevalence of thyroid autoimmunity. Endocrine 42, 252-265 (2012).

[3] Silvia Martina Ferrari, Ilaria Ruffilli, Giusy Elia, Francesca Ragusa, Sabrina Rosaria Paparo, Armando Patrizio, et al. Chemokines in hyperthyroidism. J Clin Transl Endocrinol 2019;16:100196.

[4] Nystrom, H. F., Jansson, S. and Berg, G. Incidence rate and clinical features of hyperthyroidism in a long-term iodine sufficient area of Sweden (Gothenburg) 2003-2005. Clin. Endocrinol. 78, 768-776 (2013).

[5] Laurberg, P., Pedersen, K. M., Vestergaard, H. and Sigurdsson, G. High incidence of multinodular toxic goitre in the elderly population in a low iodine intake area versus high incidence of Graves' disease in the young in a high iodine intake area: Comparative surveys of thyrotoxicosis epidemiology in East-Jutland Denmark and Iceland. J. Intern. Med. 229, 415-420 (1991).

[6] Zimmermann MB, Boelaert K. Iodine deficiency and thyroid disorders. Lancet Diabetes Endocrinol 2015; 3: 286-295.

[7] Smith TJ, Hegedüs L. Graves' disease. N Engl J Med 2016;375:1552e65.

[8] Laurberg, P. et al. Iodine intake as a determinant of thyroid disorders in populations. Best Pract. Res. Clin. Endocrinol. Metab. 24, 13-27 (2010).

[9] Shapira Y, Agmon-Levin N, Shoenfeld Y. Defining and analyzing geo epi-demiology and human autoimmunity. J Autoimmun 2010;34:J168e77.

[10] McGrogan A, Seaman HE, Wright JW, et al. The incidence of autoimmune thyroid disease: A systematic review of the literature. Clin Endocrinol 2008;69:687e96.

[11] M Tellez, J Cooper, C Edmonds. Graves' ophthalmopathy in relation to cigarette smoking and ethnic origin. Clin Endocrinol (Oxf). 1992 Mar;36(3):291-294.

[12] Perros, P. et al. Graves' orbitopathy as a rare disease in Europe: A European Group on Graves' Orbitopathy (EUGOGO) position statement. Orphanet J. Rare Dis. 12, 72 (2017).

[13] Joy U L Staniforth, Senarath Erdirimanne, Guy D Eslick. Thyroid carcinoma in Graves' disease: A meta-analysis. Int J Surg. 2016 Mar;27:118-125.

[14] Suzanne P MacFarland, Andrew J Bauer, N Scott Adzick, Lea F Surrey, Jessica Noyes, Ken Kazahaya, et al. Disease Burden and Outcome in Children and Young Adults With Concurrent Graves' Disease and Differentiated Thyroid Carcinoma. J Clin Endocrinol Metab 2018 Aug 1;103(8):2918-2925.

[15] Brix TH, Hegedüs L. Twins as a tool for evaluating the influence of genetic susceptibility in thyroid autoimmunity. Ann Endocrinol 2011;72:103e7

[16] Jean-Louis Wémeau, Marc Klein, Jean-Louis Sadoul, Claire Briet, Fritz-Line Vélayoudom-Céphise. Graves' disease: Introduction, epidemiology, endogenous and environmental pathogenic factors. Ann Endocrinol (Paris). 2018 Dec;79(6):599-607.

[17] Hanna J Lee, Cheuk Wun Li, Sara Salehi Hammerstad, Mihaela Stefan,

Yaron Tomer. Immunogenetics of autoimmune thyroid diseases: A comprehensive review. J Autoimmun 2015;64:82e90.

[18] Roberto Vita, Daniela Lapa, Francesco Trimarchi, Giuseppe Vita, Poupak Fallahi, Alessandro Antonelli. Certain HLA alleles are associated with stress-triggered Graves' disease and influence its course. Endocrine 2017;55:93e100.

[19] Bartłomiej Kisiel 1, Tomasz Bednarczuk, Grazyna Kostrzewa, Joanna Kosińska, Piotr Miśkiewicz, Maria Teresa Płazińska, ET AL. Polymorphism of the oestrogen receptor beta gene (ESR2) is associated with susceptibility to Graves' disease. Clin Endocrinol (Oxf). 2008 Mar;68(3):429-34.

[20] Sarah Santiloni Cury, Miriane Oliveira, Maria Teresa Síbio, Sueli Clara, Renata De Azevedo Melo Luvizotto, Sandro Conde, et al. Gene expression of estrogen receptor-alpha in orbital fibroblasts in Graves' ophthalmopathy. Arch Endocrinol Metab. 2015 Jun;59(3):273-276.

[21] Pfeilschifter, J. and Ziegler, R. (1996) Smoking and endocrine ophthalmopathy: Impact of smoking severity and current versus lifetime cigarette consumption. Clinical Endocrinology, 45, 477-481.

[22] Holm, I.A., Manson, J.E., Michels, K.B. et al. (2005) Smoking and other lifestyle factors and the risk of Graves' hyperthyroidism. Archives of Internal Medicine, 165, 1606-1611.

[23] Asvold, B.O., Bjoro, T., Nilsen, T.I. et al. (2007) Tobacco smoking and thyroid function: A population-based study. Archives of Internal Medicine, 167, 1428-1432.

[24] Belin, R.M., Astor, B.C., Powe, N.R. et al. (2004) Smokers have high serum antithyroid antibody and thyrotropin concentrations less often and low serum thyrotropin concentrations more often than nonsmokers. Journal of Clinical Endocrinology and Metabolism, 89, 6077-6086.

[25] Mehran, L., Amouzgar, A., Delshad, H. et al. (2012) The association of cigarette smoking with serum TSH concentration and thyroperoxidase antibody. Experimental Clinical Endocrinology and Diabetes, 120, 80-83.

[26] Strieder, T.G.A., Prummel, M.F., Tijssen, J.G.P. et al. (2003) Risk factors for and prevalence of thyroid disorders in a crosssectional study among healthy female relatives of patients with autoimmune thyroid disease. Clinical Endocrinology, 59, 396-401.

[27] Bulow Pedersen, I., Laurberg, P., Knudsen, N. et al. (2008) Smoking is negatively associated with the presence of thyroglobulin autoantibody and to a lesser degree with thyroid peroxidase autoantibody in serum: A population study. European Journal of Endocrinology, 158, 367-373.

[28] Belin, R.M., Astor, B.C., Powe, N.R. et al. (2004) Smokers have high serum antithyroid antibody and thyrotropin concentrations less often and low serum thyrotropin concentrations more often than nonsmokers. Journal of Clinical Endocrinology and Metabolism, 89, 6077-6086.

[29] Jorde, R. and Sundsfjord, J. (2006) Serum TSH levels in smokers and non-smokers. The 5th Tromso study. Experimental Clinical Endocrinology and Diabetes, 114, 343-347.

[30] Silvia Martina Ferrari 1, Poupak Fallahi 1, Alessandro Antonelli 1, Salvatore Benvenga. Environmental Issues in Thyroid Diseases. Front Endocrinol (Lausanne). 2017 Mar 20;8:50.

[31] Kassem Sharif, Abdulla Watad, Louis Coplan, Benjamin Lichtbroun, Alec Krosser, Michael Lichtbroun et al. The role of stress in the mosaic of autoimmunity: An overlooked association. Autoimmun. Rev. 17, 967-983 (2018).

[32] La Rocca, C., Carbone, F., Longobardi, S. and Matarese, G. The immunology of pregnancy: Regulatory T cells control maternal immune tolerance toward the fetus. Immunol. Lett. 162, 41-48 (2014).

[33] Stagnaro-Green, A. et al. A prospective study of lymphocyte-initiated immunosuppression in normal pregnancy: Evidence of a T-cell etiology for postpartum thyroid dysfunction. J. Clin. Endocrinol. Metab. 74, 645-653 (1992).

[34] Menconi, F., Hasham, A. and Tomer, Y. Environmental triggers of thyroiditis: Hepatitis C and interferon-alpha. J. Endocrinol. Invest. 34, 78-84 (2011)

[35] Bartalena, L., Bogazzi, F. and Martino, E. Amiodaroneinduced thyrotoxicosis: A difficult diagnostic and therapeutic challenge. Clin. Endocrinol. 56, 23-24 (2002).

[36] Basaria, S. and Cooper, D. S. Amiodarone and the thyroid. Am. J. Med. 118, 706-714 (2005)

[37] Edmunds MR, Mellington F, Ford RL, et al. Clinical challenges of thyroid eye disease in HIV-positive patients on highly active antiretroviral therapy. J Clin Endocrinol Metab. 2015;100(3):779-787.

[38] Pariani N, Willis M, Muller I, et al. Alemtuzumab-induced thyroid dysfunction exhibits distinctive clinical and immunological features. J Clin Endocrinol Metab. 2018;103(8):3010-3018.

[39] Morganstein DL, Lai Z, Spain L, et al. Thyroid abnormalities following the use of cytotoxic T-lymphocyte antigen-4 and programmed death receptor protein-1 inhibitors in the treatment of melanoma. Clin Endocrinol. 2017;86(4):614-620.

[40] Yamauchi I, Sakane Y, Fukuda Y, et al. Clinical features of nivolumab-induced thyroiditis: A case series study. Thyroid. 2017; 27(7):894-901.

[41] Azmat U, Liebner D, Joehlin-Price A, et al. Treatment of ipilimumab induced Graves' disease in a patient with metastatic melanoma. Case Rep Endocrinol. 2016;2016:2087525.

[42] M P Mourits et al. Clinical activity score as a guide in the management of patients with Graves' ophthalmopathy. Clin Endocrinol (Oxf). 1997 Jul;47(1):9-14.

[43] Perini, N., Santos, R. B., Romaldini, J. H. and Villagelin, D. Thyroid acropachy: A rare manifestation of Graves' disease in joints. AACE Clin. Case Rep. 5, e369–e371 (2019)

[44] de los Santos ET, Starich GH, Mazzaferri EL 1989 Sensitivity, specificity, and cost-effectiveness of the sensitive thyrotropin assay in the diagnosis of thyroid disease in ambulatory patients. Arch Intern Med 149:526-532.

[45] Douglas S. Ross, Henry B. Burch, David S. Cooper, M. Carol Greenlee, Peter Laurberg, Ana Luiza Maia et al. 2016 American Thyroid Association Guidelines for Diagnosis and Management of Hyperthyroidism and Other Causes of Thyrotoxicosis. Thyroid. 2016 Oct;26(10):1343-1421.

[46] Shigemasa C, Abe K, Taniguchi S, Mitani Y, Ueda Y, Adachi T, Urabe K, Tanaka T, Yoshida A, Mashiba H 1987 Lower serum free thyroxine (T4) levels in painless thyroiditis compared with

Graves' disease despite similar serum total T4 levels. J Clin Endocrinol Metab 65: 359-363.

[47] Abraham-Nordling M, Torring O, Hamberger B, Lundell G, Tallstedt L, Calissendorff J, Wallin G 2005 Graves' disease: A long-term quality-of-life follow up of patients randomized to treatment with antithyroid drugs, radioiodine, or surgery. Thyroid 15:1279-1286.

[48] Van Dijke, C. P., Heydendael, R. J. and De Kleine, M. J. Methimazole, carbimazole, and congenital skin defects. Ann. Intern. Med. 106, 60-61 (1987).

[49] Yang, J. et al. Analysis of 90 cases of antithyroiddrug-induced severe hepatotoxicity over 13 years in China. Thyroid 25, 278-283 (2015).

[50] Wang, M. T., Lee, W. J., Huang, T. Y., Chu, C. L. and Hsieh, C. H. Antithyroid drug-related hepatotoxicity in hyperthyroidism patients: A population-based cohort study. Br. J. Clin. Pharmacol. 78, 619-629 (2014).

[51] Watanabe, N. et al. Antithyroid drug-induced hematopoietic damage: A retrospective cohort study of agranulocytosis and pancytopenia involving 50,385 patients with Graves' disease. J. Clin. Endocrinol. Metab. 97, E49–E53 (2012).

[52] Nakamura, H., Miyauchi, A., Miyawaki, N. and Imagawa, J. Analysis of 754 cases of antithyroid drug-induced agranulocytosis over 30 years in Japan. J. Clin. Endocrinol. Metab. 98, 4776-4783 (2013).

[53] Geffner, D. L. and Hershman, J. M. βadrenergic blockade for the treatment of hyperthyroidism. Am. J. Med. 93, 61-68 (1992).

[54] Stan MN, Durski JM, Brito JP, Bhagra S, Thapa P, Bahn RS 2013 Cohort study on radioactive iodine-induced hypothyroidism: Implications for Graves' ophthalmopathy and optimal timing for thyroid hormone assessment. Thyroid 23:620-625.

[55] Traisk F, Tallstedt L, Abraham-Nordling M, et al. Thyroid-associated ophthalmopathy after treatment for Graves' hyperthyroidism with antithyroid drugs or iodine-131. J Clin Endocrinol Metab. 2009;94(10):3700-3707.

[56] Tallstedt L, Lundell G, Torring O, et al. Occurrence of ophthalmopathy after treatment for Graves' hyperthyroidism. The Thyroid Study Group. N Engl J Med. 1992;326(26):1733-1738.

[57] Bartalena L, Chiovato L, Vitti P: Management of hyperthyroidism due to Graves' disease: Frequently asked questions and answers (if any). J Endocrinol Invest 2016; 39: 1105-1114.

[58] Erbil Y, Ozluk Y, Giris M, Salmaslioglu A, Issever H, Barbaros U, Kapran Y, Ozarmagan S, Tezelman S: Effect of lugol solution on thyroid gland blood flow and microvessel density in the patients with Graves' disease. J Clin Endocrinol Metab 2007; 92: 2182-2189.

[59] Sosa JA, Bowman HM, Tielsch JM, Powe NR, Gordon TA, Udelsman R: The importance of surgeon experience for clinical and economic outcomes from thyroidectomy. Ann Surg 2008; 228: 320-330.

[60] Wilmar M. Wiersinga. Smoking and thyroid. Clinical Endocrinology (2013) 79, 145-151).

[61] Salvi M, Vannucchi G, Beck-Peccoz P. Potential utility of rituximab for Graves' orbitopathy. J Clin Endocrinol Metab. 2013;98(11):4291-4299.

[62] Cooper DS, Laurberg P. Hyperthyroidism in pregnancy. Lancet Diabetes Endocrinol 2013; 1: 238-249.

[63] Leslie De Groot 1, Marcos Abalovich, Erik K Alexander, Nobuyuki Amino, Linda Barbour, Rhoda H Cobin. et al. Management of thyroid dysfunction during pregnancy and postpartum: an Endocrine Society clinical practice guideline. J Clin Endocrinol Metab 2012; 97: 2543-2565.

[64] Fatourechi, V. Pretibial myxedema: Pathophysiology and treatment options. Am. J. Clin. Dermatol. 6, 295-309 (2005).

[65] Paul Sanders, Stuart Young, Jane Sanders, Katarzyna Kabelis, Stuart Baker, Andrew Sullivan. etal. Crystal structure of the TSH receptor (TSHR) bound to a blocking-type TSHR autoantibody. J Mol Endocrinol. 2011 Feb 15; 46(2):81-99.

[66] Patrick Marcinkowski, Inna Hoyer, Edgar Specker, Jens Furkert, Claudia Rutz, Martin Neuenschwander. etal. A New Highly Thyrotropin Receptor-Selective Small-Molecule Antagonist with Potential for the Treatment of Graves' Orbitopathy. Thyroid. 2019 Jan; 29(1):111-123.

Chapter 3

Graves' Disease: Hyperthyroidism, Symptoms, Causes and Treatment

Paula Aragão Prazeres de Oliveira,
Beatriz Nayara Muniz de Oliveira,
Eduarda da Silva Souza Paulino,
Fernanda Carolinne Marinho de Araujo
and Paula Gabriele Tabosa Lyra

Abstract

DG presents with three main presentations: hyperthyroidism with diffuse goiter, infiltrative ophthalmopathy and pre-tibial myxedema. Patients with Graves' Disease can rarely develop severe hyperthyroidism. The hyperthyroidism of Graves' Disease is characterized immunologically by the lymphocytic infiltration of the thyroid gland and by the activation of the immune system with elevation of the circulating T lymphocytes. In GD, goiter is characteristically diffuse. May have asymmetric or lobular character, with variable volume. The clinical manifestations of hyperthyroidism are due to the stimulatory effect of thyroid hormones on metabolism and tissues. Nervousness, eye complaints, insomnia, weight loss, tachycardia, palpitations, heat intolerance, damp and hot skin with excessive sweating, tremors, hyperdefecation and muscle weakness are the main characteristics. In the laboratory diagnosis, biochemical and hormonal exams will be done to assess thyroid hormones and the anti-thyroid antibodies. Additionally, imaging tests may be performed, such as radioactive iodine capture in 24 hours, ultrasonography, thyroid scintigraphy and fine needle aspiration. It is necessary to make the differential diagnosis of Graves' Disease for thyrotoxicosis, subacute lymphocytic thyroiditis and toxic nodular goiter. The treatment of DG aims to stop the production of thyroid hormones and inhibit the effect of thyroid hormones on the body. Hyperthyroidism caused by DG can be treated in the following ways: it may be the use of synthetic antithyroid medicines, thionamides, MMI being a long-term medicine, it allows a single daily dose, and adherence to treatment occurs, a disadvantage is that it cannot be used in pregnant women; beta-blockers, preferably used in the initial phase of DG with thionamides; radioactive iodine therapy (RAI), being the best cost–benefit and preventing DG recurrence; finally the total thyroidectomy, causing the withdrawal of the thyroid gland. Therefore, it should be discussed with the patient what is the best treatment for your case, with a view to the post and against each approach. If the patient develops Graves ophthalmopathy, in lighter cases the artificial tears should be used, and in more severe cases can be used as treatment, corticosteroids, orbital decompression surgery, prisms and orbital radiotherapy. In addition, the patient should keep their body healthy, doing exercise and healthy eating, following the guidance of their doctor.

Keywords: Graves' Disease, Hyperthyroidism, Goiter, Thyroid hormones

1. Introduction

GD presents with three main presentations: hyperthyroidism with diffuse goiter, infiltrative ophthalmopathy and dermopathy (pretibial myxedema). Patients with Graves' Disease rarely may develop severe hyperthyroidism (thyroid storm or thyrotoxic crisis) [1]. Consider tests for thyroid dysfunction for people if there is a clinical suspicion of thyroid disease, but bear in mind that only an isolated symptom may not be associated with this disease [2].

2. Hyperthyroidism

Graves' Disease hyperthyroidism is characterized immunologically by lymphocytic infiltration of the thyroid gland and by activation of the immune system with elevation of circulating T lymphocytes, appearance of autoantibodies that bind to the TSH receptor (TRAb) and that stimulate glandular growth and function [3–5]. The reasons for triggering this autoimmune process have not yet been fully understood, but factors such as susceptibility genetics, constitutional factors such as sex hormones and changes in immune function, and factors environmental factors (stress, iodine intake and the action of infectious agents) [6, 7].

From a clinical point of view, the hyperthyroidism of Graves' Disease is characterized by diffuse enlargement and hyperactivity of the gland thyroid, associated or not with infiltrative ophthalmopathy and, more rarely, localized myxedema. Excess thyroid hormones can lead to the development of serious complications such as congestive heart failure, cardiomyopathy and arrhythmias, mainly atrial fibrillation (10–30%). It is also associated with increased bone resorption, increased calcium and phosphorus excretion in urine and faeces, with a consequent decrease in bone mineral density and risk of fractures in women elderly [1, 3].

Symptoms of Graves' Disease	
Nervousness	Fatigue
Excessive sweating	Increased evacuations
Heat intolerance	Menstrual disorders
Palpitation	Increased appetite

3. Dermopathy (pretibial myxedema)

It affects only 5 to 10% of patients with GD and is almost associated with ophthalmopathy (usually severe) and high levels of TRAb [8]. Exceptionally, it has seen in euthyroid patients with GD [1] or with Hashimoto's thyroiditis [9]. It consists of within the thickening of the skin, particularly within the pretibial area, because of the buildup of the glycosaminoglycans. The evidence is shown in plaques and on them; the skin is type of thickened, with the looks of orange rind and violet color. Sometimes a Dermopathy involves the entire lower leg and should reach the feet. Rarely (less than 1% of cases), it can be seen in other places (hands or shoulders), especially after prolonged trauma [8, 10]. Very rarely, pretibial myxedema is the initial manifestation of GD [1, 11].

4. Goiter

In GD, goiter is characteristically diffuse. May have asymmetric or lobular character, with variable volume. In some patients, there is thrill and murmur over the gland, produced by increased flow of blood, this finding being exclusive to the disease. Any patient with diffuse goiter and hyperthyroidism has GD until they prove the opposite [4, 12]. In the elderly, when present, the goiter tends to be small [1].

5. Ophthalmopathy

The clinical manifestations of hyperthyroidism are due to the stimulatory effect of thyroid hormones on metabolism and tissues. Nervousness, eye complaints, insomnia, weight loss, tachycardia, palpitations, heat intolerance, damp and hot skin with excessive sweating, tremors, hyperdefecation and muscle weakness are the main characteristics [13, 14].

In GD, goiter is singularly diffuse, being present in 97% of cases. Asymmetric or lobular, with variable volume. In some patients, an exclusive finding of the disease is that the increase in blood flow brings the presence of thrill and murmur over the gland. Any patient with diffuse goiter and hyperthyroidism has GD until proven otherwise. In the elderly, when present, the goiter tends to be small [15, 16].

Ophthalmopathy or orbitopathy has an equivalent autoimmune pathogenesis as GD hyperthyroidism and may exacerbate both hypo and thyroid hyperfunction. Antibodies react by causing intraorbital auto-aggression, as in tissue thyroid. Ophthalmopathy can precede hyperthyroidism (20% of the time), succeed it (40%) or appear concomitantly with it (40%) [1, 15].

The cases during which ophthalmopathy, transiently or permanently, isn't in the course of hyperthyroidism are called Graves' euthyroid disease. Clinically evident ophthalmopathy occurs in up to 50% of patients with GD. It stems from the thickening of the muscles extraocular and increased retrobulbar fat, which results in a rise in intraorbital pressure. Consequently, protrusion of the eyeball (proptosis or exophthalmos) and decreased venous drainage may occur, leading to periorbital edema, conjunctival edema and conjunctival hyperemia [16, 17].

The most common ocular manifestations in the GD are the eyelid retraction, the stare or frightened look and the sign of lid-lag (delay in lowering the upper eyelid when the eyeball is moved down). Nevertheless, they occur in any sort of thyrotoxicosis, as they're consequent to adrenergic hyperactivity. On the opposite hand, the finding of periorbital edema and exophthalmos practically confirms the diagnosis of GD. Additionally, diplopia can occur in 5 to 10% of patients, because of the functional impairment of the musculature extrinsic ocular. Ophthalmoplegia and eyelid ptosis also can occasionally be seen. Finally, severe cases, there could also be dysfunction of the nervus opticus, defects in the visual fields, disturbance of vision in color or loss of vision [1, 15–18].

GD exophthalmos is typically bilateral, but it can be unilateral. During this situation, it must be differentiated from a tumor retrobulbar or arteriovenous malformation using computerized tomography or resonance imaging. The most effective way to verify the existence of the property and establish its magnitude is by using Hertel's exophthalmometer. A measurement greater than 20 mm in Caucasians is taken into account abnormal, 18 mm between Orientals and 22 mm in blacks. However, caution is required in borderline interpretations of up to

2 mm. Proposals are often selected as mild (increase of 3 to 4 mm), moderate (5 to 7 mm) and severe (>7 mm) [1, 16, 18].

6. Laboratory diagnosis

6.1 Biochemical and hormonal exams

6.1.1 Thyroid function tests

For adults when secondary thyroid dysfunctions are not suspected, it is appropriate to consider measuring thyroid-stimulating hormone (TSH) itself, then if the TSH is above the reference range, measure free thyroxine (FT4) in the same sample. If the TSH is below the reference range, measure FT4 and free triiodothyronine (FT3) yet in the same sample. In addition, consider measuring both TSH and FT4 for adult patients when secondary thyroid dysfunction (pituitary disease) is suspected in children and young people. If the TSH is below the reference range, measure FT3 in the same sample. Consider repeating the tests for thyroid dysfunction if symptoms worsen or new symptoms develop (but just 6 weeks from the most recent test) [2].

6.1.2 Antithyroid antibodies

The antibodies are often classified a minimum of three general types. Thyroid stimulating antibodies (TSAb, sometimes TSI) interact with the TSH receptor during a positive functional manner and initiate the adenylyl cyclase function and the phospholipase A2 function of the receptor, causing all aspects of thyroid stimulation [12, 19].

Functionally, this is probably identical to the effects induced by TSH itself. Other antibodies can interact with the receptor in a slightly different manner, presumably by binding to different epitopes on the receptor, and can block the binding of TSH to the receptor while not themselves stimulating function. These antibodies are known as thyroid stimulation blocking antibodies, or TBAb [19, 20].

A third set of antibodies can bind to the receptor but neither stimulate nor inhibit its function. These are known as thyrotropin binding immunoglobulins. They are commonly recognized by assays which detect their ability to interfere with the binding of TSH to the receptor, and are identified as TRAb, or TBII [19]. Probably all patients with Graves' Disease have a mixture of all of these antibodies. If TSAb predominates, thyroid stimulation occurs and, if the activity is sufficient, the patient may become hyperthyroid and be characterized as having Graves' Disease. If the antibodies block the action of TSH, they may induce hypothyroidism, in which case the patient might be characterized as having Hashimoto's thyroiditis or idiopathic myxedema [12, 20].

Among patients with GD, up to 50% have anti-thyroglobulin (anti-Tg) antibodies and up to 90% have antibodies antithyroperoxidase (anti-TPO), at lower titers than those observed in Hashimoto's thyroiditis [21]. Although TSH anti-receptor antibodies (TRAb) can be found in normal individuals (exceptionally), in Hashimoto's thyroiditis (in 6 to 60%) and in painless subacute thyroiditis or postpartum thyroiditis (in 5 to 15%), its occurrence in hyperthyroid patients is highly specific for GD (present in 90 to 100% of cases) [13, 14].

A recent meta-analysis showed high sensitivity (97.1 to 97.4%) and specificity (98.3 to 99.2%) for the second and third TRAb assays generations. According to these data, the probability of a TRAb-positive individual having GD is 1,367 to 3,420 times higher (depending on the type of assay) compared to a TRAb-negative individual [1, 22]. In Europe, around 85% of specialists measure TRAb in the initial diagnostic assessment of GD [23]. A similar approach is reported in Japan and Korea [18, 24]. In Brazil and the USA [16, 18] the guidelines still recommend prioritizing the dosage of TRAb in some specific situations, such as: 1- In the diagnosis of euthyroid GD; 2- in the diagnosis of apathetic hyperthyroidism; 3- In the distinction between GD and postpartum thyroiditis or subacute lymphocytic thyroiditis; 4- In assessing the risk of recurrence of hyperthyroidism after discontinuation of thionamide treatment (elevated titers increase the risk of relapse); and 5- In pregnant women with GD [1].

TRAb at elevated titers at the end of pregnancy implies an increased risk of neonatal hyperthyroidism. On the other hand, its negativity favors the interruption of treatment, aiming to decrease the risk of fetal hypothyroidism [1, 14].

6.1.3 Hematological and biochemical parameters

In GD, leukopenia (common), hypercalciuria and hypercalcemia (occasional), elevated transaminases and hyperbilirubinemia (in the most severe cases). Reduction of total cholesterol and LDL-cholesterol can also be found [1].

6.2 Medical imaging

6.2.1 Radioactive iodine capture in 24 hours (RAIU/24H)

The uptake of radioactive iodine in 24 hours appears high in basically 100% of cases of GD, generating the possibility of its distinction with cases of thyroid acid and thyroid oxycosis secondary to lymphocytic subacute thyroid, in which the RAIU/24 h has low or absent characteristics. In addition the RAIU/24H should only be requested when there is diagnostic doubt between the GD and the mentioned pathologies. A path to differentiation is thyroid ultrasonography with color Doppler or specification of TRAb levels (lower accuracy) [1, 25–29].

6.2.2 Ultrasonography

Ultrasonography has similar sensitivity to RAIU/24 h for the diagnosis of GD (95.4% vs. 97.4%, respectively). Advantages of ultrasonography are absence of exposure to radiation, greater precision within the detection of possible thyroid nodules and cost low. Additionally, color Doppler ultrasonography can differentiate GD (diffusely enlarged hypoechogenic gland) from thyrotoxicosis induced by follicular destruction (reduced glandular volume and blood flow) [1, 30, 31].

6.2.3 Thyroid scintigraphy

Scintigraphy with radioactive iodine (123I or 131I) or technetium should be performed in patients with nodules identified at ultrasonography, to assess whether such nodules are "hot" or "cold" [1].

In clinical practice thyroid scintigraphy is most ordinarily used to differentiate between subacute thyroiditis and Graves' Disease. Additionally, patients with congenital hypothyroidism, functioning thyroid nodule, suspected ectopic thyroid, thyroid carcinoma, and midline neck swelling (thyroglossal cyst) also require thyroid scintigraphy [1].

6.3 Fine needle aspiration

It will be indicated when normal thyroid nodules or hypocaptants are found on scintigraphy. It's been suggested by some studies that such nodules would be at higher risk for malignancy in patients with GD, however newer studies haven't confirmed this possibility [32, 33].

6.4 Differential diagnosis

6.4.1 Graves' Disease versus other causes of thyrotoxicosis

Hyperthyroidism can have several etiologies. In the distinction between these etiologies, some data clinical and laboratory tests are often useful, for instance, the presence of infiltrative ophthalmopathy or pretibial myxedema in patients with hyperthyroidism is sufficient to verify the diagnosis of Graves' Disease (GD) [1, 32]. Furthermore, any patient with diffuse toxic goiter, until proven otherwise, has GD. However, within the absence of ophthalmopathy and dermopathy, the involvement of other pathologies in the genesis of thyrotoxicosis may be considered, especially subacute thyroiditis lymphocytic (TSL) and toxic nodular goiter, the likelihood of TSL, although low, is higher in patients with goiters small, mild and short-lived [1, 32].

Rarely, Graves' Disease and toxic nodular goiter coexists, characterizing the Marine-Lenhart syndrome [1]. This possibility should be suspected whenever the treatment of hyperthyroidism requires high doses of synthetic antithyroid drugs or when relapse happens soon after suspension of an equivalent. In patients with thyrotoxicosis and low 131I uptake, additionally to subacute thyroiditis, other diagnostic considerations include factitious thyrotoxicosis (using thyroid hormones), functioning metastasis from follicular carcinoma and also the rare struma ovary (ovarian teratoma with ectopic thyroid issues), in the latter situation, there's increased RAIU within the pelvic region [34, 35].

6.5 Atypical presentations of Graves' Disease

Occasionally, GD can manifest itself during a very atypical way, making diagnosis difficult. Sometimes she goes with marked muscle atrophy and wishes to be differentiated from a primary nervous disorder. In the elderly, as mentioned, we are able to find apathetic hyperthyroidism, during which the classic manifestations of GD are usually absent, with predominance of cardiac symptoms. Thus, GD should be considered in any patient with atrial fibrillation or heart failure without apparent cause and/or refractory to the standard treatment [1, 36, 37]. GD should also be considered in cases of amenorrhea or infertility, since some young women may present these problems as a manifestation hyperthyroidism. GD can rarely happen, especially in Eastern and Latino men, with a sudden flaccid paralysis and hypokalemia (periodic hypokalemic thyrotoxic paralysis). Such paralysis is typically resolvable spontaneous, are often the initial manifestation of hyperthyroidism and may be treated by potassium supplementation and use of beta-blockers. It's cured by the right treatment of hyperthyroidism [1, 36, 37].

6.6 Treatment

Hyperthyroidism due to Graves' Disease is treated with one among the subsequent approaches: synthesis antithyroid drugs (thionamides), surgical removal of the thyroid gland (total thyroidectomy), or RAI-induced shrinkage of the thyroid tissue [1, 18, 21]. These options have advantages and drawbacks, they ought to always be presented to the patient, if he has the ability to discern [1, 21]. Treatment should be individualized based on the clinical characteristics, age, etiology, size of goiter, concurrent comorbidities, patient's preference, and special situations like pregnancy [3].

6.7 Medical treatment

6.7.1 Synthesis antithyroid drugs (thionamides)

The available antithyroid drugs are methimazole (MMI), also called thiamazol, carbimazole and propylthiouracil (PTU) [3, 18]. The use of thionamide antithyroid drugs as an initial treatment varies according to geographic location, they are the foremost common treatment of GD in Asia, Europe and Latin America. However, radioiodine is used more often than medications in the United States [21, 38]. These drugs are actively transported into the thyroid where they inhibit iodide oxidation and organification by inhibiting thyroid peroxidase and therefore the coupling of the iodotyrosine to synthesise T4 and T3 [38, 39]. The long duration of MMI (up to 24 hours or more) makes it possible to administer it during a single daily dose, which facilitates the most effective adherence to the treatment [40].

The PTU should be administered, at least initially, in two to three daily doses [1, 41]. Nonetheless, a divided dose could also be more effective initially within the most severe cases. Compared to PTU, MMI makes it possible to get euthyroidism more frequently and faster, additionally being better tolerated and causing less hepatotoxicity [36, 41, 42]. The current guidelines of the American Thyroid Association and also the latest consensus of the Brazilian Society of Endocrinology and Metabology recommends that you must always choose MMI as the first option. Two exceptions to the this rule are the first trimester or pregnancy and severe intolerance to MMI [36, 37].

6.8 Mechanism of action

The mechanism of action of those drugs is the inhibition of synthesis of thyroxine (T4) and triiodothyronine (T3) in the follicular cells, for interference with the organization (formation of MIT and DIT) and coupling (joining MIT and DIT to make T3 and T4) of iodotyrosine, by blocking thyroid peroxidase, and enzyme responsible for the iodination of tyrosine residues in the thyroglobulin [40, 42]. Additionally, PTU, but not methimazole, inhibits the peripheral conversion of T4 to T3, with a consequent drop by serum T3 levels and increased reverse T3 when utilized in high doses (> 600 mg/day) [1]. There's, however, little evidence that this effect is clinically relevant, except possibly in patients with severe thyrotoxicosis [32]. The antithyroid drugs negatively impact the activity and numbers of intrathyroidal T cells, the aberrant thyrocyte expression of MHC class II, also because of the generation of reactive oxygen species, lipid peroxidation, and subsequent oxidative damage [2, 43].

6.9 Posology

For dosage for hyperthyroidism, the severity will follow, the MMI dose is 10 to 40 mg/day, the PTU dose is 100 to 400 mg/day, these are the initial portions. When a more severe case occurs the recommended is a higher MMI dosage of 30 to 40 mg/day, causing faster normalization of thyroid hormones, however, bringing side effects on a larger scale [44, 45].

After treatment, the patient has to be monitored every 4 to 6 weeks, achieving eutyroidism, the dose is gradually decreased, obtaining the lowest possible dose for the patient, in addition, the medical consultations should be quarterly. Usually the preservation dose is 5 to 10 mg/day of MMI, since OCT is 50 to 100 mg/day 2 times/day. Carbimazole corresponds to more than 140% of methimazole relative to dosage. It is important to monitor serum TSH levels, since they are suppressed even after a few months after euthyroidism, being essential to see when there is biochemical hypothyroidism. Therefore, the dosage of TSH at initiation of treatment with tionamides is limited [44, 45].

One type of scheme used in the former was blocking and replacement, an L-thyroxine adjustment and high doses of TAD, however, causes a greater danger of adverse effects. Occasionally combined therapy is used when metimanzol maintenance therapy is difficult to titrate, so 10 mg/day of MMI is used in combination with 12.5 to 25 μg/day of L-thyroxine [44, 45].

6.10 Effectiveness of treatment

Among patients who tolerate and take thionamides properly, the overwhelming majority will achieve hormonal normalization, but recurrences are frequent. Relapses are common in the first year, especially in the first six months post-treatment suspension. They rarely manifest after 4 to 5 years. Patients at increased risk of recurrence are those with severe hyperthyroidism, larger goiter, orbitopathy, duration of treatment <12 months, elevated T3:T4 ratio, TSH persistently suppressed and, above all, high concentrations of TRAb at the beginning or at the end of treatment [1, 21, 30, 40, 46]. In case of recurrence, a second course of treatment with DAT could also be attempted, but usually opts for an additional sort of therapy, preferably radioactive iodine [1, 25].

7. Factors affecting the long-term response to thionamides

One factor may be time, there are still conflicts about the appropriate duration of therapy, but it seems to be 12 to 18 months. Patients treated for one semester have less favorable results when compared to those treated for 1 to 2 years [47, 48].

A metanalysis was performed and one of the interpretations of the study was that the rate of remission in adults does not improve when treatment is performed for a period longer than one and a half years. Another factor is the dose of thionamide. According to studies, the definitive remission rate appears to be similar with the use of low or high doses of TAD. On the other hand the higher doses are indicated for patients with more severe hyperthyroidism, and through their use it was also possible to observe the reach of euthyroidism more quickly [10, 14]. Classically, it is known through studies that children and adolescents compared to adults have considerably lower remission rates [49, 50].

Another factor was demonstrated by most of the reverse relationship studies between the initial size of the bucket and the possibility of remission. Patients with large buoyancy (≥ 80 g) are the least likely to relapse, the same occurring in cases with persistently suppressed TSH at the end of treatment [51]. It also has TSH anti-receptor antibody factor (TRAb); their levels at diagnosis and end of treatment are linked to higher relapse rate compared to low expression of these antibodies [52].

Thyroid function at baseline levels of T3 > 500 ng/dl are associated with increased likelihood of disease reappearance [51, 53]. And a very high rate of relapse of hyperthyroidism occurred in the postpartum period in women who were in remission during pregnancy; a higher probability was also related to ophthalmopathy, as was the use of iodine or drugs that have it in their composition. Some studies have also found smokers, mostly male, as part of this higher-risk group. Patients with a high chance of recurrence should be evaluated more frequently and shorter intervals after stopping antithyroid drugs (TDD). On the other hand, mild disease carriers, small bullets and negative TRAb have a remission rate > 50%, making the use of TDD potentially more favorable in this patient group [1, 8, 14, 53–55].

8. Long-term thionamide treatment

In cases of patients, from young people to the elderly, who do not opt for definitive therapies in the face of the reappearance of the disease, such as surgery or radioiodine, it is reasonable to consider other treatment routes, such as long-term maintenance [14, 50, 55, 56].

Researchers examined studies in the Ovid MEDLINE, Ovid Embase and Scopus databases, on GD until 2020, and evaluated the effectiveness of long-term antithyroid drugs in achieving and maintaining euthyroidism compared to the state of euthyroidism during the treatment of hypothyroidism after ablative therapies. They cited a retrospective study that concluded that long-term antithyroid drugs were effective in maintaining euthyroidism. And it has been seen that the risk of hypothyroidism is greater after treatment with radiation compared to antithyroid drugs. Bearing in mind that when considering a health-related quality of life, long-term antithyroid drugs are possibly an economical alternative, despite the fact that radioactive iodine is considered the most affordable first-line treatment [57].

9. Adverse effects of thionamide

The effects are most common in the first half of treatment. The most common are allergic in origin such as itching, rash, fever and even arthralgia. And also very frequent epigastralgia. Subdivisions in two groups: mild reactions (allergic reactions, gastric intolerance, neutropenia, fever, hair loss/alopecia, anaemia and decreased or even palate loss) and severe reactions (thrombocytopenia, medullary aplasia, cholestatic hepatitis, agranulocytosis, hepatocellular necrosis, hypoglycemia, ANCA-positive vasculitis, polyarteritis and glomerulonephritis [30, 50].

In cases of mild side effects the switch to another thioamide can be done cautiously or even the concomitant use of an antihistamine solves the rashes within a few days. Patients who develop severe reactions such as vasculitis, hepatitis or agranulocytosis should no longer be medicated with another compound in the same group [55, 58].

They may possibly also have cramps, muscle pain, edema, general fatigue and toxic psychosis rarely occurs. Other serious adverse reactions include polyarthritis, lomerulonephritis and lupus-simile syndrome, more common with PTU than with MMI [55, 58].

10. Beta blockers

Especially useful in the initial phase of GD treatment with amides, when euthyroidism has not yet been achieved. Its main indication is the elderly with symptomatic thyrotoxicosis and other thyrotoxic patients with high resting heart rate or who have a presence of cardiovascular disease. Caution should be paramount as high doses can cause a decrease in serum T3 levels. Usually the medication is stopped in the third or fourth week. There is also an option to use selective B-1 drugs [24, 30, 51].

10.1 Potassium iodide

Since the arrival of antithyroid drugs, iodine has ceased to be used as primary therapy for GD. Its main limitation is the escape of the inhibition of the synthesis of thyroid hormones by iodine, a phenomenon referred to as the by Wolff-Chaikoff [1, 32, 41].

10.2 Radioactive iodine (radioiodine)

Radioiodine is definitely administered orally, in solution or capsules, and has low cost. This treatment is proper to patients with persistent hyperthyroidism after completion of a 12–18 month first course of antithyroid drugs therapy, those with a recurrence or relapse of thyrotoxicosis, individuals with poor compliance on ATD, patients with major ATD-induced of effects and subjects who choose this approach. It is often used either as initial therapy or after treatment with medication. Antithyroid drugs, when used, are generally discontinued for 3 to 7 days before radioiodine therapy, since the effectiveness of radioiodine could even be diminished when antithyroid drugs are given concurrently [59]. Compared to other sorts of treatment of GD, 131I is taken into account to be the foremost cost-effective [3, 41, 60, 61]. The goal of radioiodine therapy is induced hypothyroidism so as to prevent a recurrence of Graves' Disease. This goal is achieved in approximately 80% of patients [58].

11. Dose

Most specialists choose to use fixed doses for their high simplicity (from 10 to 20 mCi. However, the dose is usually calculated in microcusts (μCi) or megabecquerels (MBq) per gram (g) of thyroid tissue, from thyroid size and in the capture of radioactive iodine of 24 hours. Generally, 160 to 200 μCi/g is recommended to leave the treatment safe and ensure it, the two squirrels being [1, 41, 56, 62].

12. Effectiveness

The rate satisfactory response to radioiodine therapy, with the resultant appearance of hypo or euthyroidism, is approximately 80 to 90% [1]. An oversized goiter with hypoechogenicity at US, the presence of anti-TPO antibodies and high doses of 131I increase the likelihood of hypothyroidism [1]. In many patients, normalization of thyroid function tests and symptoms occurs within the period of 4 to 8 weeks. Hypothyroidism can appear after 4 weeks, but more commonly it occurs between 2 and 6 months [1, 21]. With the use of fixed or calculated doses, the efficacy appears to be an equivalent [3, 21]. Higher doses provide success earlier and, generally, more expressive therapeutic, lower doses (< 10 mCi), tend to result in failure rates and more pronounced recurrence [3, 21, 63].

13. Factors that influence the response to radio

Among the varied factors which will interfere with the response to 131I, the quantification of the goiter appears to be the foremost important. Smaller goiters are the ones that respond best and those the most often progress to hypothyroidism, especially with fixed doses. Also it had been demonstrated that patients with HLA-DR3 would have greater resistance to radioiodine therapy [23, 32, 40]. Clinical features most related to therapeutic failure include: male gender, smoking, large goiter (> 50 g): RAIU/24 h very high (>90%) and a marked increase in T3 levels (> 500 ng/ml) [64]. Persistence of levels of elevated TRAb and increased thyroid blood flow at Doppler also increases the likelihood of relapses [1].

14. Complications

Hypothyroidism is the main adverse effect of radioiodine therapy, being the frequency in the short term, depending on the dosage used, and may be more than 12 to 20 mCi than with 8 to 10 mCi. However, the amount of patients with hypothyroidism does not depend on the dose of 131I, reaching a minimum of 80% of these adequately treated patients. A frequency of hypothyroidism is observed in about 50% in the first year, followed by 5% per year, at doses between 12 and 15 mCi. However, hypothyroidism due to 131I may be transient, occurring in about 25% of patients who acquired hypothyroidism in the first 6 months after dosing. If the patient is severely symptomatic, L-thyroxine and discontinue treatment 6 months later, checking the maintenance of the disease. Hypothyroidism may develop or persist after one year, it is almost always permanent. In addition, one of the complications of radioiodine therapy is actinic thyroid or radiation, transient and occurs in approximately 3% of treated patients. It may cause pain in the anterior cervical region, lasting up to 4 weeks, and sometimes exacerbation of hyperthyroidism due to the release of t3 and t4 into the bloodstream. Elevation of thyroid hormones is reported in up to 10% of patients and should result in actinic thyroiditis or increased TRAb, observed 3 to 6 months after taking 131I [1, 14, 39].

15. Radioiodine and thyroid eye disease

When radioiodine therapy (RAI) is used, in a delimited group as in smokers, an adverse effect is thyroid eye disease. This issue may occur because of glucocorticoid therapy and the next conditions are considered; smoking, active ophthalmopathy or severe hyperthyroidism. Moreover, in these cases, prior to RAI, the correct is to achieve euthyroidism with thionamide, preferably MMI, possessing the most prolonged radioprotective effect on propylthiouracil. However, for patients with severe DG and risk for vision disorders, radiotherapy is not recommended by choosing thioamides. Different corticotherapy regimens, such as prednisone 0.2 mg/kg/day, were analyzed one day after administration of radioactive iodine and held the dosage for 6 months, this decreased the dosage and discontinued at most within two months. There is evidence that thyroid eye disease may worsen in patients who may develop hypothyroidism after treatment. Therefore, in the face of thyroid hypofunction tests, revising the introduction of L-thyroxine early. Soon after 7 days of radiotherapy in patients with registered hyperthyroidism, MMI should be reintroduced [1, 14, 24, 65, 66].

16. Preparation for radioactive iodine with thionamides

The danger of worsening hyperthyroidism or thyrotoxic crisis triggering induced 131I is <1%. In Brazil and Europe, radioiodine without prior treatment with thioamides is usually common, not in the USA. However, this should be avoided in cardiopathic patients with severe hyperthyroidism and the elderly. Due to the assumed radioprotective effect of PTU, preference should be given to MMI, therefore, it should be administered until it reaches euthyroidism, with the drug discontinuation 5 to 7 days prior to the 131I dose, its reintroduction 4 to 7 days after it. In addition, patients using PTU, a 25% increase in radioiodine dose is recommended. Another important point is that patients with an iodine allergy have no contraindication for 131I [1, 14].

17. Contraindications

The use of 131I in pregnant or lactating patients is contraindicated. Women or men who intend to have children within the next 6 months are also advised not to be given radioactive iodine. However, there is insufficient evidence of the risk of teratogenicity with radioiodine. Other equivalent contraindications are: severe inflectional ophthalmopathy and patient refusal [3, 14, 57, 66].

18. Radioiodine and thyroid nodules

Radioiodine treatment is indicated for ablation of autonomous tissue and reduction of thyroid volume. There is disagreement whether nodules have a greater chance of malignancy in GD cases. It is then suggested that non-functioning nodules >1 to 1.5 cm undergo a fine needle suction puncture (PAAF) prior to administration of I [14].

19. Monitoring after radioactive iodine

Thyroid function should be monitored 1–2 months after radioactive iodine therapy. Some suggest that it be checked after 15 days and then monthly or every 2 months; Such guidance is aimed at the early detection of hypothyroidism, especially in patients at risk of developing or worsening orbitopathy. If the patient is still thyrotoxic within two months of therapy, thyroid function should be monitored every 4–6 weeks until the patient is euthyroid or hypothyroid, remember that it may take up to 6 months or more for TSH to normalise. Substitution of levothyroxine should be initiated as soon as hypothyroidism occurs before laboratory tests proving the condition, immediately introducing L-thyroxine replacement. Patients with relapse or persistent hyperthyroidism after 6 months may re-receive radioactive iodine or those with minimal response to treatment ≤3 months [14, 50, 56].

20. Thyroidectomy

Thyroidectomy is the oldermost treatment for GD. The main objective is the rapid and definitive control of effects of excess thyroid hormones. That is achieved by removing all or almost all of the functioning tissue of the thyroid gland. Indications for surgery in the treatment of GD do not are well established in the literature, being classified by some authors in absolute and relative indications. The indications considered absolute are large goiter with compressive symptoms, suspicious nodule or malignant, pregnant woman who does not get control with DAT, refusal of treatment with 131I, woman planning pregnancy within six to 12 months and intolerance to DAT. At relative indications are large goiter, ophthalmopathy severe, poor adherence and lack of response to treatment with DAT [56, 62, 67].

The standard procedure is total thyroidectomy (TT), which provides a cure rate of around 100% for hyperthyroidism of the DG [14, 65]. The risk of recurrence is almost 0% after TT, while subtotal thyroidectomy (TST) implies a probability of 5 to 20% (8%, on average) of persistence or recurrence of hyperthyroidism in 5 years [65]. Furthermore, with the exception of hypothyroidism early, as rates of complications with TT and TST may be comparable when the patient is operated on by a surgeon experienced (more than 100 thyroidectomies/year): transient hypocalcemia, 9.6 vs. 7.4%; definitive hypoparathyroidism, 1.6 vs. 1.0%; recurrent laryngeal injury, 0.9 vs. 0.7%, respectively [65]. In a recent meta-analysis and systematic review, the risk for hypoparathyroidism (transient or permanent) survived the older ones with TT. In a few centers, there is underwent an endoscopic thyroidectomy [38].

21. Preoperative management and follow-up of patients who receive thyroidectomy

Before surgery, patients should be euthyroid. Pretreatment with ATD reduces the risk of thyroid storm precipitated by surgery, and β blockers control hyperthyroid symptoms. Pretreatment with inorganic iodide, such as potassium iodide (50 mg iodide, three times daily, for 7–10 days before surgery) can also be considered in patients with Graves' Disease [67]. Inorganic iodide reduces thyroid hormone release and thyroid vascularity [68], which in turn decreases intraoperative blood loss. After surgery, levothyroxine replacement should be started and TSH concentration monitored 6–8 weeks after surgery. Oral calcium and calcitriol supplementation can be used before surgery and according to postoperative serum calcium concentrations [69].

22. Side effects

Surgical complications are rare, occurring in 1–3% of patients [60]. The most frequent complication is hypocalcemia due to permanent hypoparathyroidism, followed by permanent recurrent laryngeal nerve injury. The risk of these complications is lower when thyroidectomy is done by a high-volume thyroid surgeon [59, 61].

Author details

Paula Aragão Prazeres de Oliveira[1*], Beatriz Nayara Muniz de Oliveira[2], Eduarda da Silva Souza Paulino[2], Fernanda Carolinne Marinho de Araujo[2] and Paula Gabriele Tabosa Lyra[2]

1 Centro Universitário Maurício de Nassau-UNINASSAU, Disciplina de Endocrinologia, Recife, Pernambuco, Brazil

2 Centro Universitário Maurício de Nassau-UNINASSAU, Medicina, Recife, Pernambuco, Brazil

*Address all correspondence to: endopaulaoliveira@gmail.com

References

[1] Endocrinologia clínica/Lucio Vilar ... [et al.] - 6. ed. - Rio de Janeiro: Guanabara Koogan, 2016. il.

[2] National Institute for Health and Care Excellence. Thyroid disease: assessment and management. Natl Inst Heal Care Excell Guidel [Internet]. 2019;(June):1-49. Available from:https://www.nice.org.uk/guidance/ng145/resources/thyroid-disease-ssessment-and-management-pdf-66141781496773

[3] Andrade VA, Gross JL, Maia AL. Iodo radioativo no manejo do hipertireoidismo da doença de Graves. Arq Bras Endocrinol Metabol. 2004;48(1):159-65.

[4] Paschke R, Ludgate M. The thyrotropin receptor in thyroid diseases. N Engl J Med 1997;337:1675-81.

[5] LiVolsi VA. Pathology. In: Braverman LE, Utiger RD, eds. Werner and Ingbar's The Thyroid. 8th ed. Philadelphia: Lippincort Williams & Wilkins 2000:488-511.

[6] Brix TH, Kyvik KO, Hegedüs L. What is the evidence of genetic factors in the etiology of Graves' disease? A brief review. Thyroid 1998;8:627-34.

[7] Tomer Y, Barbesino G, Greenberg DA, Concepcion E, Davies TF. Mapping the major susceptibility loci for familial Graves' and Hashimoto's diseases: evidence for genetic heterogeneity and gene interactions. J Clin Endocrinol Metab 1999;84:4656-64.

[8] Schwartz KM, Fatourechi V, Ahmed DD et al. Dermopathy of Graves' disease (pretibial myxedema): long-term outcome. J Clin Endocrinol Metab. 2002; 87:438-46.

[9] Cannavo SP, Borgia F, Vaccaro M et al. Pretibial myxoedema associated with Hashimoto's thyroiditis. J Eur Acad Dermatol Venereol. 2002; 16:625-7.

[10] Mandel SJ, Reed Larsen P et al. Thyrotoxicosis. In: Melmed S et al. (Ed.). Williams textbook of endocrinology. 12th ed. Philadelphia: Elsevier Saunders, 2012. p. 362-405.

[11] Georgala S, Katoulis AC, Georgala C et al. Pretibial myxedema as the initial manifestation of Graves' disease. J Eur Acad Dermatol Venereol. 2002; 16:380-3.

[12] Groot LJ De. Graves' Disease and the Manifestations of Thyrotoxicosis. Http://WwwEndotextOrg/ [Internet]. 2015;(April):1-77. Available from: http://creativecommons.org/licenses/by-nc-nd/2.0/

[13] Brent GA. Graves' Disease. 2008;2594-605.

[14] Weetman AP. Medical progress: Graves' disease. N Engl J Med. 2000; 343:1236-48.

[15] Greenspan S, Resnick NM. Geriatric endocrinology. In: Greenspan F, Gardner DG (Ed.). Basic & clinical endocrinology. 7th ed. McGraw-Hill Co., 2004. p. 842-66.

[16] Bahn RS. Graves' ophthalmopathy. N Engl J Med. 2010; 362:726-38.

[17] Bartalena L, Wiersinga WM, Pinchera A. Graves' ophthalmopathy: state of the art and perspectives. J Endocrinol Invest. 2004;27:295-301.

[18] Burch HB. Overview of the clinical manifestations of thyrotoxicosis. In: Braverman LE (Ed.). Werner & Ingbar's the thyroid.

[19] Kahaly George J., Diana Tanja. Receptor Antibody Functionality and Nomenclature. Frontiers in Endocrinology.8th ed. 2017; 1664-2392.

[20] Eckstein AK, Plicht M, Lax H, Neuhauser M, Mann K, Lederbogen S, Heckmann C, Esser J, Morgenthaler NG.Thyrotropin receptor autoantibodies are independent risk factors for Graves' ophthalmopathy and help to predict severity and outcome of the disease. J Clin Endocrinol Metab. 2006 Sep;91(9):3464-70.

[21] DeGroot LJ. Graves' Disease and the Manifestations of Thyrotoxicosis. In: DeGroot LJ et al. (Ed.). Endotext [Internet]. South Dartmouth (MA): MDText.com, Inc.; 2000-2015 Jul 11.

[22] Tozzoli R, Bagnasco M, Giavarina D et al. TSH receptor autoantibody immunoassay in patients with Graves' disease: improvement of diagnostic accuracy over different generations of methods. Systematic review and meta-analysis. Autoimmun Rev. 2012; 12:107-13.

[23] Kahaly GJ, Bartalena L, Hegedus L. The American Thyroid Association/ American Association of Clinical Endocrinologists guidelines for hyperthyroidism and other causes of thyrotoxicosis: a European perspective. Thyroid. 2011; 21:585-91.

[24] Yamashita S, Amino N, Shong YK. The American Thyroid Association and American Association of Clinical Endocrinologists hyperthyroidism and other causes of thyrotoxicosis guidelines: viewpoints from Japan and Korea. Thyroid 2011; 21: 577-80.

[25] Satapathy SK, Sanyal AJ. Epidemiology and natural history of nonalcoholic fatty liver disease. Semin Liver Dis. 2015; 35:221-35.

[26] Angulo P. Nonalcoholic fatty liver disease. N Engl J Med. 2002; 346:1221-31.

[27] Marchesini G, Bugianesi E, Forlani E et al. Nonalcoholic fatty liver, steatohepatitis, and the metabolic syndrome. Hepatology. 2003; 37:917-23.

[28] Younossi ZM, Venkatesan C. A 2012 clinical update for internists in adult nonalcoholic fatty liver disease. Panminerva Med. 2012; 54:29-3

[29] Fazel Y, Koenig AB, Sayiner M et al. Epidemiology and natural history of non-alcoholic fatty liver disease. Metabolism. 2016 Jan 29. [Epub ahead of print.]

[30] Bahn RS, Burch HB, Cooper DS et al. Hyperthyroidism and other causes of thyrotoxicosis: management guidelines of the American Thyroid Association and American Association of Clinical Endocrinologist. Endocr Pract. 2011; 17:456-520.

[31] Paula FJA, Foss MC. Hipocalcemia, hipoparatireoidismo, pseudo-hipoparatireoidismo e pseupseudo-hipoparatireoidismo. In: Coronho V et al. (Ed.). Tratado de endocrinologia e cirurgia endócrina. Rio de Janeiro: Guanabara Koogan, 2001. p. 649-59.

[32] Klubo-Gwiezdzinska J, Wartofsky L. Thyroid emergencies. Med Clin North Am. 2012; 96:385-403.

[33] Shoback DM. Hypocalcemia management. In: De Groot LJ, Beck-Peccoz P, Chrousos G et al. (Ed.). Endotext [Internet]. South Dartmouth (MA): MDText.com, Inc., 2000-2015 Apr 12.

[34] Mirrakhimov AE. Hypercalcemia of malignancy: an update on pathogenesis and management. N Am J Med Sci. 2015; 7:483-93

[35] Body JJ. Hypercalcemia of malignancy. Semin Nephrol. 2004; 24:48-54.

[36] Jublanc C, Bruckert E. Adrenal insufficiency of the adult. Rev Med Interne. 2016 Mar.

[37] Arlt W, Allolio B. Adrenal insufficiency. Lancet. 2003; 361:1881-93.

[38] De Leo S, Lee SY, Braverman LE. Hyperthyroidism. Lancet. 2016;388(10047):906-18.

[39] Cooper DS. Antithyroid drugs. *N Engl J Med.* 2005;352:905-17. [PubMed] [Google Scholar]

[40] Motivala S, Gologorsky Y, Kostandinov J et al. Pituitary disorders during pregnancy. Endocrinol Metab Clin North Am. 2011; 40:827-36.

[41] Nayak B, Burman K. Thyrotoxicosis and thyroid storm. Endocrinol Metab Clin North Am. 2006; 35:663-86.

[42] Soares DV, Conceição FL, Vaisman M. Clinical, laboratory and therapeutics aspects of Sheehan's syndrome. Arq Bras Endocrinol Metabol. 2008; 52:872-8.

[43] Humar M, Dohrmann H, Stein P, et al. Thionamides inhibit the transcription factor nuclear factor-kappaB by suppression of Rac1 and inhibitor of kappaB kinase alpha. J Pharmacol Exp Ther. 2008;324(3):1037-44.

[44] Mandel SJ, Reed Larsen P et al. Thyrotoxicosis. In: Melmed S et al. (Ed.). Williams textbook of endocrinology. 12th ed. Philadelphia: Elsevier Saunders, 2012. p. 362-405

[45] Marinò M, Latrofa F, Menconi F et al. Role of genetic and non-genetic factors in the etiology of Graves' disease. J Endocrinol Invest. 2015; 38:283-94.

[46] Bajwa SJ, Jindal R. Endocrine emergencies in critically ill patients: challenges in diagnosis and management. Indian J Endocrinol Metab. 2012; 16:722-7.

[47] Groot LJ De. Graves ' Disease and the Manifestations of Thyrotoxicosis. Http://WwwEndotextOrg/ [Internet]. 2015;(April):1-77. Available from: http://creativecommons.org/licenses/by-nc-nd/2.0/

[48] Brent GA. Graves ' Disease. 2008;2594-605.

[49] SPANOU Ioanna, CHRISTIDI Foteini, LIAKAKIS Georgios, RIZONAKI Konstantina, BOUGEA Anastasia, ANAGNOSTOU Evangelos et al. Subtipos de cefaleia primária e disfunção tireoidiana: existe alguma associação ?. Arq. Neuro-Psiquiatr. [Internet]. 20 de novembro de 2020 [citado em 20 de março de 2021]; 78 (11): 695-699. Disponível em: http://www.scielo.br/scielo.php?script=sci_arttext&pid=S0004-282X2020001100695&lng=en. Epub 30 de outubro de 2020.

[50] Burch HB, Cooper DS. Management of Graves disease. A Review. JAMA. 2015; 314:2544-54.

[51] Monzani F, Del Guerra P, Caraccio N et al. Appearance of Graves' disease after percutaneous ethanol injection for the treatment of hyperfunctioning thyroid adenoma. J Endocrinol Invest. 1997; 20:294-8.

[52] Brent GA. Clinical practice. Graves' disease. N Engl J Med. 2008; 358:2594-605.

[53] Antonelli A, Ferrari SM, Ragusa F, Elia G, Paparo SR, Ruffilli I, et al. Graves' disease: Epidemiology, genetic and environmental risk factors and viruses. Best Pract Res Clin Endocrinol Metab. 2020;34.

[54] Leslie WD, Ward L, Salamon EA, Ludwig S, Rowe RC, Cowden EA. A randomized comparison of radioiodine doses in Graves' hyperthyroidism. J Clin Endocrinol Metab 2003;88:978-83

[55] Pearce EN, Braverman LE. Hyperthyroidism: advantages and

disadvantages of medical therapy. Surg Clin North Am. 2004; 84:833-47.

[56] Ross DS. Radioiodine therapy for hyperthyroidism. N Engl J Med. 2011; 364:542-50.

[57] Cruz Júnior Antônio Fiel, Takahashi Míriam Hideco, Albino Cláudio Cordeiro. Tratamento clínico com drogas antitireoidianas ou dose terapêutica de iodo-131 no controle do hipertireoidismo na doença de graves: avaliação dos custos e benefícios. Arq Bras Endocrinol Metab [Internet]. 2006 Dec [cited 2021 Mar 20]; 50(6): 1096-1101. Available from: http://www.scielo.br/scielo.php?script=sci_arttext&pid=S0004-27302006000600017&lng=en.

[58] Cooper DS: Antithyroid drugs. N Engl J Med 2005,352(9):905-917. 10.1056/NEJMra042972

[59] Hauch A, Al-Qurayshi Z, Randolph G, Kandil E. Total thyroidectomy is associated with increased risk of complications for low- and high-volume surgeons. Ann Surg Oncol 2014; 21: 3844-52

[60] Pradeep PV, Agarwal A, Baxi M, Agarwal G, Gupta SK, Mishra SK. Safety and effi cacy of surgical management of hyperthyroidism: 15-year experience from a tertiary care center in a developing country. World J Surg 2007; 31: 306-12, discussion 313.

[61] Kandil E, Noureldine SI, Abbas A, Tufano RP. The impact of surgical volume on patient outcomes following thyroid surgery. Surgery 2013; 154: 1346-52, discussion 1352-53.

[62] Sztal-Mazer S, Nakatani VY, Bortolini LG et al. Evidence for higher success rates and successful treatment earlier in Graves' disease with higher radioactive iodine doses. Thyroid. 2012; 22:991-5.

[63] Westphal SA. Unusual presentations of hypothyroidism. Am J Med Sci. 1997; 314:333-7.

[64] De Groot LJ, Bartalena L. Thyroid Storm. In: De Groot LJ, Beck-Peccoz P, Chrousos G et al. (Ed.). Endotext [Internet]. South Dartmouth (MA): MDText.com, Inc., 2000-2015 Apr 12

[65] Maia AL, Scheffel RS, Meyer EL et al.; the Brazilian Society of Endocrinology and Metabolism. The Brazilian consensus for the diagnosis and treatment of hyperthyroidism: recommendations by the Thyroid Department of the Brazilian Society of Endocrinology and Metabolism. Arq Bras Endocrinol Metabol. 2013; 57: 205-32.

[66] Hegedus L. Treatment of Graves' hyperthyroidism: evidence based and emerging modalities. Endocrinol Metab Clin North Am. 2009; 38:355-71.

[67] Shinall MC Jr, Broome JT, Baker A, Solorzano CC. Is potassium iodide solution necessary before total thyroidectomy for Graves disease? Ann Surg Oncol 2013; 20: 2964-67

[68] Erbil Y, Ozluk Y, Giriş M, et al. Eff ect of lugol solution on thyroid gland blood fl ow and microvessel density in the patients with Graves' disease. J Clin Endocrinol Metab 2007; 92: 2182-89.

[69] Bahn Chair RS, Burch HB, Cooper DS, et al, and the American Thyroid Association and American Association of Clinical Endocrinologists. Hyperthyroidism and o ther causes of thyrotoxicosis: management guidelines of the American Thyroid Association and American Association of Clinical Endocrinologists. Thyroid 2011; 21: 593-646

Section 2

Pathophysiology of Graves' Disease

Chapter 4

Graves' Disease: Pathophysiology, Genetics and Management

Mosin S. Khan, Suhail S. Lone, Sunia Faiz, Iqra Farooq and Sabhiya Majid

Abstract

Graves' Disease is an autoimmune disorder in which hyperthyroidism (over active thyroid) is caused by the autoantibodies against the TSH receptor. It is mainly characterized by the appearance of goiter. The symptoms are wide ranging as thyroid hormone affects many body systems. It is common in women and in people with age below than 40. Graves' Disease is caused by a combination of genetic and environmental factors while genetics being the main cause. Graves' Disease is not a single gene defect but has a complex pattern of inheritance. Today it is clear that genetic predisposition to Graves' Disease is caused by multiple genes. HLA gene is one the most studied gene predisposing to Graves' Disease. Lot of polymorphisms in this gene has been to be associated with the disease. Lymphoid tyrosine phosphatase encoded by the gene PTPN22 has been found to increase the risk of many autoimmune diseases including Graves' Disease. The best documented association of *PTPN22* variants to autoimmune disorders including GD is rs2476601 (C1858T). Other genes associated with the risk of GD are thyrotropin receptor (TSHR), thyroglobulin gene, FCRL3, SCGB3A2, and CTLA4. This chapter will discuss in detail the genetics, pathophysiology, diagnosis and treatment of Graves' hyperthyroidism.

Keywords: Graves' Disease, GD, HLA region, PTPN22, CD40, CTLA4, CD152, TSHR, Tg, FCRL3, SCGB3A2

1. Introduction

Graves' Disease (GD) was named after *Robert J. Graves,* who first recognized this disease in the 19th century as a syndrome with enlarged and overactive thyroid gland (hyperthyroidism due to circulating autoantibodies), an high heart rate, and eye abnormalities (**Figure 1**). On the quality of life, GD has unpropitious effects [1], as a consequence of somatic and psychiatric symptoms, an inability to work and is connected with an increased risk of death [2]. The autoimmune basis of the GD results from complex interactions between different factors which include genetic, endogenous and environmental factors, and this is compulsory for current understanding of this disease [3, 4]. The circulating antibodies (IgG) that binds and activates the G-protein–coupled thyrotropin receptor leads to hyperthyroidism in this disease [5]. In this disease the G-protein–coupled thyrotropin receptor after getting activated stimulates follicular cell growth and excessive development which results in the enlargement of thyroid gland and also increase in thyroid hormone production and the fraction of triiodothyronine (T3) relative to thyroxine (T4) in

IntechOpen

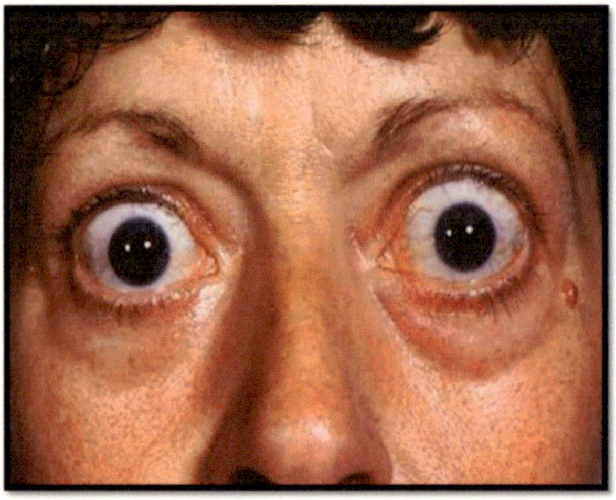

Figure 1.
Graves' Disease.

thyroid secretion [6]. In GD the suppressed serum thyrotropin level and elevated levels of serum T4 and T3 are revealed by the thyroid functioning tests. A term known as *subclinical hyperthyroidism* is referred when serum thyrotropin level is low as compared to normal serum levels of T4 and T3 [7].

2. Epidemiology

GD with an annual incidence of 20 to 50 cases per 100,000 persons is the most common cause of hyperthyroidism [8]. The incidence of GD peaks between 30 to 50 years of age, but people can be affected at any age. The lifetime risk for women is 3% and for men it is 0.5%. The risk of GD is not influenced by Long-term variations in iodine intake, but rapid repletion can transiently increase the incidence. The GD–associated incidence of ophthalmopathy is 16 cases per 100,000 in women and in men it is 3 cases per 100,000 annually. It is more common in whites than in Asians [9]. Older men develop severe ophthalmopathy more likely than younger persons [10]. Subtle abnormalities are revealed in 70% of patients by orbital imaging with GD [11]. In up to 50% of patients in specialized centres, clinically consequential ophthalmopathy is detected with GD, and as a consequence of corneal breakdown or optic neuropathy in 3 to 5% of such patients, sight is threatned [12]. The thyroid levels remain normal or autoimmune hypothyroidism develops either in 10% of the persons with ophthalmopathy [10–12]. In the *Whickham study* a population-based survey in England, the annual incidence of Graves' Disease was approximately 80 per 100,000 women, with most other surveys reporting incidence rates ranging from 15 to 50 per 100,000 persons per year while as the annual incidence in English men was approximately eight to ten fold lower than women (10 per 100,000) in keeping with gender differences seen in other thyroid diseases [13]. The incidence of Graves' hyperthyroidism in area of particularly high iodine intake (Japan), has been reported to be as high as 200 cases per 100,000 general population [14]. Similarly, following the introduction of iodine supplementation, an increases in the apparent incidence of GD have been reported, although in an area of mild to moderate iodine deficiency (Switzerland), a 33% reduction in the incidence of GD was associated with iodine supplementation [15].

3. Pathophysiology of Graves' Disease

In GD, four standard thyroid antigens: thyroglobulin, thyroid peroxidase, sodium-iodide symporter and the thyrotropin receptor are recognized to direct B and T lymphocyte-mediated autoimmunity. However, the primary auto antigen of GD is the thyrotropin receptor itself and is responsible for the manifestation of hyperthyroidism. In this disease, the antibody and cell-mediated thyroid antigen-specific immune responses are properly defined. The development of hyperthyroidism in healthy subjects by transferring thyrotropin receptor antibodies in serum from patients with GD and the passive transfer of thyrotropin receptor antibodies to the foetus in pregnant women are the direct proof of an autoimmune disorder that is mediated by means of autoantibodies. By circulating autoantibodies against the thyrotropin receptor, the thyroid gland is under continuous stimulation, and because of the increased production of thyroid hormones pituitary thyrotropin secretion is suppressed [16]. In the immunoglobulin G1 subclass, the stimulating activity of thyrotropin receptor antibodies is found mostly. The release of thyroid hormone and thyroglobulin that is mediated via 3,'5′-cyclic adenosine monophosphate (cyclic AMP) are caused by these thyroid-stimulating antibodies, and they also stimulate iodine uptake, protein synthesis, and thyroid gland growth. In the etiology of hyperthyroidism in GD the anti-thyroglobulin, anti-sodium-iodide symporter, and anti-thyroid peroxidase antibodies seem to have a very little role. However, against the thyroid, these are markers of autoimmune disease. In persons with autoimmune thyroid disease, intrathyroidal lymphocytic infiltration is the initial histologic abnormality which has a direct correlation with thyroid antibodies' titer [17, 18]. In addition to autoantigens, the cells of thyroid produce specific immune mediators such as cytokines and Fas which are involved in various immune process including complement legislation and T cell adhesion. Those individuals who are suffering from Graves' Disease have lesser percentage of CD4 lymphocytes in thyroid as compared to their peripheral blood. In addition, the CD4 reduction in these patients may also be related to the elevated Fas expression in intrathyroidal CD4 T lymphocytes. *CD40, CTLA-4, thyroglobulin, TSH receptor,* and *PTPN22* are several autoimmune thyroid disease susceptibility genes that have been identified. Either to GD or *Hashimoto thyroiditis*, some of these susceptibility genes are unique, while others confer susceptibility to both conditions. With environmental factors or activities to precipitate the onset of GD the genetic predisposition to thyroid autoimmunity might also interact [17–19]. The RNASET2-FGFR1OP-CCR6 region at 6q27 and an intergenic region at 4p14 are two new susceptibility loci that had been found [20]. Moreover, thyroid-stimulating hormone receptor and major histocompatibility complex class II versions have strong associations with thyroid stimulating hormone receptor autoantibodies (TRAb)-positive GD [21]. Compared with healthy controls, GD patients have higher rate of peripheral blood mononuclear cell conversion into $CD34^+$ fibrocytes. The production of inflammatory cytokines like Inter-leukin 6 (IL-6) and TNF-alpha by these cells after piling up in orbital tissues also contribute to the pathophysiology of thyroid eye disease (opthalmopathy) [22]. In a whole genome association study of more than 1500 individuals suffering from Graves' Disease and equal controls, six susceptible loci which are (*CTLA4; cytotoxic T-lymphocyte-associated protein 4, MHC; major histocompatibility complex, FCRl3; Fc receptor-like protein 3, TSHR; thyroid stimulating hormone receptor, RNASET2-FGFR1OP-CCR6 region at 6q27, and an intergenic region at 4p14*) have been discovered to be associated with GD. **Figure 2** describes the pathophysiology of Graves' Disease [23].

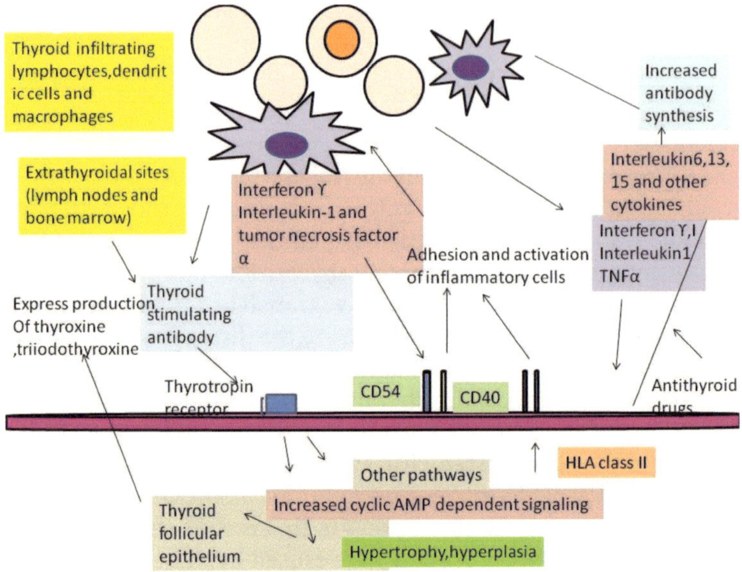

Figure 2.
Pathophysiology of Graves' Disease.

4. Genetics of Graves' Disease

GD is a complex autoimmune disorder which affects the functioning of the thyroid gland, which is the butterfly shaped gland in the lower neck. Specific antibodies targetting the thyrotropin receptor are found in about 95% of patients with GD. GD is thought to result from a combination of environmental and genetic factors most of which are unknown. A number of genes predispose to the GD which include *HLA region*, *protein tyrosine phosphatase-22 (PTPN22)*, *cluster of differentiation 40(CD40)*, *the cytototoxic T lymphocyte- Associated factor4 (CTLA4 or CD152)*, *thyrotropin receptor (TSHR)*, *thyroglobulin (Tg)*, *FCRL3 (FC receptor-like-3)*, *Secretoglobulin 3A2 (SCGB3A2) gene* encoding secretory uteroglobin- related protein 1 (UGRP) and many others. The role of these genes in the pathophysiology of GD is discussed below:

4.1 HLA region

Human leukocyte antigen (HLA) region (6p21) within the human genome codes for 252 expressed loci including numerous key immune response genes is the most gene dense region [24]. This region contains the highest degree of polymorphism within the genome and is divided into different classes which includes the extended class I, classical class I, classical class III, classical class II and extended class II [24] (**Figure 3**). The densest linkage disequilibrium (LD) is also shown by this gene, extending up to 540 kb [25], which compares with distances of between 1 and 173 kb seen in the rest of the genome [26]. When trying to tease out the exact site of etiological variants, the degree of LD within the region is challenging. Most studies highlights the importance on the role of HLA class II encoded HLA-DR and –DQ molecules, which present exogenous antigens for recognition by CD4+ T helper (Th) cells. Including GD, strong associations of *HLA* with almost all autoimmune disorders have been detected. Many studies regarding association of *HLA* alleles with GD have been done. Among different ethnic populations, association of *HLA* alleles with GD varies like *HLA-B*08, DR3* and *DQA1*05:01* are associated with a

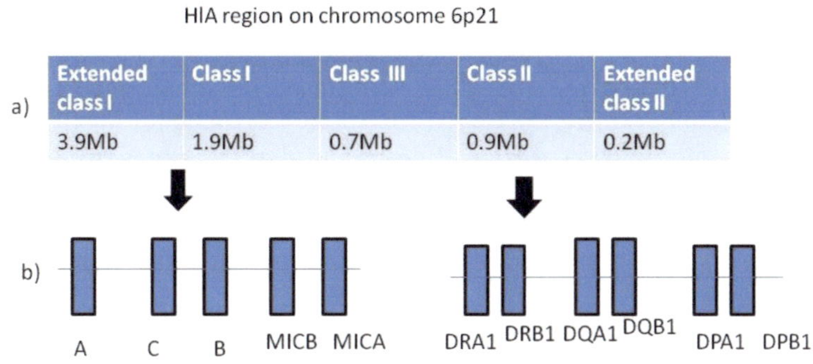

Figure 3.
HLA region on chromosome 6p21. a) nucleotide length of genes of HLA, b) regions of HLA genes.

high risk of GD, and *HLA-DRB1*07:01* is a protective allele against GD in Caucasian populations [27]. *HLA* alleles have been shown to predispose certain groups of people to the disease and vary regionally. British Caucasians showed role of HLA class II alleles DRB1-0304, DQB1-02, and DQA1-0501 [28]. The *HLA* complex shows strong linkage disequilibrium. In Caucasians populations, It is found that there is strong linkage disequilibrium between the genes that codes DR and DQ molecules therefore the existence of a particular DRB1 variant to a larger degree determines DQA1 and DQB1 alleles. *DRB1*03:01-DQA1*05:01-DQB1*02:01 (DR17, DQ2)* and *DRB1*04:01- DQA1*03:01-DQB1*03:02 (DR4, DQ8)* are HLA haplotype combinations in GD sibling pairs. The maximum risk related to this disease is associated with *DR17, DQ2 while as the HLA-DRB1*07 (DR7)* is protective for Graves' Disease. The recessive inheritance of MHC related susceptibility is favored by the distribution of *HLA-B8* genotypes and it is in close accord with Hardy–Weinberg equilibrium proportions. The possibility that an individual will be affected with GD depends on sex, *HLA* genotype, and family history. 14.9% of DR3-positive women with an affected first-degree relative are liable to be affected [29]. *HLA Class I* is also linked with GD, the disease may be mainly associated with alleles of *HLA class I*, in particular *HLA-C*07* whereas *C*03* and *C*16* provides protection [30]. *HLA-DPB1*05:01* was the main gene predisposing to GD. Other alleles included *B*46:01, DRB1* 15:02* and *16:02* whereas *DRB1*12:02* and *DQB1*03:02* provide protection. The association of *DQA1*05:01* with GD was not supported by Linkage Disequilibrium patterns observed in Asians [31]. Peptides derived from TSHR are the cause of association with HLA and development of immune response. Other cause is owing to thymic selection affecting positive and negative selection of T cell clones with regulatory or effector functions. Moreover, impact on NK cell repertoire through interactions with killer immunoglobulin-like receptors (KIR) and/or serving directly as a source of auto antigens after misfolding and presentation by HLA class II molecules [30]. Development of Graves' Disease is related to HLA-DR3. The extracellular domain (ECD) of human TSH receptor (hTSH-R) is a crucial antigen in Graves' Disease. hTSH-R peptide 37 (amino acids 78-94) is an important immunogenic peptide [32]. HLA is the cause of many diseases, the disease occurred at an earliest age in HLA-DR3 positive patients and important link between exophthalmos and either exophthalmos and/or soft tissue modifications were found with DR3. HLA-DR3 positive patients were found to be more resilient to radioiodine therapy than patients negative for these antigens [33]. It has been hypothesized that arginine at position 74 of the HLA- DRB1 chain has role in GD pathogenesis. But the most common residues at position 74 of *DRB1*15:01* and *DRB1*16:02* reported in our association study are both alanine and it is considered to be neutral for GD risk [34]. On the other hand, HLA region is linked to GD susceptibility in both

Caucasian and Chinese Han populations [35]. The associated alleles vary from those in Causacians. *HLA-DPB1*05:01* is the major gene of GD in our population, *B*46:01, DQB1*03:02, DRB1*15:01* and *DRB1*16:02* were closely linked with GD [31]. As per the other meta-analysis study, the *HLA-B*46* allele is a risk factor for GD in Asian populations. The distribution of *HLA-B*46* and *HLA-B*08* vary between European and Asian populations. The allelic frequency of *HLA-B*08* is around 12%, while the allelic frequency is 0.3 to 0.5% in most Asian populations. By contrast, the allelic frequency of *HLA-B*46* is 3.9 to 8.6% in Asian populations and almost zero in Europe populations [35]. **Figure 4** depicts the classical HLA Class I and II pathways.

4.2 Protein tyrosine phosphatase-22 (PTPN22)

Protein tyrosine phosphatase, non-receptor type 22 (lymphoid) is also known as PTPN22. This in humans is encoded by the *PTPN22 gene* [36]. This gene has various variants. The mutations of this gene are associated with increase or decrease in the risk of autoimmune diseases. In many autoimmune diseases, this gene has been found strongly associated after HLA [37]. *rs2476601 (C1858T) is* the best known association of *PTPN22* variants to autoimmune condition including GD. This SNP (R620W) located in the P1 proline - rich motif of *PTPN22* binds with strong affinity to the SH3 domain of tyrosine kinase, Csk. This mutation disrupts the interaction between *PTPN22* and *Csk* [38] and also increases phosphatase activity which inturn suppresses the TCR signaling more efficiently than the wild type [39]. A role of *PTPN22* in T-cell regulation has been found by the results of knocking out the murine homolog of *PTPN22,* which lowered thresholds for T-cell-receptor signaling and inhibited production of IL-2 in these animals [40]. This *PTPN22 620 W* substitution, a gain of function mutation resulting in the reduction of phosphorylation of key signaling molecules and associated downregulation of TCR signaling which inturn leads to the inhibition of expansion of T cells, weakening of the positive selection in the thymus, and decreasing the antibodies' titer by reducing the activity of helper T lymphocytes [41]. Association between the GD and *PTPN22 620 W* polymorphism has been demonstrated in several studies among Caucasians

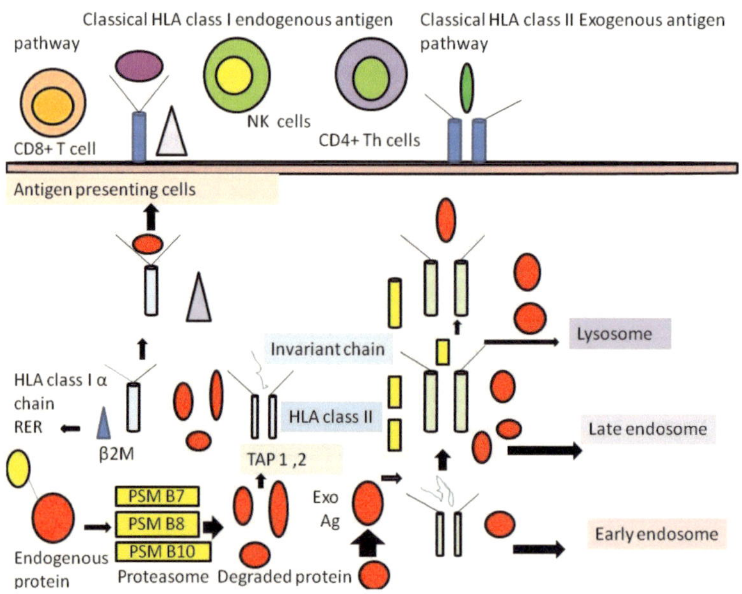

Figure 4.
Classical HLA class I and II pathways.

with odds ratio as OR 1.5-1.9 [42], which makes *PTPN22 620 W* polymorph one of the strongest known genetic factors influencing to autoimmune diseases. In polish population a gene dose-dependent effect of *PTPN22* 'T' allele on the age of onset of GD has been found [42] but that was not replicated in a cohort study done in UK [43]. The other available results have shown that the *PTPN22* locus contains other functionally important variants, particularly those conferring protection.

4.3 Cluster of differentiation 40 (CD40)

The Cluster of Differentiation (CD) are cell surface proteins with each of them assigned a specific number thereby allowing cell phenotypes to be recognized. Surface expression of a particular CD molecule is functional for the characterization of cell phenotypes. These molecules can act either as receptors or ligands. Some CD proteins though do not play role in cell signaling, but do have other functions, such as cell adhesion. CD for humans is numbered upto 371 with their specific functions. CD40 is a costimulatory protein found on the antigen- presenting cells and results in their activation. The binding of CD154 (CD40L) on helper T cells to CD40 activates antigen presenting cells and induces a variety of downstream effects. Deficiency can lead to Hyper-IgM syndrome type3. It is located on chromosome 20 in humans and chromosome 2 in mouse. Disruption of the CD40- CD40L co-stimulatory pathway has been found in many autoimmune diseases, including GD. on the basis of a genome-wide linkage study in GD, *CD40* has been associated with GD as a positional candidate which implicated 20q11 chromosomal region, designated GD-2, as harboring a susceptibility locus [44]. C/T polymorphism (rs1883832) located at position −1 relative to translation start site affects the initiation step of translation as it has a direct effect on kozak sequence. The C allele of *rs1883832* has been found to confer risk of GD among Caucasians whereas the results from in vitro transcription/translation system suggested that this allele predisposes to GD by increasing the efficiency of translation of CD40 mRNA [44]. There is a close association between GD and C variant of *rs1883832* as supported by studies in the Japanese population although in this population the effect may be constrained to patients with the late onset of disease [45] and/or to the CC and CT genotypes, signifying a dominant rather than a recessive model of inheritance [45]. Recently, siRNA mediated inhibition of CD40 expression was evaluated for potential to prevent development of GD in mice immunized with adenovirus expressing human TSHR A subunit. In spite of successful lowering of CD40 expression, no effect on the rate of disease induction was observed [46].

4.4 The cytotoxic T lymphocyte-associated factor 4 (CTLA4 Or CD152)

It is a protein receptor that functions as an immune checkpoint and down-regulates immune responses. It is constitutively expressed in regulatory T cells but only upregulated in conventional T cells after activation; a phenomenon which is particularly notable in cancers [47]. It is homologous to the T-cell co-stimulatory protein, CD28, and both molecules bind to CD80 and CD86, also called B7-1 and B7-2 respectively, on antigen-presenting cells. CTL4-4 binds CD80 and CD86 with greater affinity and avidity than CD28 thus enabling it to outcompete CD28 for its ligands. CTLA4 transfers an inhibitory signal to T cells, [48] whereas CD28 transmits a stimulatory signal [48]. CTLA4 is also found in regulatory T cells and thereby contributing to their inhibitory function. CTLA4 consists of four exons encoding different functional domains such as a leader sequence and extracellular, transmembrane as well as cytoplasmic domains. The most reliable associations with GD within *CTLA4* locus were found with three polymorphisms: the

AT-microsatellite polymorphism (ATn) at the 3'untranslated region (3'UTR) of the gene [49]. It has been proposed that this AT-repeat allele decreased the` stability of *CTLA4* mRNA thus dampening the inhibitory function of the protein and thus diminishing the control of T-cell proliferation [50]. The *second* polymorphism implicated was *rs231775 (A49G)* in the signal peptide causing a substitution of Thr to Ala [51]. This amino acid change could influence post-translational processing leading to inefficient glycosylation of the autoimmunity predisposing variant [52]. Another widely studied genetic polymorphism in *CTLA4 gene* is *rs3087243 (CT60)* located downstream from the 3'UTR of the *CTLA4* [53]. After taking into account the CT60 genotype, Examination of full-length (flCTLA-4) and sCTLA-4 expression revealed a lower expression of sCTLA-4 in persons homozygous for the G allele [54]. But, in a larger Swedish study this result was not replicated which also did not find any association between concentration of serum sCTLA4 and disease status or CT60 genotype [54]. Lately, in Japanese patients a noteworthy association with CTLA4 CT60 was found for GD with OR=2.97. The present state of knowledge does not specify evidently the mechanism behind the association of *CTLA4* with GD. However, *CTLA4* polymorphism is consistently associated with thyroid autoimmune diseases in the majority of populations.

4.5 The thyrotropin receptor (TSHR)

The thyrotropin receptor (TSHR) responding to thyrotropin (thyroid-stimulating hormone, TSH) is a Gs-protein coupled receptor and stimulates the production of thyroxin (T4) and triiodothyronine (T3). It is primarily found on the surface of the thyroid epithelial cells [55], but also found on adipose tissue and fibroblasts. A G protein signal cascade is activated upon the binding of circulating ligand TSH which activates adenylyl cyclase that synthesizes cAMP from ATP and subsequently resulting in increased intracellular levels of cAMP. cAMP functions as a secondary messenger and activates all functional aspects of the thyroid cells which include thyroglobulin synthesis, iodine pumping, endocytosis, iodination, proteolysis, thyroid peroxidase activity and hormone release. *TSHR gene* is located on 14q31 [56] and consists of 13 exons [57]. The TSHR is among the susceptibility genes of GD because it encodes for a protein that is both responsible for the clinical manifestations of the disease and is the direct target of the autoimmune response in GD. The anti-TSHR antibodies in serum are the main serological manifestations of GD. Indeed, TSHR- stimulating antibodies (TSAbs) are present in nearly all cases of GD and severity of the disease correlates with TSAbs levels. One of the first non-MHC genes to be tested for association with the disease was TSHR. Three germline missence mutations (a substitution of aspartic acid (D) for histidine (H) in position 36 *(D36H)*; a substitution of a proline (P) for threonine (T) in position *52(P52T)*, and a substitution of aspartic acid (D) for glutamic acid (E) in position *727 (D727E)* were primarily described in individuals suffering from GD and proposed to be associated with the disease [3]. Of these three, *D36H* and *P52T* are the two mutations which are located in the putative ligand binding region of the extracellular domain of the TSHR, while the third one, *D727E* lies within the intracellular domain of the receptor.

4.6 FCRL3 (FC receptor-like-3)

Fc receptor-like protein 3 is a protein that in humans is encoded by *FCRL3 gene* [58]. It is located on 1q23.1. This gene located on q arm of chromosome 1st is one of the several Fc receptors like glycoproteins which encode a member of the IR superfamily. The encoded protein plays a role in regulation of the immune system and in its cytoplasmic domain it contains immunoreceptor-tyrosine activation motifs and immunoreceptor-tyrosine inhibitory motifs. Rheumatoid arthritis, autoimmune thyroid disease, and systemic lupus erythematosus have been associated in the mutation of this gene [58]. FCRL3 is a novel immunoregulatory gene believed to perform similar functions as FC gamma receptors due to high structural homology between them. FCRL3 gene polymorphism is related to the susceptibility to GD with regional and ethnic variability [59]. A SNP at the position *-169A/G (rs7528684)* in promoter of *FCRL3* gene has been found to be associated with GD. Correlation of this SNP to serum levels of FT3, FT4, TSH and TRAb, gender, age, TpoAb, TgAb, severity of goiter and presence or absence of exophthalmos in GD have been widely investigated [59]. There is an association of anther SNP *rs3761959* (tagging rs7528684) with GD. Overall the available data suggest that genetic polymorphism(s) modifying susceptibility for GD do exist in the *FCRL3* region but the primarily associated variant(s) remain(s) to be found [60].

4.7 Secretoglobin 3A2 (SCGB3A2) gene

This gene is present on chromosome 5 in humans and chromosome 18 in mouse. It is a homodimeric protein thought to play a role in the modulation of inflammation and tumorigenesis. SCGB3A2 is a member of secretoglobin superfamily, a family of small, secreted proteins found in animals exclusively of mammalian lineage. *SCGB3A2* mRNA is predominantly expressed in the lung with low levels of expression in the thyroid. Variants in the promoter of the *SCGB3A2* gene encoding secretory uteroglobin-related protein 1 (UGRP1) have been found associated with GD in an extensive study of a total of ~2500 patients and controls from the Chinese population who aimed to explain signals in the chromosomal region 5q12-q33 obtained in previous studies using linkage analysis [61–63]. Song *et al.* reported the strongest association of GD with *rs1368408 (112G/A, OR=1.28, P=1.43x10-6)* and *SNP75 (-623~-622 AG/-T, OR=1.32, P=7.62x10-5)* [60, 61]. Association between GD and the A allele of *rs1368408* (OR=1.18, P=0.007) was independently confirmed in a similarly sized UK cohort [64]. Recently, further evidence for association between rs1368408 and GD was provided by a study in a Russian cohort (~1500 cases and controls, OR=1.33, P=2.910-5) [60]. It should be noted that a relatively early study in a Chinese population did not observe the effect of *rs1368408,* although this might have been caused by low power due to limited numbers of subjects (~200 cases and controls) [62]. Till present it is still not clear how variants in *SCGB3A2* predispose to GD.

There are other genes which have strong association with GD such as cytokine genes: *IL3, IL4, IL5, IL9, IL13* and the *ADRB2* gene encoding beta-2-Adrenergic receptor [65–67] were all associated with GD.

5. Diagnosis of Graves' Disease

The diagnosis to confirm the cause of Graves' hyperthyroidism is based on the clinical and biochemical manifestations of hyperthyroidism and on the clinical and laboratory features. For the presence of hyperthyroidism, measurement of serum thyrotropin is a useful screening test, because the secretion of thyrotropin is reduced by very small increase in thyroid secretion, so by the measurement of serum free thyroxine the diagnosis of hyperthyroidism must be confirmed [68]. Patients may have only increased secretion of triiodothyronine in the earliest stage of Graves' hyperthyroidism; therefore, patients with normal serum free thyroxine concentrations and low serum thyrotropin concentrations, serum free triiodothyronine should be measured. Because of the use of certain drugs and increase in thyroid hormone–binding proteins, measurements of serum total thyroxine and triiodothyronine are less reliable as it can cause high values [69]. In patients with hyperthyroidism and a diffuse goiter, the signs of ophthalmopathy or dermopathy are sufficient to confirm the diagnosis of GD. In patients with GD, other autoimmune disorders occur more frequently (Type 1 diabetes mellitus, Addison's disease, Vitiligo, Pernicious anemia Alopecia areata, Myasthenia gravis, Celiac disease) and their presence therefore supports this diagnosis. Occasionally, in patients with pre-existing nodular goiter, GD occurs which causes confusion. The presence of a high serum concentration of thyroid peroxidase antibody which is present in about 75 percent of patients with Graves' hyperthyroidism, or a thyroid radionuclide scan demonstrating a diffuse goiter provides evidence of GD, when the diagnosis is unclear clinically. Occasionally, to distinguish between Graves' hyperthyroidism and thyrotoxicosis caused by painless, destructive (autoimmune) thyroiditis, thyroid radionuclide studies may be indicated especially in women post-partum. Patients may have a small diffuse goiter with painless thyroiditis, like those with GD. However, it is very unlikely that thyrotoxicosis due to painless thyroiditis will last longer than two months [70].

5.1 Measurement of thyrotropin-receptor antibodies in serum

It is largely a matter of individual preference, whether serum thyrotropin-receptor antibodies should be measured in the differential diagnosis of GD, some argue that a test for the antibodies should be done routinely, and others that a diagnosis of GD can nearly always be inferred correctly on the basis of the clinical findings. The immunoglobulin-mediated inhibition of the binding of radiolabeled thyrotropin to thyrotropin receptors is most widely used assay for thyrotropin-receptor antibodies and is positive approximately in 80% of individuals suffering for Graves' hyperthyroidism [2]. Up to 99% sensitivity is shown by newer assays. Even though a positive result might specify the occurrence of either thyroid- stimulating antibodies or thyrotropin-receptor– blocking antibodies, it is rational to conclude that a positive test in the individual suffering from hyperthyroidism is owing to thyrotropin-receptor–stimulating antibodies. With time as the mechanism of the interactions of antibodies with the thyrotropin receptor improves, it would be possible to develop simple, precise immunoassays for thyroid-stimulating antibodies for routine use. The antibodies identified by bioassays that measure the synthesis of cAMP in retort to the stimulation of thyrotropin receptors are only thyroid-stimulating antibodies — for instance, in cells transfected with thyrotropin receptor— but such assays are relatively expensive and not widely available [71].

5.2 Computed tomography (CT) or magnetic resonance imaging (MRI)

CT and/or MRI of the orbits is indicated if there is any uncertainty about the cause of ophthalmopathy, particularly in a patient with unilateral exophthalmos, to rule out a retrobulbar tumor or arteriovenous malformation. Approaches used in assessing the activity of ophthalmopathy are very helpful in determining which individuals will be benefitted from immunosuppressive treatment. Measurement of the relaxation time for extraocular muscles on T2-weighted MRI, Clinical activity scores (CAS), and orbital scanning with indium In 111 pentetreotide [54] have all been suggested for this purpose but have not been fully assessed. These above tests are not needed for the majority of individuals, who have only mild or moderate Graves' ophthalmopathy [72].

6. Therapy for Graves' Disease

According to age, severity of hyperthyroidism, goiter size, presence and degree of ophthalmopathy, as well as patient's personal preference, GD treatment should be tailored in each individual patient. Medical treatment with anti-thyroid medicine (thionamides) is usually suggested in all patients to revive euthyroidism at first. Once euthyroidism is achieved, the long strategy comprises many choices, including relatively long-term (usually twelve to twenty four months) course of anti-thyroid drugs, radioactive iodine or surgery. Beta-blockers, if not inadvisable are time and again used prior to restoration of euthyroidism to reduce the symptoms of thyrotoxicosis. The thyroid hormone formation is blocked by specific thionamides or antithyroid drugs (propylthiouracil and methimazole). These drugs prevent the thyroid hormone production by inhibiting iodine organification and coupling of iodotyrosines. Treatment of this disease with these drugs is usually well tolerated. Some of the side effects like skin rash and, hardly Granulopenia, Hepatits and Arteritis may occur. Methimazole is currently most well liked over propylthiouracil, owing to the proof of a lower prevalence of severe side-effects, particularly hepatitis [73], with the exception of the first trimester of pregnancy, when propylthiouracil is preferred due to the increased rate of congenitalmal formations, especially aplasia cutis, which has been reported with the utilization of methimazole [74]. Due to the high probability of recurrence of hyperthyroidism after the withdrawal of therapy, this method is not suggested to individuals having large goiters. Contrary, in individuals with thyroid eye disease (ophthalmopathy), we tend to like a surgical removal of all or part of the thyroid gland (thyroidectomy), radioiodine ablation, or both owing to the pathogenetic role of cross-reactive antigens between the thyroid and orbital tissues [75]. In some centers, the methimazole is used at higher doses than desirable amounts needed to correct hyperthyroidism in coalition with thyroid hormone for block and replacement treatment. This tactic relies on plausible immunosuppressive methimazole action, which still has not been incontestable in studies related to humans [76]. Radioiodine is ideally administered after the accomplishment of euthyroidism with the help of anti-thyroid drugs. Hypothyroidism is induced to attain a stable remission of GD, this is the goal of the treatment. To calculate the appropriate radioactive iodine dose to be given, 24 hour radioactive iodine uptake is usually performed before treatment and used together with gland volume. However, a fixed radioiodine dose may also be given without interfering with the outcome [77]. Radioiodine treatment, when using appropriate dose, within 1 to 6 months in the majority of patients (about 80%), it leads to hypothyroidism. Those Patients having large goiter the radioiodine therapy should not be used as it has low success rate unless repeated treatments are planned. It has been seen that radioiodine has acute side effects which are mild, well tolerated and generally self-limiting. Radioactive therapy for the treatment of hyperthyroidism sometimes causes a transitory pain and swelling of the neck and subsequently requires a treatment with oral glucocorticoids. During this process, for a short period of time the symptoms of thyrotoxicosis may exacerbate due to the release of preformed thyroid hormones. After radioiodine treatment, a transient worsening or more rarely, the fresh appearance of thyroid eye disease may occur, but it can be easily prevented by the administration of oral prednisone after radioiodine for 8–12 weeks. After radioiodine therapy in adults with Graves, there is no evidence of an increased risk of thyroid cancer and other solid tumors as well as of leukemia [78]. No major studies are available in children unfortunately. So, radioiodine treatment is not recommended before the age of 18–20 years. With the exception of a transitory decrease in testosterone levels in men, no effects on the reproductive system in male and female have been described [79]. A patient with a large goiter has been indicated by Thyroidectomy. The surgical procedures most commonly recommended in patients with GD are near total thyroidectomy (NT) or total thyroidectomy (TT), consisting in the removal of most or all visible thyroid tissue, respectively. Both procedures result in hypothyroidism. Recurrence of hyperthyroidism is extremely rare. The rate of post-operative complications (e.g. surgical hypoparathyroidism, laryngeal nerve paralysis) is not increased compared with that observed using other less aggressive surgical procedures [80]. Briefly, the treatment of choice depends on the seriousness and activity of GD. In individuals with moderately severe thyroid eye disease, the usage of intravenous glucocorticoids is the first-line treatment and if this intravenous glucocorticoids treatment fails, orbital decompression is performed [81]. And this rehabilitative surgery (orbital decompression, muscle or eyelid surgery) must be considered when the eye disease is inactive. No major treatments are required for the majority of patients having a mild ophthalmopathy, and patients are given local measurement (e.g. eye lubricants, sun glasses) or, based on a recent study, selenium [82].

7. Conclusion

Since the incidence of Graves' Disease is increasing at pace and already told in the above chapter that it has an unpropitious effects on the quality of life as it causes weight loss, fatigue irritability, goiter (swelling in the thyroid gland) and much more. It also affects skin and eyes the conditions called Graves' dermopathy and Graves' ophthalmopathy respectively. As explained earlier this disease is thought to result from a combination of environmental and genetic factors most of which are unknown. So it is necessary to understand those factors, which will help us in the better management of this disease in future.

Author details

Mosin S. Khan*, Suhail S. Lone, Sunia Faiz, Iqra Farooq and Sabhiya Majid
Department of Biochemistry, Government Medical College Srinagar and Associated Hospitals, Srinagar, Kashmir, India

*Address all correspondence to: mosinsaleemkhan@gmail.com

References

[1] Kahaly GJ, Petrak F, Hardt, et al. Psychosocial morbidity of Graves' orbitopathy. Clinical Endocrinology. 2005; 63(4): 395-402.

[2] Terry JS and Laszlo H. Graves' Disease. N Engl J Med. 2016; 375 (16):1552-1565.

[3] Tomer Y. Mechanisms of autoimmune thyroid diseases: From genetics to epigenetics. Annual Review of Pathology: Mechanisms of Diseas.2014; 9: 147-156.

[4] Brix TH, Kyvik KO, Christensen, et al. Evidence for a major role of heredity in GD. A population-Based Study of Two Danish Twin Cohorts. J Clin Endocrinol Metab. 2001; 86(2): 930-934.

[5] Anthony PW. Graves' Disease. The New England Journal of Medicine. 2000; 343(17): 1236-1248.

[6] Girgis CM, Champion BL, Wall JR. Current concepts in GD.Therapeutic Advances in Endocrinology and Metabolism. 2011; 2(3): 135-144.

[7] Anthony. Subclinical hyperthyroidism. N Engl J Med. 2001; 345: 512-516.

[8] Zimmermann MB and Boelaert K. Iodine deficiency and thyroid disorders. The Lancet Diabetes and Endocrinology. 2015; 3(4): 286-295.

[9] Sagili VBR, Anu Jain, SB Yadav, et al. Prevalence of Graves' ophthalmopathy in patients with GD presenting to a referral centre in north India. Indian J Med Res. 2014; 139(1):99-104.

[10] Rebecca SB. Graves' Ophthalmopathy. N Engl J Med. 2010; 362(8):726-38.

[11] Villadolid MC, Yokoyama N, Izumi M. Untreated GD patients without clinical ophthalmopathy demonstrate a high frequency of extraocular muscle (EOM) enlargement by magnetic resonance. Journal of Clinical Endocrinology and Metabolism. 1995; 80(9): 2830-2833.

[12] Luigi B and Maria LT. Graves' Ophthalmopathy. N Engl J Med. 2009; 360 (10):994-1001.

[13] McIver B and Morris JC. The pathogenesis of GD. Endocrinology and Metabolism Clinics of North America. 1998; 27(1): 73-89.

[14] Sarıtas A, Sarıtas PU, Kurnaz MM et al. Spectrum and Prevalence of Thyroid Disorders in Patients Admitted to the Anaesthesiology Outpatient Clinic for Surgery. 2015;43(4): 240-245.

[15] Bg B and Lichiardopol C. Iodine Deficiency, Still a Global Problem. Curr Health Sci J. 2017; 43(2): 103-111.

[16] Morshed SA, Latif R, Davies TF. Characterization of thyrotropin receptor antibody induced signaling cascades. Endocrinology. 2009; 150(1):519-529.

[17] Jacobson EM and Tomer Y. The CD40, CTLA-4, thyroglobulin, TSH receptor, and PTPN22 gene quintet and its contribution to thyroid autoimmunity: Back to the future. Journal of Autoimmunity. 2007; 28 (2-3): 85-98.

[18] Iwama S, Ikezaki A, Kikuoka N, et al. Association of HLA-DR, –DQ genotype and CTLA-4 gene polymorphism with GD in Japanese children. Hormone Res. 2005; 63:55-60.

[19] Nagata K, Nakayama Y, Higaki K, et al. Reactivation of persistent Epstein-Barr virus (EBV) causes secretion of thyrotropin receptor antibodies (TRAbs) in EBV-infected B

lymphocytes with TRAbs on their surface.Autoimmunity. 2015; 48(5):328-335.

[20] Chu X, Pan CM, Zhao SX, et al. A genome-wide association study identifies two new risk loci for GD. Nature Genetics. 2011; 43(9): 897-901.

[21] Bell L, Hunter AL, Kyriacou A, et al. Clinical diagnosis of Graves' or non-Graves' hyperthyroidism compared to TSH receptor antibody test. Endocrine Connections. 2018; 7(4):504-510.

[22] Douglas RS, Afifiyan NF, Hwang CJ, et al. Increased generation of fibrocytes in thyroid-associated ophthalmopathy. Journal of Clinical Endocrinology and Metabolism. 2010; 95 (1):430-438.

[23] Rafał P, Konrad S, Tomasz B. The Genetic Basis of Graves' Disease. Curr Genomics. 2011; 12(8): 542-563.

[24] Horton R, Wilming L, Rand V, et al. Gene map of the extended human MHC. Nat Rev Genet. 2004; 5: 889-899.

[25] Shiina T, Inoko H, Kulski JK, et al. An update of the HLA genomic region, locus information and disease association. Tissue Antigens 2004; 64: 631-649.

[26] Simmonds MJ, Gough SC. Genetic insights into disease mechanisms of autoimmunity. Br Med Bull. 2004; 71: 93-113.

[27] Yanagawa T, Mangklabruks A, Chang YB. Human histocompatibility leukocyte antigen-DQA1*0501 allele associated with genetic susceptibility to Graves' disease in a Caucasian population. J Clin Endocrinol Metab. 1993; 76: 1569-1574.

[28] Joanne Heward, Amit Allahabadia, Jacquie Daykin, et al. Linkage Disequilibrium between the Human Leukocyte Antigen Class II Region of the Major Histocompatibility Complex and Graves' Disease: Replication Using a Population Case Control and Family-Based Study. *The Journal of Clinical Endocrinology & Metabolism. 1998; 83:3394-3397.*

[29] Stenszky V, Kozma L, Balazs C, et al. The genetics of Graves' disease. HLA and disease susceptibility. J Clin Endocrinol Metab. 1985; 61: 735-740.

[30] Gough SCL and Simmonds MJ. The HLA Region and Autoimmune Disease: Associations and Mechanisms of Action. Curr Genomics. 2007; 8(7):453-465.

[31] Chen PL, Fann CS, Chu CC, et al. Comprehensive genotyping in two homogeneous Graves' Disease samples reveals major and novel HLA association alleles. PLoS ONE. 2011; 6: e16635.

[32] Pearson TA and Manolio TA. How to interpret a genome-wide association study. JAMA. 2008; 299: 1335-1344.

[33] Ban Y , Davies TF , Greenberg DA , et al. Arginine at position 74 of the HLA-DR β1 chain is associated with Graves' disease. Genes & immunity. 2004; 5: 203-208.

[34] Brix TH, Kyvik KO, Christensen K, et al. Evidence for a major role of heredity in Graves' disease: a population-based study of two Danish twin cohorts. J. Clin. Endocrinol. Metab. 2001; 86: 930-934.

[35] Cohen S, Dadi H, Shaoul. Cloning and characterization of a lymphoid-specific, inducible human protein tyrosine phosphatase. Blood. 1999; 93: 2013-24.

[36] Lee YH, Rho YH, Choi SJ, Ji, et al. The PTPN22 C1858T functional polymorphism and autoimmune diseases--a meta-analysis. Rheumatology. 2007; 46: 49-56.

[37] Begovich, AB, Carlton VEH, Honigberg LA, et al. A missense

single-nucleotide polymorphism in a gene encoding a protein tyrosine phosphatase (PTPN22) is associated with rheumatoid arthritis. Am J Hum Genet. 2004; 75: 330-337.

[38] Rieck M, Arechiga A, Onengut Gumuscu S, et al. Genetic variation in PTPN22 corresponds to altered function of T and B lymphocytes. J Immunol. 2007; 179: 4704-4710.

[39] Stanford SM, Mustelin TM, Bottini N. Lymphoid tyrosine phosphatase and autoimmunity: human genetics rediscovers tyrosine phosphatases. Semin Immunopathol. 2010; 32: 127-136.

[40] Hasegawa K, Martin F, Huang G, et al. Pest domain-enriched tyrosine phosphatase (PEP) regulation of effector/memory t cells. Science. 2004; 303: 685-689.

[41] Zhebrun D, Kudryashova Y, Babenko A, et al. Association of PTPN22 1858T/T genotype with type 1 diabetes, Graves' disease but not with rheumatoid arthritis in Russian population. Aging (Albany, NY). 2011 ; 3(4): 368-373.

[42] Zeitlin AA, Heward JM, Brand OJ, et al. Use of Tag single nucleotide polymorphisms (SNPs) to screen PTPN21: no association with GravesGÇÖ disease. Clin Endocrinol. 2006; 65: 380-384.

[43] Ban Y, Tozaki T, Taniyama M, et al. Association of the protein tyrosine phosphatase nonreceptor 22 haplotypes with autoimmune thyroid disease in the Japanese population. Thyroid. 2010; 20(8): 893-9.

[44] Ye F, Shi B, Wu, et al. Experience with lentivirus-mediated CD40 gene silencing in a mouse model of Graves' disease. J. Endocrinol. 2011; 208: 285- 291.

[45] Qureshi OS, Zheng Y, Nakamura K, et al. Trans-endocytosis of CD80 and CD86: a molecular basis for the cell-extrinsic function of CTLA-4. Science. 2011; 332: 600-603.

[46] Syn NL, Teng MW, Mok TS et al. De-novo and acquired resistance to immune checkpoint targeting. The lancet.Oncology. 2017; 18:731-741.

[47] Waterhouse P, Penninger JM, Timms E.et al. Lymphoproliferative disorders with early lethality in mice deficient in CTLA4. Science. 1995; 270: 985-8.

[48] Jermendy A, Szatmári, Laine AP, et al. The interferon-induced helicase IFIH1 Ala946Thr polymorphism is associated with type 1 diabetes in both the high-incidence Finnish and the medium-incidence Hungarian populations. Diabetologia. 2010; 53: 98-102.

[49] Enevold C, Oturai AB, Sorensen PS, et al. Multiple sclerosis and polymorphisms of innate pattern recognition receptors TLR1-10, NOD1-2, DDX58, and IFIH1. J. Neuroimmunol. 2009; 212: 125-131.

[50] Daroszewski J, Pawlak E, Karabon L, et al. Soluble CTLA-4 receptor an immunological marker of Graves' disease and severity of ophthalmopathy is associated with CTLA-4 Jo31 and CT60 gene polymorphisms. Eur. J. Endocrinol. 2009; 161: 787-793.

[51] Anjos S, Nguyen A, Ounissi-Benkalha H, et al. A common autoimmunity predisposing signal peptide variant of the cytotoxic T-lymphocyte antigen 4 results in inefficient glycosylation of the susceptibility allele. J. Biol. Chem. 2002; 277: 46478-46486.

[52] Petrone A, Giorgi G, Galgani A, et al. CT60 single nucleotide

polymorphisms of the cytotoxic Tlymphocyte-associated antigen-4 gene region is associated with Graves' disease in an Italian population. Thyroid. 2005; 15: 232- 238.

[53] Mayans S, Lackovic K, Nyholm C, et al. CT60 genotype does not affect CTLA-4 isoform expression despite association to T1D and AITD in northern Sweden. BMC. Med. Genet. 2007; 8: 3.

[54] Takahashi M and Kimura A. HLA and CTLA4 polymorphisms may confer a synergistic risk in the susceptibility to Graves' disease. J. Hum. Genet. 2010; 55: 323-326.

[55] Brand OJ, Barrett JC, Simmonds MJ, et al. Association of the thyroid stimulating hormone receptor gene (TSHR) with Graves' disease. Hum Mol Genet. 2009; 18: 1704- 1713.

[56] Ploski R, Brand OJ, Jurecka-Lubieniecka B, et al. Thyroid stimulating hormone receptor (TSHR) intron 1 variants are major risk factors for Graves' disease in three European Caucasian cohorts. PLoS ONE. 2010; 5: e15512.

[57] Davis RS, Wang YH, Kubagawa H. Identification of a family of Fc receptor homologs with preferential B cell expression. Proc Natl Acad Sci USA. 2001; 98: 9772-7.

[58] Sgarbi JA, Kasamatsu TS, Matsumura LK. Parity is not related to autoimmune thyroid disease in a population-based study of Japanese-Brazilians. Thyroid. 2010; 20: 1151-1156.

[59] Chistiakov DA, Voronova NV, Turakulov RI, et al. The -112G > A polymorphism of the secretoglobin 3A2 (SCGB3A2) gene encoding uteroglobin-related protein 1 (UGRP1) increases risk for the development of Graves' disease in subsets of patients with elevated levels of immunoglobulin. E. J. Appl. Genet. 2011; 52: 201-207.

[60] Song HD, Liang J, Shi JY, et al. Functional SNPs in the SCGB3A2 promoter are associated with susceptibility to Graves' disease. Hum. Mol. Genet. 2009; 18: 1156-1170.

[61] Areschoug T and Gordon S. Scavenger receptors: role in innate immunity and microbial pathogenesis. Cell Microbiol. 2009; 11: 1160-1169.

[62] Jin Y, Teng W, Ben S, et al. Genome-wide scan of Graves' disease: evidence for linkage on chromosome 5q31 in Chinese Han pedigrees. J. Clin. Endocrinol. Metab. 2003; 88: 1798-1803.

[63] Simmonds MJ, Yesmin K, Newby PR, et al. Confirmation of association of chromosome 5q31.33 with United Kingdom caucasian graves' disease. Thyroid. 2010; 20: 413-417.

[64] Thakur SA, Beamer CA, Migliaccio CT, et al. Critical role of MARCO in crystalline silica-induced pulmonary inflammation. Toxicol. Sci. 2009; 108: 462-471.

[65] Zhu W, Liu N, Zhao Y, et al. Association analysis of polymorphisms in IL-3, IL-4, IL-5, IL-9, and IL-13 with Graves' disease. J. Endocrinol. Invest. 2010; 33: 751-755.

[66] Chu X, Dong Y, Shen M, et al. Polymorphisms in the ADRB2 gene and Graves disease: a casecontrol study and a meta-analysis of available evidence. BMC Medical Genetics. 2009; 10:26.

[67] Jacqueline J, Antonio CB, Andrew JB, et al. Guidelines for the Treatment of Hypothyroidism: Prepared by the American Thyroid Association Task Force on Thyroid Hormone Replacement. Thyroid. 2014; 24(12): 1670-1751.

[68] Garber JR, Cobin RH, Gharib H, et al. Clinical practice guidelines for hypothyroidism in adults: Cosponsored by the american association of clinical endocrinologists and the American thyroid association. Endocrine Practice. 2012; 18: 988-1028.

[69] Stan MH, Garrity JH, Bahn RS. The evaluation and treatment of graves Ophtalmologie. Med Clin North Am. 2012; 96(2): 311-328.

[70] Matthews DC and Syed AA. The role of TSH receptor antibodies in the management of GD. European Journal of Internal Medicine. 2011; 22: 213-216.

[71] Streetman DD and Khanderia U. Diagnosis and treatment of GD. Annals of Pharmacotherapy. 2003; 37: 1100-1109.

[72] Prummel MF, Bakker A, Wiersinga WM, et al. Multi-center study on the characteristics and treatment strategies of patients with Graves' orbitopathy: The first European Group on Graves' Orbitopathy experience. European Journal of Endocrinology. 2003; 148: 491-495.

[73] Orgiazzi J. Antithyroid drugs. Encyclopedia of Endocrine Diseases. 2018; 683-687.

[74] De Groot L, Abalovich M, Alexander EK, et al. Management of thyroid dysfunction during pregnancy and postpartum: An endocrine society clinical practice guideline. Journal of Clinical Endocrinology and Metabolism. 2012; 97: 2543-2565.

[75] Louvet C, De Bellis A, Pereira B, et al. Time course of Graves' orbitopathy after total thyroidectomy and radioiodine therapy for thyroid cancer. Medicine. 2016; 95: e5474.

[76] Menconi F, Marcocci C, Marinò M. Diagnosis and classification of GD.AutoimmunityReviews. 2014; 13(4-5): 398-402.

[77] Leslie WD, Ward L, Salamon, EA, Ludwig S, Rowe RC, Cowden EA. A randomized comparison of radioiodine doses in graves' hyperthyroidism. Journal of Clinical Endocrinology and Metabolism. 2003; 88(3): 978-983.

[78] Bonnema SJ and Hegedüs. Radioiodine therapy in benign thyroid diseases: Effects, side effects, and factors affecting therapeutic outcome. Endocrine Reviews. 2012; 33(6): 920-980.

[79] Leo SD, Lee SY, Braverman LE. Hyperthyroidism. Lancet. 2016; 388(10047): 906-918.

[80] Nawrot I, Pragacz A, Pragacz K, et al. Total thyroidectomy is associated with increased prevalence of permanent hypoparathyroidism. Medical Science Monitor. 2014; 20: 1675-1681.

[81] Bartalena L, Baldeschi L, Dickinson A, et al. Consensus statement of the European Group on Graves' orbitopathy (EUGOGO) on management of GO. European Journal of Endocrinology. 2008; 158(3): 273-285.

[82] Marcocci C, Kahaly GJ, Krassas GE, et al. Selenium and the Course of Mild Graves' Orbitopathy. New England Journal of Medicine. 2011; 364(20): 1920-1931.

Chapter 5

Autoimmune Mechanism and Recurrence Risk in Graves' Disease

Vasudha Bakshi and Gollapalli Rajeev Kumar

Abstract

Graves' Disease (GD) is an autoimmune thyroid disorder where autoantibodies are produced against TSH (Thyroid Stimulating Hormone) receptor causing thyrotoxicosis. It is characterized by goiter, ophthalmopathy, and occasionally pretibial myxedema. The autoimmune mechanism causing disease is not well understood and it is complex. It involves multifactorial etiology involving environmental and genetic factors. Smoking and positive family history contributing to the development of GD. GD can be diagnosed based on the clinical manifestation and demonstrating low concentration of TSHs, high TRab (Thyroid Stimulating Hormone receptor autoantibodies), and high FT4 (Free thyroxine) concentration. Current treatment options aimed at stable restoration of euthyroidism by following different modalities of suppressing thyroid gland using antithyroid drugs, removing/ablating thyroid gland by surgery, and radioactive iodine treatment with iodine- 131.

Keywords: Graves' Disease, Thyroid Stimulating Hormone, Thyroid Stimulating Hormone receptor autoantibodies, Free thyroxine

1. Introduction

In this particular, Graves' Disease (GD) an autoimmune disorder, caused by excessive secretion of the glandular thyroid hormones by the thyroid follicles, which is related to the progressive hyperthyroidism condition. It is found to be the main cause of hyperthyroidism. The annual incidence has been reported of about 14–50 cases per 100,000 populations [1]. The disease may affect at any age and the incidence increases with age. The peak incidence of GD is between 30 and 50 years. It is generally accepted that younger patients have a severe immune system disorder where GD is predominantly found [1]. Few studies showed that younger patients are having poorer responses to ATD and poor prognosis with recurrent risk [2–4]. The lifetime risk of getting Graves' Disease is roughly 6 times higher in women than in men [1]. The exact mechanism of affecting the different gender is not known but believed to be associated with different sex hormones. Females are being affected more and the strongest risk factor contributed to the development of GD is estrogen. Estrogen influences B- cell functioning and regulates the immune system [5]. In GD patients, elevated estradiol relates to TRAb (TSH receptor antibody) positivity [6]. The risk of recurrence of GD after the withdrawal of the anti-thyroid drugs (ATG) is majorly seen in male GD patients [7, 8]. Large goiter with severe immune disorders and genetic aspects are associated with the development of GD in males. Genetic factors associated with GD are cytotoxic T-associated lymphocyte factor-4 (CTLA4) rs231779 and rs231775, especially Thyroglobulin (Tg) and TSHR polymorphisms are linked with relapse in GD after the withdrawal of ATD. At four weeks following the completion of a randomized tobacco trial of ATD, the TRAb level was significantly higher in smokers than in nonsmokers [9–11]. Smoking promotes elevated levels of TRAb contributed to the development of GD. A number of factors recognized against GD includes stress, sex and sex hormones, pregnancy, infection, other autoimmune diseases, iodine and other potential environmental factors such as radiation have been recognized against Graves' Disease. The resulting breakdown in thyroid tolerance would lead to errors in multiple protective immune mechanisms. It is noted that sera of Graves's patients may contain the "predominant Hashimoto" thyroglobulin (Tg) and thyroid peroxidase antibodies (TPO Abs). Antibodies toward Hashimoto bind to the TSH receptor while, rather than promoting TSH action, block the growth of TSH action during illness and have seen positive results throughout the thyroid condition of Graves' Disease [12].

2. Clinical features of Graves' Disease condition

Symptoms of hyperthyroidism associated with thyrotoxicosis are nervousness, overactivity, insomnia, palpitations, mental confusion, weight loss and prominent signs of thyrotoxicosis are tachycardia, atrial fibrillation, hyperreflexia systemic hypertension, warm moist skin, hyperactivity, and tremors. The clinical features predominantly observed in GD are orbithopathy, pretibial myxedema, and goiter.

The pathogenesis of ophthalmopathy includes the immune response to a TSH receptor–like protein in orbital connective tissue initiates cytokine formation further promoting production by orbital fibroblasts of hydrophilic glycosaminoglycan, resulting in high osmotic pressure, fluid accumulation, and clinical ophthalmopathy. Eye muscle antigens include the flavoprotein (Fp) subunit of mitochondrial succinate dehydrogenase, G2s and the FOX P1 protein, a winged helix transcription factor, and their respective antibodies are clinically useful markers in the diagnosis of GD. The respective roles of the connective tissue response and eye muscle antibodies involved in the pathogenesis are under investigation.

3. Pathogenesis

Autoimmune thyroid diseases are the most prevalent organ- specific which includes Graves' Disease (GD) and Hashimoto's Thyroiditis (HT). The hyperactivity of the thyroid gland is due to the production of thyroid stimulating antibodies (autoantibodies) and are known to recognize and activate thyroid stimulating hormone receptor. The autoantibodies produced by TSHR increase the growth and functioning to thyroid follicular cells resulting over production of T3 and T4. It has been suggested by the studies that a genetic clonal lack of suppressor T cells may be responsible for the inappropriate and unregulated production of TSH receptor antibody [13].

3.1 Autoimmunity mechanism

The pathological process involved in Graves' Disease is similar to other autoimmune disease but a unique aspect found in the majority of patients is TSHR antibodies which cannot be found in normal individuals. The characterization of the autoimmunity process includes a lymphocytic infiltrate seen at the target organ and the presence of antigen-reactive T and B cells against thyroid antigens. As in all autoimmune diseases it is observed when self-tolerance is broken; T cells identify self-antigens, and B cells produce antibodies targeting host cells. Many cell self-specific T cells escape thymic deletion; however, additional mechanisms like clonal anergy and peripheral suppression normally prevent reactions to auto antigen. B cells which recognize a specific cell auto antigen in the lymphoid organs are taken into T lymphocyte areas; B lymphocytes normally kill by apoptosis if they are not activated by T available cells while B lymphocytes, binding soluble self-antigen, are anergised; they down- regulate expression of membrane IgM and live for a short period. B cells are inactivated by T-cells available for support. An additional B cell tolerance mechanism includes allelic exclusion and clonal ignorance in receptor and autoreactive B cell receptor (BCRs).

3.2 The thyroid antigens

3.2.1 Tg and TPO

Thyroglobulin (Tg) is 660 kDa, a dimeric glycoprotein secreted by the follicular cells of the thyroid gland and acts as a substrate for the synthesis of T3 and T4. Besides, it stores an inactive form of thyroid hormone and iodine in the lumen of the thyroid follicle. The antibodies produced in response to Tg induce massive destruction of the thyroid gland but few studies propose to show high levels of Tg do not *perse* induce antibody production. Thyroid hormones are synthesized on the Tg with the help of thyroid peroxidase (TPO). TPO is an enzyme Anti-thyroglobulin antibody (ATA) and TPO- specific T cells are often found in GD patients. Tg antibodies recognize the confirmation of a large fragment of Tg [14]. These are directed against the same epitopes which are mainly observed in GD. Antibodies against TPO are involved in complement/antibody-mediated cell toxicity and target toward conformational epitopes.

3.2.2 GD auto antigen and TSH receptor antibodies

The auto antigen which is mainly expressed in Graves' Disease is thyroid stimulating hormone receptor (TSHR). It is a G protein coupled receptor with 7 trans membrane spanning domains expressed in thyroid gland but also in adipose cells, fibroblasts, bone cells including heart cells [15]. Binding to circulating TSH, a G-Protein signal activates adenylcyclase cascade events and intracellular levels of c AMP increases. Rise in c AMP activates all the functional activities of thyroid cell which includes iodine pumping; synthesis of thyroglobulin, iodination, endocytosis, and proteolysis; activity involving thyroid peroxidases; and hormone release. Literatures suggest that there may be a shedding of the TSHR ectodomain [16–18] even though it has not been confirmed in vivo.

The presence of TSHR-Antibodies (TSHR-Abs) [19] is the most unusual feature of most GD-patients. The early analysis of TSHR-Abs [20] represents the most accurate definition of their features, which resulted by analysis of monoclonal antibodies to the TSHR from various sources, including human, mouse and hamster: mouse and hamster antibodies are secondary to TSHR [21–23]. Three types of TSHR-Ab are identified among autoimmune-thyroid patients and similar diseases are observed in immunized rodents; stimulating, blocking, and so-called "neutral." TSHR-Abs that has proved to be beyond neutral in their biological activity has been characteristic of the TSHR ectodomain's cleavage. Stimulating Antibodies (Stimulating Abs) induce cAMP production and inhibit any simultaneous activation of the thyroid function that bind to naturally conformed TSHR. TSHR blocking antibodies, its main bioactivity of this is to prevent TSH receptor binding in a manner that may cause thyroid problems, and also it act as weak TSH agonists. Such blocking antibodies depend on conformation, and others are very similar to the decreased TSHR antigen and/or linear peptides. At the end, neutral TSHR antibodies may not prevent or stimulate cAMP production or TSH adhering. Neutral TSHR-antibodies bind only to linear epitopes and are targeted against the "unique region" located in receptor among specific amino acids 316–366 [24]. In GD patients, the presence of different ratios with high-affinity TSHR-Abs contributes to the clinical phenotype. Therefore, a function-based classification of these antibodies appears more relevant than their ability or failure to influence the binding of TSHs or cAMPs.

3.3 Different epitopes of TSHR Abs

3.3.1 Monoclonal antibodies against TSHR

Any monoclonal antibody raised to TSHR protein or antigen includes synthesized peptides and recombinant ones, that have been shown to be neutralizing in mechanism. Only natural intact TSH receptors or genetic immune are used to stimulate thyroid-stimulating antibodies and establish an animal hyperthyroidism model [25–28]. Monoclonal antibodies, such as MS-1, have been raised in hamsters utilizing rare B cells that secrete TSHR-enhancing antibodies [29]. Rodents and humans have been used to identify blocking and neutral monoclonal antibodies (mAbs).

3.3.2 Stimulating TSHR-Ab epitopes

Part of the TSHR ectodomain has also been crystallized with the support of appropriate stimulating monoclonal fragment TSHR Fab bound in situ [30]. Many amino acids have a large section of the concave surface of the TSHR ectodomain that has been identified as important for antibody binding, in the leucin-rich repeat region (LRR). Reviewing recent studies particularly at conformational epitopes using mass spectrometry [29] have shown that epitopes exist outside the LRR for blocking and stimulating monoclonal antibodies. The prominent region exist at N terminal region of the extracellular domain (ECD) has been well demonstrated and also at the residues in the "hinge" region [31].

3.3.3 Blocking TSHR-Ab epitopes

TSHR antibodies block epitopes are widely distributed compared to stimulating antibodies. Thus, blocking TSHR monoclonal antibodies (TSHR-mAbs) have been shown to have binding affinities to independent or confirmational epitopes [32]. In patients with GD or HT, TSHR autoantibodies showed themselves to compete in N-terminal TSHR beta subunit (aa382–415), with a blocking TSHR-mAb. Blocking hypothyroid antibodies therefore is heterogeneous in nature and this repertoire of anti-bodies involves multiple epitopes. Crystallization and modeling of human and mouse blocking TSHR Abs attempting to block and these TSHR-Abs strongly proposed that the N-terminal and the leucine-rich binding are linked [33, 34].

3.3.4 Cleavage TSHR-Ab epitopes

Peptide binding (ELISA) and the monoclonal competition of antibodies in patients with Graves' Disease is shown throughout cleavage (aaa 316–366) (competitive inhibition assay by FACS). The tissues of the TSHR are strongly related. The main linear epitopes in animal GD models are known in the area of cleavage [35].

Such antibodies are not competitive to TSH-borne binding in the cleaved area and are therefore often called "neutral."

3.4 TSHR-mAb induced signal transduction

Through the stimulation of agonist, TSH and TSHR-Abs the TSH receptor seems to be active and enhanced. Intracellular signal transmissions spread through classical GPCR effector proteins with the Gαq and Gαs interaction with the recipient directly.

Docking Gαs into the activated receptor results in an increased adenylatecyclasis activity generated by the cAMP, direct activation of protein kinase A (PKA) and cAMP element-binding protein (CREB). Gαq docking involves PI3 and DAG formation and further activation of Ca2+ and protein kinase C (PKC). Enables Erk1/2 and p90RSK subsequently. Stimulating TSH-mAb has shown to act in a dose-dependent and time-dependent manner via the Gαq-PKC-Akt cascade, and the rat thyroid model (FrTL-5) was found to be relevant on PKA signaling [36, 37]. Monoclonal antibodies, which are frequently detected by point-of-care tests, were also demonstrated to activate non classical TSH receptor pathways, though this was reported as only a few of the studies have shown this. Certain neutral antibodies are not found to increase cAMP, but could signal by means of Akt, c-Raf/ERK1/2/p90RSK, PKC, and PKA/CREB [37].

3.5 Apoptosis in GD

Apoptosis is absolutely essential for the development of the aggressive immune system. The initial theories about thyroidectomy-induced autoimmunity postulated that antibody and T cell-mediated destruction of the thyroid contributed to the death of thyrocytes. In the ensuing years, it is discovered that apoptosis had a part in GD [38]. Apoptosis provided a new insight into autoimmune target destruction, further implying the participation in possible pathogenesis of thyroid autoimmunity from death-controlled receptors and cytokine-related apoptotic pathways. An abnormally increased level of CD4(+) regulatory T cells break host immune tolerance and initiate T-reg apoptosis [39] and, in this way, foster abnormal T-mediated immune activation in patients with GD. Bcl-2 regulatory protein family is recently linked to the pathogenesis of GD [40] looked at apoptotic proteins, and observed a relation to the expression of the Bcl-2 regulatory family in the thyroid follicular cells in GD [41]. Furthermore, the researchers suggested that an increase in apoptotic molecules (Fas/FasL and caspase 8) are present on T and B lymphocytes in GD and HT patients, demonstrating involvement in GD pathogenesis. It is clear to describe in apoptosis, death receptors/ligands play a regulatory role, but caspase-independent mechanisms can also coexist and contribute to GD thyroid cell death.

3.6 Apoptosis and thyrocyte oxidative stress induced by TSHR antibodies

The induction of cell proliferation via stimulating- monoclonal antibodies (mAbs) shown in thyrocyte stimulation studies with TSHR-mAbs that have been conducted with cAMP. Some neutral monoclonal antibodies (mAbs) have been identified as stimulating multiple stress signals and apoptosis induced. These antibodies are responsible for activation of multiple oncogenes, including p53, p73 and Reactive oxygen species (ROS). In addition, endoplasmic reticulum stress protein (gp98) is induced and the expression of heat shock proteins (p27 and p107), hemaoxygenase (HO) and superoxide dismutase (SOD) is further activated and supported.These data support stress signals in the thyroid cells of Graves' Disease.

A morphologic staining (annexin V and propidium iodide) and a quantitative flow cytometry test [42] confirmed the cell death caused by apoptosis, and is likely to confirm the previously described histological evidence that thyroid tissue apoptosis is found in GD patients. These observations have revealed that stress signaling cascades have been involved although oxidative stress alone or cell-specific signaling molecules induced such apoptosis remain unclear. These results also indicated the ability of neutral TSHR monoclonal antibodies (TSHR-mAbs), which is known to activate inborn and bystander immune reactivity via DNA release from apoptotic cells [43], to aggravate the local infiltration in a thyroid. This same phenomenon may be associated with Graves' orbitopathy as these cells were abundantly expressed by activation-induced fibroblast death.

3.7 Humoral immunity

The GD Rodents have shown humoral immunity against other TSHR-immunized antigens, unless outbred animals like hamsters have been used, to show intrathyroid infiltrate. This implies that GD is an intricate genetic disorder, usually associated with autoimmune thyroiditis. AITD is not known for the presence of pendrin antibodies, sodium iodides symporters [44, 45], thyroxine, triiodothyronin [46], tubulin, megalin, calmo-modulin and DNA, or DNA-related proteins [47–49]. The IGF-1 receptor is widespread in B cells and in fibroblast from GD patients, although over-expressed. In activation of the thyrocyte, synergism between antibodies to TSHR and the IGF-1 receptor was suggested. That requires further research as TSH and IGF-1 or insulin are commonly known to induce proliferation of thyroid cells.

4. Diagnosis

Diagnosis of GD is complex and difficult. The combined effect of several symptoms and symptoms leads the doctor to suspect the thyroid irregularity. Comprehensive history such as intake or exposure to iodine, drugs, thyroid and autoimmune history and physical exam, vital signs such as pulse rate measurement, blood pressure measurement, respiratory and body weight. Moreover, the presence or absence of a thyroid tenderness, symmetry and nodularity should also be evaluated; pulmonary, cardiac and neuromuscular function and the presence of eye signs or pretibial myxedema. Because hyperthyroidism is frequently associated with low or undetectable levels of TSH, it is an easy biochemical diagnosis to make if thyrotoxicosis is found. T4 and T3 are usually high, but are relatively higher in GD serumT3 than T4. The T4 and T3 concentration levels are usually high. In mild forms of hyperthyroidism and during earliest phases of DG only serum T3 levels can be enhanced (T3 toxicosis). The removal of the lid, anxiety, an increase in neck volume, signs of involvement with the eye and the history of autoimmune disease in the family also distinguish GD from other types of hyperthyroidism (e.g., toxin goiter, toxic adenoma) (e.g., silent or subacute thyroiditis, exogenous thyroid hormone use). Serum measurement of the TSH-receptor automatic antibody (TRAb) helps confirm diagnosis. New bioassays for the thyroid stimulant immunoglobulin (TSI) especially aid in the measurement of TSI's ability to increase the intracellular cAMP level by detecting stimulating antibodies. Radioactive Iodine uptaking (RAIU), despite a clinical examination, thyroid function evaluation and TRAb detection should only be carried out when the diagnosis is unclear. The pattern for iodine uptake in GD is diffuse if no coexisting nodules or fibrosis do not occur. Technetium

99 can be of assistance. Increased color Doppler flow supports thyroid hyperactivity diagnosis. In case of thyroid nodularity in the neck or in a thyroid scintigram, thyroid scan must be conducted.

5. The factors that influence the recurrence in GD patients

5.1 Biochemical parameter

The severity is linked to recurrence risk in ATD-treated GD patients. Partly the biochemical parameters help to determine the seriousness of GD. The parametric increase of serum T3, which is affected by increased intrathyroid type 1 deiodinase activity, is significant in untreated GD. Independent GD factors influenced free thyroxine-to-free triiodothyronine ratio (FT3 andFT4) is predictive for the ATD treatment outcome for patients with GD. Hyperthyroidism symptoms observed after the treatment with beta-blockers. Patients with a higher T3/FT3 or FT3/T4 serum ratio have been found to be more at recurrence, requiring a longer and more additional dose in the treatment. The risk of relapsed treatment is increased for patients with a higher serum T3 and FT3/FT4 ratio. When a patient has a high T3/T4 ratio, therapy should be continued for at least one year after the ATD has been removed. Serum thyroid-stimulating hormone (TSH) should be measured. However, as it is known, the thyroid hormone has a negative feed-back influence on the TSH. Thus, prior research has established that drug discontinuation is associated with elevated levels of TSH. These findings suggest that treatment with a prolonged ATD may be indicated for GD patients who do not normalize their thyroid-stimulating hormone levels quickly.

5.2 Immune parameters

The GD is the result of hyper-activation by TRAb of the TSH receptor in follicular thyroid cells. In approximately 95% of newly diagnosed GD patients, TRAb is positive and higher TRAb levels are indicative of serious immune disorder. Recent times have demonstrated TRAb as a helpful and qualitative prognostic indicator for ATD therapy. At the time of GD diagnosis, patients with high TRAb levels had a considerably higher recurrence risk, while TRAb patients were often more likely to get long-term recovery. Switching from positive to negative TRAb in GD patients involves a reduced immune disorder after ATD therapy. In the prognosis of GD patients, TRAb levels were also observed at ATD withdrawal. Recurrence risk was noted to be increased in TRAb-positive GD during the time of drug discontinuation. New assays can be used to distinguish the stimulating (stimulating) and blocking (disturbing) effects of medications on antigen responses. Thyroid stimulating antibodies (TSAb) antibodies are found to be predominant in GD patients. Recently, the value of TRAb for patients on GD treatments for recurrence risk with prediction has been shown to be greater than that of GD, particularly TSAb. GD patients with thyroiditis from Hashimoto appear to be remission after Hashimoto's thyroiditis due to advanced harm. The prevalence of peroxidase/peroxidase antibodies is highest in people with Hashimoto's thyroiditis. Few studies have analyzed whether the existence of Thyroid peroxidase antibodies (TPOAb) and Thyroglobulin antibodies (TgAb) autoantibodies is linked to the risk of a subsequent relapse in those with GD. People with GD may also show low TPOAb and TgAb levels, and in such cases, the clinical and laboratory findings are not completely consistent with the diagnosis of Hashimoto's disease.

5.3 Goiter size

A major clinical manifestation found in GD patients is the large goiter. Previous studies show a large predictor of increased risk of recurrence in GD patients after the removal of ATD, goiter size. Findings from 5 years of trail follow-up have shown that the rate of remission for normal or mild-goiter patients is higher than for large-goiter patients. GD patients with significantly lower goiter sizes tend to have higher rates of remission after ATD treatment. Enlarged goiter size at the time of GD diagnosis and drug withdrawal is associated with a higher recurrence risk of GD.

5.4 Graves' orbitopathy

At the time of diagnosis of GD, Graves' orbitopathy is observed in 35% of patients. Sometimes, the presence of the Graves orbitopathy indicated that the immune system gets worsen. Previous studies show that the risk of GD recurrence after withdrawal of ATD in patients with Graves' orbitopathy is higher [38]. An Eckstein et al. study even found that GD patients with severe Graves' orbitopathy only received a 7% remission rate. Although the recurrence rate is higher, the ATD treatment remains a preferred therapeutic option for GD patients with orbitopathy of Graves because Graves's orbitopathy improves as well as a steady eutyroid status achieved and reduces inflammatory markers of the TRAb. Recent studies have demonstrated that the continuous low dose of ATD has helped to improve GD disease in Graves orbitopathy patients.

5.5 Genetic factors

Genetic factors plays a key role in the pathogenesis of GD and increase the risk of recurrence to the development of GD. Several studies supports both cytotoxic T-lymphocyte-associated factor 4 (CTLA4) rs231775 and rs231779 polymorphisms were strongly associated with recurrence of GD even after ATD withdrawal in Asians, while there is no association in Caucasians for developing GD. In Caucasian patients with GD, the recurrence risk after ATD withdrawal was observed with the polymorphisms of HLA DQA2, HLA DRB1∗03, and HLA DQB1∗02. The HLA region majorly contains immune response genes and tHLA polymorphisms might also influence the outcome of GD patients by regulating the immune system.

5.6 Environmental factors

GD starts with some environmental factors in the predisposed genetic association in individuals. Stress is one of the important environmental considerations, and a majority of the studies have supported the association between stress and recurrence in GD patients after ATD therapy. The overall stress score for large life events was significantly higher in the recurrence group in a prospective study that examined the recurrence risk of GD in patients than in the remission. Another trial showed that the recurrence group was more stressful than the remission patients, and that the total number of stressful events is linked to the number of the recurrence. Psychosocial stress is an important part of a stressful event. It is worth mentioning. Previous trials showed that the risk of GD recurrence is higher than that of GD patients without such a disease for patients with psychiatric disorders as depression and hypochondriasis. Therefore, reducing stress is an essential way of improving the prognosis of ATD-treated GD patients. Another ecological factor is iodine intake.

The synthesis of the thyroid hormone is based on Iodine. Increased content of iodine in thyrocytes has promoted degradation of ATD and reduced uptake of ATD. The supplementation of iodine increased the GD recurrence rate. After ATD withdrawal hyperthyroidism in euthyroid GD patients arose when pharmaceutical doses of iodine were taken. Epidemiologic studies have shown, however, that in iodine-adequate countries, recurrence rates in GD patients do not exceed those in iodine-deficient areas following ATD withdrawal.

6. Conclusion

Autoimmunity is a collection of heterogeneous disorders which is controlled by complex genetic and environmental factors. In GD, the prominent antigen responsible is TSHR and the studies of extra thyroidal TSHR expression in different variety of cell types and immune cells has added to the complexity of the disease and also introduced a variety of potential new mechanisms that may be involved. A common approach of GD is that TSHR-Abs promote the disease by enhancing thyroid antigen expression. Precision medicine's promise is still important in the future. The chapter has personalized diagnostic and therapeutic approaches will encompass both a patient's genomic makeup and their environmental factors.

Acknowledgements

This work was supported by the management, faculty and staff of Anurag University, Hyderabad, India.

Conflicts of interest

The authors declare that they have no conflicts of interest.

Author details

Vasudha Bakshi* and Gollapalli Rajeev Kumar
School of Pharmacy, Anurag University, Hyderabad, India

*Address all correspondence to: vasudhapharmacy@cvsr.ac.in

References

[1] IreneCampi, MarioSalviEncyclopedia of Endocrine Diseases (Second Edition)Volume 4, 2018, Pages 698-701

[2] X. G. Vos, E. Endert, A. H. Zwinderman, J. G. Tijssen, and W. M. Wiersinga, "Predicting the risk of recurrence before the start of antithyroid drug therapy in patients with Graves' hyperthyroidism," The Journal of Clinical Endocrinology and Metabolism, vol. 101, no. 4, pp. 1381-1389, 2016.

[3] T. Yamada, T. Aizawa, Y. Koizumi, I. Komiya, K. Ichikawa, and K. Hashizume, "Age-related therapeutic response toantithyroid drug in patients with hyperthyroid Graves' disease," Journal of the American Geriatrics Society, vol. 42, no. 5, pp. 513-516, 1994

[4] A. Allahabadia, J. Daykin, R. L. Holder, M. C. Sheppard, S. C. Gough, and J. A. Franklyn, "Age and gender predict the outcome of treatment for Graves' hyperthyroidism," The Journal of Clinical Endocrinology and Metabolism, vol. 85, no. 3, pp. 1038-1042, 2000.

[5] J. A. Da Silva, "Sex hormones, glucocorticoids and autoimmunity: facts and hypotheses," Annals of the Rheumatic Diseases, vol. 54, no. 1, pp. 6-16, 1995

[6] L. O. Chailurkit, W. Aekplakorn, and B. Ongphiphadhanakul, "The relationship between circulating estradiol and thyroid autoimmunity in males," European Journal of Endocrinology, vol. 170, no. 1, pp. 63-67, 2014

[7] P. Anagnostis, F. Adamidou, S. A. Polyzos et al., "Predictors of long-term remission in patients with Graves' disease: a single center experience," Endocrine, vol. 44, no. 2, pp. 448–453, 2013

[8] F. Magri, F. Zerbini, M. Gaiti et al., "Gender influences the clinical presentation and long-term outcome of Graves' disease," Endocrine Practice, vol. 22, no. 11, pp. 1336-1342, 2016

[9] P. W. Wang, I. Y. Chen, S. H. Juo, E. Hsi, R. T. Liu, and C. J. Hsieh, "Genotype and phenotype predictors of relapse of Graves' disease after antithyroid drug withdrawal," European Thyroid Journal, vol. 1, no. 4, pp. 251-258, 2013.

[10] J. Y. Hsiao, M. C. Hsieh, K. J. Tien, S. C. Hsu, S. J. Shin, and S. R. Lin, "Association between a C/T polymorphism in exon 33 of the thyroglobulin gene is associated with relapse of Graves' hyperthyroidism after antithyroid withdrawal in Taiwanese," Journal of Clinical Endocrinology and Metabolism, vol. 92, no. 8, pp. 3197-3201, 2007.

[11] D. Glinoer, "Clinical epidemiology of Graves' disease: a multicentric prospective study in Belgium," Revue Médicale de Bruxelles, vol. 21, no. 4, pp. 296-299, 2000

[12] Tamai H, Kasagi K, Takaichi Y, Takamatsu J, Komaki G, Matsubayashi S, et al. Development of spontaneous hypothyroidism in patients with Graves' disease treated with anti-thyroidal drugs: clinical, immunological and histological findings in 26 patients. J ClinEndocrinolMetab 1989;69:49-53.

[13] Volpe R. The immunoregulatory disturbance in autoimmune thyroid disease. Autoimmunity 1988;2:55-72

[14] Latrofa F, Ricci D, Grasso L, Vitti P, Masserini L, Basolo F, et al. Characterization of thyroglobulin epitopes in patients with autoimmune and non-autoimmune thyroid diseases using recombinant human monoclonal

thyroglobulin autoantibodies. J ClinEndocrinolMetab. 2008; 93(2):591-596. Epub 2007/11/22. [PubMed: 18029466]

[15] Bahn RS, Dutton CM, Natt N, Joba W, Spitzweg C, Heufelder AE. Thyrotropin receptor expression in Graves' orbital adipose/connective tissues: potential autoantigen in Graves' ophthalmopathy. J ClinEndocrinolMetab. 1998; 83(3):998-1002. [PubMed: 9506762]

[16] Chazenbalk GD, Pichurin P, Chen CR, Latrofa F, Johnstone AP, McLachlan SM, et al. Thyroidstimulating autoantibodies in Graves disease preferentially recognize the free A subunit, not the thyrotropinholoreceptor. J Clin Invest. 2002; 110(2):209–

[17] [PubMed: 12122113] 21. Kajita Y, Rickards CR, Buckland PR, Howells RD, Rees SB. Analysis of thyrotropin receptors by photoaffinity labelling. Orientation of receptor subunits in the cell membrane. Biochem J. 1985; 227(2):413-20. [PubMed: 2988500]

[18] Loosfelt H, Pichon C, Jolivet A, Misrahi M, Caillou B, Jamous M, et al. Two-subunit structure of the human thyrotropin receptor. ProcNatl AcadSci USA. 1992; 89(9):3765-3769. [PubMed: 1570295]

[19] Vlase, H.; Davies, TF. Insights into the molecular mechanisms of the autoimmune thyroid diseases.. In: Eisenbarth, GS., editor. Endocrine and organ specific autoimmunity. R.G. Landes Co.; CA: 1999. p. 98-132.

[20] Adams DD, Purves HD. Abnormal responses in the assay of thyrotropin. ProcUnivOtago Med School. 1956; 34:11-12

[21] Ando T, Davies TF. Monoclonal antibodies to the thyrotropin receptor. ClinDevImmunol. 2005; 12:137-143. [PubMed: 16050145]

[22] Ando T, Latif R, Pritsker A, Moran T, Nagayama Y, Davies TF. A monoclonal thyroid-stimulating antibody. J Clin Invest. 2002; 110:1667-1674. [PubMed: 12464672]

[23] Ando T, Latif R, Davies TF. Antibody-induced modulation of TSH receptor post-translational processing. J Endocrinol. 2007; 195:179-186. [PubMed: 17911409]

[24] Ando T, Latif R, Daniel S, Eguchi K, Davies TF. Dissecting linear and conformational epitopes on the native thyrotropin receptor. Endocrinology. 2004; 145:5185-5193. [PubMed: 15297445]

[25] Costagliola S, Many MC, Denef JF, Pohlenz J, Refetoff S, Vassart G. Genetic immunization of outbred mice with thyrotropin receptor cDNA provides a model of Graves' disease. J Clin Invest. 2000; 105:803-811. [PubMed: 10727449]

[26] Sanders J, Allen F, Jeffreys J, Bolton J, Richards T, Depraetere H, Nakatake N, Evans M, Kiddie A, Premawardhana LD, Chirgadze DY, Miguel RN, Blundell TL, Furmaniak J, Smith BR. Characteristics of a monoclonal antibody to the thyrotropin receptor that acts as a powerful thyroid-stimulating autoantibody antagonist. Thyroid. 2005; 15:672-682. [PubMed: 16053383]

[27] Muehlberg T, Gilbert JA, Rao PV, McGregor AM, Banga JP. Dynamics of thyroid-stimulating and - blocking antibodies to the thyrotropin receptor in a murine model of Graves' disease. Endocrinology. 2004; 145:1539-1545. [PubMed: 14764633]

[28] Sanders J, Allen F, Jeffreys J, Bolton J, Richards T, Depraetere H, Nakatake N, Evans M, Kiddie A, Premawardhana LD, Chirgadze DY,

Miguel RN, Blundell TL, Furmaniak J, Smith BR. Characteristics of a monoclonal antibody to the thyrotropin receptor that acts as a powerful thyroid-stimulating autoantibody antagonist. Thyroid. 2005; 15:672-682. [PubMed: 16053383]

[29] Latif R, Teixeira A, Michalek K, Ali MR, Schlesinger M, Baliram R, Morshed SA, Davies TF. Antibody protection reveals extended epitopes on the human TSH receptor. PLoS One. 2012; 7:e44669. [PubMed: 22957097]

[30] Sanders J, Chirgadze DY, Sanders P, Baker S, Sullivan A, Bhardwaja A, Bolton J, Reeve M, Nakatake N, Evans M, Richards T, Powell M, Miguel RN, Blundell TL, Furmaniak J, Smith BR.Crystal Structure of the TSH Receptor in Complex with a Thyroid-Stimulating Autoantibody. Thyroid. 2007; 17:395-410. [PubMed: 17542669]

[31] Chazenbalk GD, Pichurin P, Chen CR, Latrofa F, Johnstone AP, McLachlan SM, Rapoport B. Thyroid-stimulating autoantibodies in Graves disease preferentially recognize the free A subunit, not the thyrotropin holoreceptor. J Clin Invest. 2002; 110:209-217. [PubMed: 12122113]

[32] Ando T, Latif R, Daniel S, Eguchi K, Davies TF. Dissecting linear and conformational epitopes on the native thyrotropin receptor. Endocrinology. 2004; 145:5185-5193. [PubMed: 15297445]

[33] Sanders P, Young S, Sanders J, Kabelis K, Baker S, Sullivan A, Evans M, Clark J, Wilmot J, Hu X, Roberts E, Powell M, Nunez Miguel R, Furmaniak J, Rees Smith B. Crystal structure of the TSH receptor (TSHR) bound to a blocking-type TSHR autoantibody. J MolEndocrinol. 2011; 46:81– 99. [PubMed: 21247981]

[34] Evans M, Sanders J, Tagami T, Sanders P, Young S, Roberts E, Wilmot J, Hu X, Kabelis K, Clark J, Holl S, Richards T, Collyer A, Furmaniak J, Smith BR. Monoclonal autoantibodies to the TSH receptor, one with stimulating activity and one with blocking activity, obtained from the same blood sample. ClinEndocrinol (Oxf). 2010; 73:404-412. [PubMed: 20550534]

[35] Davies TF, Ando T, Lin RY, Tomer Y, Latif R. Thyrotropin receptor-associated diseases: from adenomata to Graves disease. J Clin Invest. 2005; 115:1972-1983. [PubMed: 16075037]

[36] Iacovelli L, Capobianco L, Salvatore L, Sallese M, D'Ancona GM, De BA. Thyrotropin activates mitogen-activated protein kinase pathway in FRTL-5 by a cAMP-dependent protein kinase Aindependent mechanism. MolPharmacol. 2001; 60:924-933. [PubMed: 11641420]

[37] Morshed SA, Latif R, Davies TF. Characterization of thyrotropin receptor antibody-induced signaling cascades. Endocrinology. 2009; 150:519-529. [PubMed: 18719020]

[38] Stassi G, De MR. Autoimmune thyroid disease: new models of cell death in autoimmunity. Nat Rev Immunol. 2002; 2(3):195-204. [PubMed: 11913070]

[39] Mao C, Wang S, Xiao Y, Xu J, Jiang Q, Jin M, et al. Impairment of regulatory capacity of CD4+ CD25+ regulatory T cells mediated by dendritic cell polarization and hyperthyroidism in Graves' disease. J Immunol. 2011; 186(8):4734-4743. Epub 2011/03/15. [PubMed: 21398613]

[40] Bossowski A, Czarnocka B, Bardadin K, Urban M, Niedziela M, Dadan J. Expression of Bcl-2 family proteins in thyrocytes from young patients with immune and nonimmune thyroid diseases. Horm Res. 2008; 70(3):155-164. Epub 2008/07/30. [PubMed: 18663316]

[41] Bossowski A, Czarnocka B, Bardadin K, Stasiak-Barmuta A, Urban M, Dadan J, et al. Identification of apoptotic proteins in thyroid gland from patients with Graves' disease and Hashimoto's thyroiditis. Autoimmunity. 2008; 41(2):163-173. Epub 2008/03/08. [PubMed: 18324486]

[42] Morshed SA, Ando T, Latif R, Davies TF. Neutral antibodies to the TSH receptor are present in Graves' disease and regulate selective signaling cascades. Endocrinology. 2010; 151(11):5537

[43] Epub 2010/09/17. [PubMed: 20844004] 62. Kawashima A, Tanigawa K, Akama T, Wu H, Sue M, Yoshihara A, et al. Fragments of genomic DNA released by injured cells activate innate immunity and suppress endocrine function in the thyroid. Endocrinology. 2011; 152(4):1702-12. Epub 2011/02/10. [PubMed: 21303947]

[44] Endo T, Kogai T, Nakazato M, Saito T, Kaneshige M, Onaya T. Autoantibody against Na+/Isymporter in the sera of patients with autoimmune thyroid disease. BiochemBiophys Res Commun. 1996; 224(1):92-95. [PubMed: 8694839]

[45] Yoshida A, Hisatome I, Taniguchi S, Shirayoshi Y, Yamamoto Y, Miake J, et al. Pendrin is a novel autoantigen recognized by patients with autoimmune thyroid diseases. J ClinEndocrinolMetab. 2009; 94(2):442-448. [PubMed: 19050049]

[46] Benvenga S, Trimarchi F, Robbins J. Circulating thyroid hormone autoantibodies. J Endocrinol Invest. 1987; 10(6):605-619. Epub 1987/12/01. [PubMed: 3326894]

[47] Tachi J, Amino N, Tamaki H, Aozasa M, Iwatani Y, Miyai K. Long term follow-up and HLA association in patients with postpartum hypothyroidism. J ClinEndocrinolMetab. 1988; 66(3): 480-484. Epub 1988/03/01. [PubMed: 3162458]

[48] Katakura M, Yamada T, Aizawa T, Hiramatsu K, Yukimura Y, Ishihara M, et al. Presence of antideoxyribonucleic acid antibody in patients with hyperthyroidism of Graves' disease. J ClinEndocrinolMetab. 1987; 64(3):405-408. Epub 1987/03/01. [PubMed: 3493254]

[49] Marino M, Chiovato L, Friedlander JA, Latrofa F, Pinchera A, McCluskey RT. Serum antibodies against megalin (GP330) in patients with autoimmune thyroiditis. J ClinEndocrinolMetab. 1999; 84(7):2468-2474. Epub 1999/07/15. [PubMed: 10404822]

Chapter 6

Thyroid Peroxidase (TPO) and Thyroid Stimulating Hormone Receptor (TSHR) Based Detection on Grave for Pregnant Women

Aulanni'am Aulanniam, Zulkarnain Zulkarnain, Djoko Wahono Soeatmadji, Dyah Kinasih Wuragil and Yudit Oktanella

Abstract

Graves' Disease is a form of specific autoimmune disorder in the thyroid organ characterized by thyroid-stimulating antibodies (TSAb). Pregnant women are the most susceptible to GD due to hormonal changes and tolerance of immune responses during pregnancy. The incidence of prematurity, low birth weight (LBW), and neonatal thyrotoxicosis risk are the most complications that can be acquired if treatment is late and inadequate. It has implications for increased fetomaternal morbidity and mortality. Apart from being a biomarker for definitive diagnosis, TSAb testing is also beneficial for assessing treatment response and predicting relapse of GD (relapse) after oral anti-thyroid treatment. GD patients with high TPOAb titers also tend to have a high relapse rate. However, the evaluation of both TSAb and TPOAb examinations during and after treatment is rarely done routinely due to the examination's high cost. This works proposed developing TSHR and TPO antigen-based rapid diagnostic tests through the immunochromatography method to address the challenges of financing and limited laboratory facilities in the area. Besides, understanding the importance of examining thyroid antibodies (TSAb and TPOAb) and interpretation in clinical practice is still a matter of debate in clinical circles, so it requires in-depth information.

Keywords: Graves' Disease, thyroid-stimulating antibodies, thyroid peroxidase, pregnant women

1. Introduction

Improved hygiene and technological advances in several developed and developing countries have implications for health improvements marked by a decrease in the population's infectious diseases. However, on the other hand, the tendency of autoimmune disease [1] and cancer [2] is increasingly being found with the availability of early detection screening tools. Genetic susceptibility, nutrition, and environmental factors are risk factors for the increasing prevalence and incidence of autoimmune diseases in the population [3, 4].

Autoimmune cases in specific thyroid organs are the second-highest after rheumatoid arthritis [1], with an incidence rate of about 2–5% affecting the world population [5]. Based on screening data from US and European populations, it was reported that autoimmune thyroid diseases such as Graves' Disease were more dominant in women than men with a ratio of 5: 1 [6, 7]. The cause of the predominant tendency of women to develop autoimmune disorders is still being debated. Several hypotheses are associated with the structure of the X chromosome and hormonal changes. Morphologically, the X chromosome is larger and contains more genes (800–900 genes) than Y chromosomes (50–60 genes). Most of the genes related to immune system response and regulators are present on the X chromosome so that women have a higher risk of developing autoimmune disorders than men who only have one X chromosome [8, 9].

2. Graves' Disease in pregnancy

Graves' Disease (GD) is a form of specific autoimmune disorder in the thyroid organ characterized by the formation of thyroid-stimulating antibodies (TSAb) and increased thyroid hormone secretion (hyperthyroidism) [10]. This disorder was first introduced by Robert James Graves in 1835, who has clinical features such as goiter, palpitations, and orbitopathy [11]. About 60–80% of hyperthyroid disorders in the population are due to GD [12], with an incidence of 1–2 cases occurring in 1000 pregnancies [13]. GD disorders can affect all age groups, both children [14], reproductive age [15], and the elderly [16], but the most incidence occurs in women aged 20–49 years [6, 17].

Pregnant women are the most susceptible to GD, which is thought to be due to decreased immune tolerance during pregnancy [18] and hormonal changes [19]. Approximately 0.4%-1.0% of women of reproductive age have GD before pregnancy, and 0.2% have it during pregnancy [13]. The American Thyroid Association (ATA) has issued recommendations for routine thyroid health screening in pregnant women, especially the first trimester of pregnancy and postpartum [20]. Besides, all women of reproductive age who are suffering from GD or have a previous history of GD are encouraged to seek counseling when planning pregnancy as an effort to improve fetomaternal health [19].

The high titer of maternal TSAb that can cross the placental barrier will manifest in impaired fetal thyroid function, increasing fetomaternal morbidity, and mortality [18, 21]. Preterm birth (prematurity) [22], low birth weight (LBW) [21, 22], and risk of neonatal thyrotoxicosis [23] are some of the frequently reported fetomaternal complications. Apart from TSAb testing, the ATA also recommends that pregnant women with a positive TPOAb be advised to evaluate serum TSH levels every four weeks during the second trimester [20].

3. TSHR and TPO as autoantigen

Genetically, polymorphisms in the thyroid-stimulating hormone receptor (TSHR) gene found on chromosome 14q31 [24–26] and the thyroid peroxidase gene on chromosome 2p25 (TPO) [27, 28] are closely related to susceptibility and severity of GD disease in various populations. Both thyroid-specific genes can act as autoantigens and are potential genetic biomarkers for GD [29, 30]. The term autoantigen indicates that a protein originates within the individual's own body, has a highly conserved structure, and is coded for genes with a low mutation rate. Thus, autoantigen is not an abnormal molecule but is coded only for genes that undergo polymorphisms in the population. Polymorphisms cause variations in protein structure and function so that they are sometimes recognized as foreign antigens that can interact with T lymphocytes and antibodies [31, 32].

Thyroid-stimulating hormone receptor (TSHR) is a protein molecule that plays a vital role in the growth and differentiation of the thyroid gland and is directly involved in signal transduction and regulation of thyroid hormone biosynthesis [33, 34]. TSHR protein is the primary autoantigen that triggers GD and is a target that is attacked by TSAb [35]. T lymphocyte immunotolerance's failure to the TSHR antigen triggers the infiltration of lymphocytes, dendritic cells, and macrophages into the thyroid follicle. Furthermore, lymphocyte infiltration triggers the secretion of several pro-inflammatory cytokines such as interleukin 1ß, IL-6, IL-12 interferon-ʏ, ligand CD40, and tumor necrosis factor-α. Presentation of TSHR peptides by dendritic cells on MHC-II molecules will activate B cells and differentiate plasma cells to synthesize and secrete TSAb into the circulation [10, 36]. TSAb protein, which mimics the action of TSH on the surface of the thyroid follicle cells, is the leading cause of thyroid hyperplasia and hyperfunctioning of T3 and T4 secretion becomes uncontrolled [37].

In the majority of people with GD, other autoantibodies can also be found, such as thyroid peroxidase antibody (TPOAb) [38, 39]. Thyroid peroxidase (TPO) is the main enzyme that assists in the biosynthesis of thyroid hormones. The TPO enzyme catalyzes the organization of iodine (iodination) and the coupling process of iodothyrosine residues in thyroglobulin [40]. In GD, the persistent lymphocyte infiltration of the thyroid follicular cells can also trigger a failure to tolerate the TPO autoantigen's immune response. About 80% of people with GD have positive TPOAb, which can activate the complement cascade, causing thyroid gland damage and dysfunction [38, 41]. Physiologically, the presence of TPOAb can also be found in normal populations around 10%-15% [42, 43], and in thyroid malignancies around 10%-20% [41].

Although both autoantibodies cross the placental barrier, only maternal TSAb titer can interfere with fetal and neonatal thyroid function. In contrast, the presence of TPOAb does not significantly affect neonatal thyroid function [20, 44]. However, monitoring of thyroid antibody titer and regular counseling is necessary during pregnancy due to complications of morbidity in the mother and infant [20, 45].

4. The role of TSAb and TPOAb in early-onset and relapse investigation

The early diagnosis of thyrotoxicosis is a challenge for clinicians because of the atypical clinical features and parallels the physiological changes in normal pregnancy [18]. Total T3, free T4, and TSH levels established during pregnancy also have different parameters or reference values from non-gravidas [46, 47]. The cause of thyrotoxicosis during pregnancy must be identified immediately, and must be able to differentiate between GD and other non-autoimmune hyperthyroidism such as gestational transient thyrotoxicosis (GTT) [13]. Although serum human chorionic gonadotropin (hCG) levels were higher in GTT patients compared to GD, this parameter is not typical in the early phase, so TSAb examination can be indicated to differentiate the cause of thyrotoxicosis [20].

The presence of TSAb in serum is a hallmark or the primary marker in the diagnosis of GD. More than 95% of the presence of TSAb can be found in serum with GD [31, 48]. The presence of TSAb can be detected in the early phase of GD before causing characteristic clinical symptoms (asymptomatic), and the titer will continue to increase if not handled adequately [44]. Apart from the diagnostic screening for GD, TSAb measurement is also useful for predicting cases of GD relapse after stopping treatment [37, 49]. The research of Kwon et al. (2016) found that only TSAb measurements could predict cases of GD relapse, while the thyrotropin-binding inhibitory immunoglobulin (TBII) examination was insensitive to relapsing GD cases [49]. Although the use of thionamide anti-thyroid drugs such as propylthiouracil (PTU) and methimazole (MMI) has an immunomodulatory effect of lowering TSAb titers [50], many reports of remission after treatment [51–54]. Carella et al. reported that TSAb titers remained positive in the majority of GD patients after 18 months of treatment with Methimazole (MMI) [51].

Increased TSAb titer also affects extrathyroid clinical manifestations, such as orbitopathy [55] and dermopathy (pretibial myxedema) [56], which can increase morbidity and decrease the quality of life for Graves sufferers. Bahn stated that TSAb titers have diagnostic value in euthyroid patients with exophthalmic [57].

In addition, TSAb measurement can also be used to determine treatment response (monitoring) and prognosis of Graves' Disease patients who have been treated with oral anti-thyroid [52, 58].

TSAb examination in pregnant women suffering from GD or post anti-thyroid treatment can predict the likelihood of neonatal thyrotoxicosis [59, 60]. Pregnant women who have high TSAb titers and persist until the third trimester require special monitoring of neonates and mothers because of their increased risk of thyrotoxicosis [37]. The results of research by Hamada et al. showed that patients with GD with a history of radioactive iodine therapy (I-131) had a higher TSAb titer during pregnancy and were at risk of delivering babies with thyrotoxicosis [61].

Positive TPO autoantibodies can also be found in GD abnormalities, even though a change in titer can predict recurrence of GD after anti-thyroid treatment [27]. TPOAb titers are less specific than TSAb in determining the diagnosis of GD. This is because, in certain levels, TPOAb titer can be found in the serum of normal individuals (euthyroid) and pregnant women without autoimmune thyroid disorders. The prevalence of both reaches 15% in the average population and 14% in pregnant women [42, 43]. This percentage affects the clinical specificity of TPOAb as a diagnostic indicator for the detection of AITD.

Interestingly, TPOAb titers were also found in people with GD, which suggests an association with the course of thyroiditis. Umar et al. found that 15–20% of Grave's patients had spontaneous hypothyroidism as a result of chronic thyroiditis (Hashimoto), and suspected that the widespread immune response in Grave's episode would trigger an increase in TPO and Tg autoantibodies, causing marked thyroiditis. With lymphocyte infiltration in thyrocytes cells [62].

5. Development of TSAb and TPOAb measurement methods

In recent decades, methods of measuring thyroid antibodies have continued to evolve, ranging from semiquantitative testing via agglutination and complement fixation tests [63, 64], to ligand-specific testing using recombinant antigens and cultured cells transfected with human TSHR [65, 66]. The hemagglutination method is rarely used and has many shortcomings in terms of specificity, sensitivity and depending on operator skills (subjective). Current examination methods have better precision because they directly measure autoantigen and autoantibody interactions with high sensitivity and specificity [67].

Currently, there are two methods that are often used to detect the presence of TSHR autoantibodies, namely (i) the TBII test (TSH Binding Inhibition Immunoglobulin), also known as the TRAb test, which is a test to assess the capacity of a patient's serum or IgG to inhibit TSH receptor binding with TSH labeled I125 or against recombinant TSHR protein expressed on CHO (Chinese Hamster Ovary) cells [37, 66]. (ii) A functional test (bioassay) to detect the presence of TSAb (stimulation) or TBAb (inhibition), using intact cells that are transfected with chimeric or human TSH receptors, which will then produce a biological response in the form of an increase in cAMP or bioreporter (luciferase) genes as markers. Biological activity against TSAb or TBAb activity in patient serum [68].

The TRAb method can detect TSHR autoantibodies that interact with the TSH receptor, regardless of their functional character (stimulation or inhibition). This method works based on competitive binding, i.e., the immunoglobulin in the patient's serum will compete with either porcine (porcine) or bovine TSH that is a radiolabeled or human monoclonal antibody (code M22) which binds to the TSH receptor (recombinant human TSHR) (**Figure 1**) [66, 67]. In its development, the third generation TRAb test uses a monoclonal antibody that binds to TSH (M22). In the research of Zöphel et al. proved that the sensitivity of using human TSHR monoclonal antibody M22 (90.3%, positive cutoff 0.32 IU / I) was better than that of bovine TSH (62.9%, positive cutoff 1.64 IU/I) [66]. The results of a meta-analysis study conducted by Tozzoli, et al. showed that the sensitivity and specificity of the third generation TRAb test (98.3% and 99.2%) were higher than the second generation (97.1% and 97.4%) [67].

The second method is bioassay (TSAb or TBAb), which uses intact cells transfected with chimeric or human TSH receptors, which will produce a biological response in the form of an increase in cAMP or a bioreporter gene (luciferase) as a biological marker of stimulating or inhibiting TSHR antibody activity in serum patient [68]. This method is a functional examination, which can technically be modified to detect the presence of TSAb or TBAb that are present together in a patient's serum. The development of a second-generation bioassay method using a mouse/human chimeric TSHR-LH receptor (MC4) can effectively eliminate the effect of TBAb. This approach demonstrates sufficient specificity and sensitivity for the diagnosis of GD and is clinically useful for monitoring the effect of anti-thyroid treatment (relapse and remission) [69].

One of the modalities of the bioassay method introduced recently and widely used in research is Thyretain, a method of measuring TSAb activity with a luciferase bioreporter using chimeric TSH-LH receptors (MC4) expressed on the surface of CHO (MC4-CHO-Luc) cells (**Figure 2**). In MC4, C-terminal TSHR

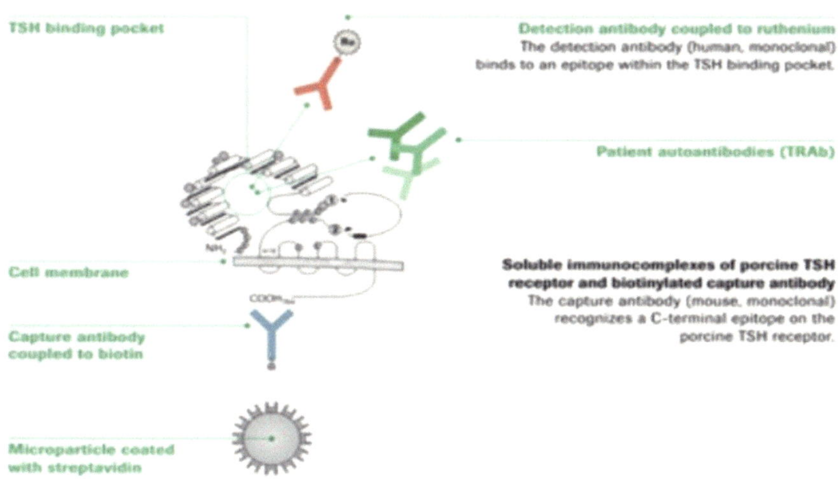

Figure 1.
Schematic illustration of TSHR autoantibodies detection with competitive binding of TSH receptor with radiolabelled or human monoclonal antibody (code: M22) [68].

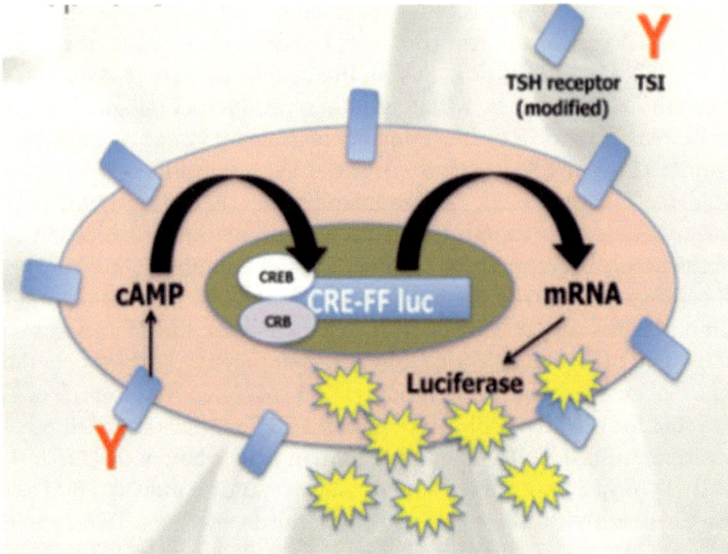

Figure 2.
Schematic illustration of measuring TSAb activity with a luciferase bioreporter chimeric TSH-LH receptor [69].

(amino acid 262–335) is substituted with amino acids 261–329 derived from the mouse LH-hCG (luteinizing hormone-choriogonadotropin) receptor. The substituted TSHR C-terminal area contains the epitope TBAb. The MC4 receptor was designed to reduce TBAb interactions when TSAb was measured, by eliminating the epitope area of TSHR using TBAb. When TSAb binds to the MC4 receptor on CHO-MC4 cells, it produces a cascade signal that stimulates increased intracellular cAMP production. Furthermore, cAMP induces activation of a promoter containing the luciferase gene CRE-luc (cAMP response element-luciferase). Luciferase activity is measured as a relative light unit, determined in cell-lysate through a luminometer [69–71].

Initially, TPO autoantibodies were detected as antibodies to thyroid microsome or AMA (anti microsomal antibody), using the semiquantitative method of erythrocyte hemagglutination and complement fixation [63]. The development of more specific detection methods is done by immunoassay or immunometric, using recombinant or purified TPO [72]. A recent study by D'Aurizio et al. evaluating and developing the diagnostic performance of third-generation immunometric methods, obtained increased sensitivity and specificity that are better than before [73].

Although many benefits can be obtained from regular TSAb and TPOAb titer checks in pregnant women who are suffering from GD or who have a history of GD before pregnancy. However, in reality, most clinicians have not routinely performed thyroid antibody tests, of course, with various considerations such as the high cost of examinations. Not all laboratory facilities can carry out TSAb examinations.

Author details

Aulanni'am Aulanniam[1*], Zulkarnain Zulkarnain[2], Djoko Wahono Soeatmadji[3], Dyah Kinasih Wuragil[4] and Yudit Oktanella[4]

1 Faculty of Life Science, University of Brawijaya, Indonesia

2 Faculty of Medicine, University of Syiah Kuala, Indonesia

3 Faculty of Medicine, University of Brawijaya, Indonesia

4 Faculty of Veterinary Medicine, University of Brawijaya, Indonesia

*Address all correspondence to: aulani@ub.ac.id

References

[1] A. Lerner, P. Jeremias, and T. Matthias, "The world incidence and prevalence of autoimmune diseases is increasing," *Int. J. Celiac Dis.*, vol. 3, no. 4, pp. 151-155, 2015, doi: 10.12691/ijcd-3-4-8.

[2] W. You and M. Henneberg, "Cancer incidence increasing globally: The role of relaxed natural selection," *Evol. Appl.*, vol. 11, no. 2, pp. 140-152, 2018, doi: 10.1111/eva.12523.

[3] K. Yamamoto and Y. Okada, "Shared genetic factors and their causality in autoimmune diseases," *Annals of the Rheumatic Diseases*, vol. 78, no. 11. pp. 1449-1451, 2019, doi: 10.1136/annrheumdis-2019-215099.

[4] M. F. Khan and H. Wang, "Environmental Exposures and Autoimmune Diseases: Contribution of Gut Microbiome," *Frontiers in Immunology*, vol. 10. 2020, doi: 10.3389/fimmu.2019.03094.

[5] A. McGrogan, H. E. Seaman, J. W. Wright, and C. S. De Vries, "The incidence of autoimmune thyroid disease: A systematic review of the literature," *Clin. Endocrinol. (Oxf).*, vol. 69, no. 5, pp. 687-696, 2008, doi: 10.1111/j.1365-2265.2008.03338.x.

[6] M. P. J. Vanderpump, "The epidemiology of thyroid disease," *Br. Med. Bull.*, vol. 99, no. 1, pp. 39-51, 2011, doi: 10.1093/bmb/ldr030.

[7] G. J. Kahaly, S. K. G. Grebe, M. A. Lupo, N. McDonald, and J. A. Sipos, "Graves' disease: Diagnostic and therapeutic challenges (multimedia activity)," *American Journal of Medicine*, vol. 124, no. 6. 2011, doi: 10.1016/j.amjmed.2011.03.001.

[8] F. Angum, T. Khan, J. Kaler, L. Siddiqui, and A. Hussain, "The Prevalence of Autoimmune Disorders in Women: A Narrative Review," *Cureus*, 2020, doi: 10.7759/cureus.8094.

[9] G. J. Yuen, "Autoimmunity in women: an eXamination of eXisting models," *Clinical Immunology*, vol. 210. 2020, doi: 10.1016/j.clim.2019.108270.

[10] T. J. Smith and L. Hegedus, "Graves' Disease," *N. Engl. J. Med.*, vol. 375, pp. 1552-1565, 2016, doi: 10.1056/NEJMra1510030.

[11] A. P. Weetman, "Graves' disease," *New England Journal of Medicine*, vol. 343, no. 17. pp. 1236-1248, 2000, doi: 10.1056/NEJM200010263431707.

[12] R. Bahn *et al.*, "Hyperthyroidism and other Causes of Thyrotoxicosis: Management Guidelines of the American Thyroid Association and American Association of Clinical Endocrinoloigists," *Endocr. Pract.*, vol. 17, no. 3, pp. 456-520, 2011, doi: 10.4158/ep.17.3.456.

[13] D. S. Cooper and P. Laurberg, "Hyperthyroidism in pregnancy," *The Lancet Diabetes and Endocrinology*, vol. 1, no. 3. pp. 238-249, 2013, doi: 10.1016/S2213-8587(13)70086-X.

[14] J. Léger, I. Oliver, D. Rodrigue, A. S. Lambert, and R. Coutant, "Graves' disease in children," *Ann. Endocrinol. (Paris).*, vol. 79, no. 6, pp. 647-655, 2018, doi: 10.1016/j.ando.2018.08.001.

[15] L. H. Zhang *et al.*, "Follow-up and evaluation of the pregnancy outcome in women of reproductive age with Graves' disease after 131 Iodine treatment," *J. Radiat. Res.*, vol. 57, no. 6, pp. 702-708, 2016, doi: 10.1093/jrr/rrw049.

[16] Y. Ueda *et al.*, "Graves' Disease in Pediatric and Elderly Patients with 22q11.2 Deletion Syndrome," *Intern. Med.*, vol. 56, no. 10, pp. 1169-1173, May 2017, doi: 10.2169/internalmedicine.56.7927.

[17] A. P. Weetman, "Thyroid disease," in *The Autoimmune Diseases*, 2019, pp. 749-767.

[18] H. V. Wright and D. J. Williams, "Thyrotoxicosis in pregnancy," *Fetal Matern. Med. Rev.*, vol. 24, no. 2, pp. 108-128, 2013, doi: 10.1017/S0965539513000077.

[19] C. T. Nguyen, E. B. Sasso, L. Barton, and J. H. Mestman, "Graves' hyperthyroidism in pregnancy: a clinical review," *Clin. Diabetes Endocrinol.*, vol. 4, no. 1, 2018, doi: 10.1186/s40842-018-0054-7.

[20] E. K. Alexander *et al.*, "2017 Guidelines of the American Thyroid Association for the Diagnosis and Management of Thyroid Disease during Pregnancy and the Postpartum," *Thyroid*, vol. 27, no. 3, pp. 315-389, 2017, doi: 10.1089/thy.2016.0457.

[21] S. Luewan, P. Chakkabut, and T. Tongsong, "Outcomes of pregnancy complicated with hyperthyroidism: A cohort study," *Arch. Gynecol. Obstet.*, vol. 283, no. 2, pp. 243-247, 2011, doi: 10.1007/s00404-010-1362-z.

[22] F. Saki, M. H. Dabbaghmanesh, S. Z. Ghaemi, S. Forouhari, G. R. Omrani, and M. Bakhshayeshkaram, "Thyroid function in pregnancy and its influences on maternal and fetal outcomes," *Int. J. Endocrinol. Metab.*, vol. 12, no. 4, p. e19378, 2014, doi: 10.5812/ijem.19378.

[23] C. Batra, "Fetal and neonatal thyrotoxicosis," *Indian J. Endocrinol. Metab.*, vol. 17, no. 7, p. 50, 2013, doi: 10.4103/2230-8210.119505.

[24] W. Qian *et al.*, "Association between TSHR gene polymorphism and the risk of Graves' disease: A meta-analysis," *J. Biomed. Res.*, vol. 30, no. 6, pp. 466-475, 2016, doi: 10.7555/JBR.30.20140144.

[25] H. Xiong *et al.*, "Genetic associations of the thyroid stimulating hormone receptor gene with Graves diseases and Graves ophthalmopathy: A meta-analysis," *Sci. Rep.*, vol. 6, 2016, doi: 10.1038/srep30356.

[26] L. Liu *et al.*, "Association between thyroid stimulating hormone receptor gene intron polymorphisms and autoimmune thyroid disease in a Chinese Han population," *Endocr. J.*, vol. 59, no. 8, 2012, doi: 10.1507/endocrj.EJ12-0024.

[27] Y. M. Choi, M. K. Kwak, S. M. Hong, and E. G. Hong, "Changes in thyroid peroxidase and thyroglobulin antibodies might be associated with Graves' disease relapse after anti-thyroid drug therapy," *Endocrinol. Metab.*, vol. 34, no. 3, 2019, doi: 10.3803/EnM.2019.34.3.268.

[28] A. Kuš *et al.*, "The association of thyroid peroxidase antibody risk loci with susceptibility to and phenotype of Graves' disease," *Clin. Endocrinol. (Oxf).*, vol. 83, no. 4, 2015, doi: 10.1111/cen.12640.

[29] R. Ploski, K. Szymanski, and T. Bednarczuk, "The Genetic Basis of Graves Disease," *Curr. Genomics*, vol. 12, no. 8, 2011, doi: 10.2174/138920211798120772.

[30] F. Ceccarelli, N. Agmon-Levin, and C. Perricone, "Genetic Factors of Autoimmune Diseases 2017," *Journal of Immunology Research*, vol. 2017. 2017, doi: 10.1155/2017/2789242.

[31] C. M. Girgis, B. L. Champion, and J. R. Wall, "Current concepts in Graves' disease," *Ther. Adv. Endocrinol. Metab.*, vol. 2, no. 3, pp. 135-144, 2011, doi: 10.1177/2042018811408488.

[32] W. M. Wiersinga, "Thyroid Autoimmunity," in *Paediatric Thyroidology*, 2012, pp. 139-157.

[33] G. Kleinau, S. Neumann, A. Grüters, H. Krude, and H. Biebermann, "Novel insights on thyroid-stimulating

hormone receptor signal transduction," *Endocr. Rev.*, vol. 34, no. 5, pp. 691-724, 2013, doi: 10.1210/er.2012-1072.

[34] G. Vassart and J. E. Dumont, "The thyrotropin receptor and the regulation of thyrocyte function and growth," *Endocr. Rev.*, vol. 13, no. 3, 1992, doi: 10.1210/edrv-13-3-596.

[35] B. Rees Smith, S. M. McLachlan, J. Ginsberg, C. Rickards, and R. Hall, "The Thyrotropin Receptor in Graves' Disease," in *Hormones in normal and abnormal human tissues Volume 2*, 2019, pp. 519-540.

[36] B. Kristensen, "Regulatory B and T cell responses in patients with autoimmune thyroid disease and healthy controls," *Dan. Med. J.*, vol. 63, no. 2, p. B5177, 2016.

[37] C. Kamath, M. A. Adlan, and L. D. Premawardhana, "The role of thyrotrophin receptor antibody assays in Graves' disease," *J. Thyroid Res.*, vol. 2012, p. 525936, 2012, doi: 10.1155/2012/525936.

[38] F. Wahab, E. Kearney, and S. Joseph, "The presence of thyroid peroxidase antibodies in Graves' disease is predictive of disease duration and relapse rates," *Endocr. Abstr.*, 2013, doi: 10.1530/endoabs.31.p367.

[39] I. Guilhem, C. Massart, J. Y. Poirier, and D. Maugendre, "Differential evolution of thyroid peroxidase and thyrotropin receptor antibodies in Graves' disease: Thyroid peroxidase antibody activity reverts to pretreatment level after carbimazole withdrawal," *Thyroid*, vol. 16, no. 10, 2006, doi: 10.1089/thy.2006.16.1041.

[40] A. Taurog, M. L. Dorris, and D. R. Doerge, "Mechanism of simultaneous iodination and coupling catalyzed by thyroid peroxidase," *Arch. Biochem. Biophys.*, vol. 330, no. 1, 1996, doi: 10.1006/abbi.1996.0222.

[41] S. Pradhan and K. Gautam, "Miscarriage and Anti TPO antibodies," *J. Pathol. Nepal*, vol. 8, no. 2, 2018, doi: 10.3126/jpn.v8i2.20894.

[42] A. Amouzegar, S. Gharibzadeh, E. Kazemian, L. Mehran, M. Tohidi, and F. Azizi, "The prevalence, incidence and natural course of positive antithyroperoxidase antibodies in a population-based study: Tehran thyroid study," *PLoS One*, vol. 12, no. 1, 2017, doi: 10.1371/journal.pone.0169283.

[43] J. G. Hollowell *et al.*, "Serum TSH, T4, and thyroid antibodies in the United States population (1988 to 1994): National Health and Nutrition Examination Survey (NHANES III)," *J. Clin. Endocrinol. Metab.*, vol. 87, no. 2, pp. 489-499, 2002, doi: 10.1210/jcem.87.2.8182.

[44] I. Bucci, C. Giuliani, and G. Napolitano, "Thyroid-stimulating hormone receptor antibodies in pregnancy: Clinical relevance," *Front. Endocrinol. (Lausanne).*, vol. 8, no. JUN, pp. 1-11, 2017, doi: 10.3389/fendo.2017.00137.

[45] G. J. Kahaly, L. Bartalena, L. Hegedüs, L. Leenhardt, K. Poppe, and S. H. Pearce, "2018 European thyroid association guideline for the management of graves' hyperthyroidism," *Eur. Thyroid J.*, vol. 7, no. 4, pp. 167-186, 2018, doi: 10.1159/000490384.

[46] C. Sriphrapradang, S. Pavarangkoon, W. Jongjaroenprasert, L. O. Chailurkit, B. Ongphiphadhanakul, and W. Aekplakorn, "Reference ranges of serum TSH, FT4 and thyroid autoantibodies in the Thai population: The national health examination survey," *Clin. Endocrinol. (Oxf).*, vol.

80, no. 5, pp. 751-756, 2014, doi: 10.1111/cen.12371.

[47] K. Lewandowski, "Reference ranges for TSH and thyroid hormones," *Thyroid Res.*, vol. 8, no. Suppl 1, p. A17, 2015, doi: 10.1186/1756-6614-8-s1-a17.

[48] L. Bell, A. L. Hunter, A. Kyriacou, A. Mukherjee, and A. A. Syed, "Clinical diagnosis of Graves' or non-Graves' hyperthyroidism compared to TSH receptor antibody test," *Endocr. Connect.*, vol. 7, no. 4, pp. 504-510, 2018, doi: 10.1530/ec-18-0082.

[49] H. Kwon *et al.*, "Usefulness of Measuring Thyroid Stimulating Antibody at the Time of Antithyroid Drug Withdrawal for Predicting Relapse of Graves Disease," *Endocrinol. Metab.*, vol. 31, no. 2, p. 300, 2016, doi: 10.3803/enm.2016.31.2.300.

[50] R. Volpe, "The Immunomodulatory Effects of Anti-thyroid Drugs are Mediated via Actions on Thyroid Cells, Affecting Thyrocyte-immunocyte Signalling A Review," *Curr. Pharm. Des.*, vol. 7, no. 6, pp. 451-460, 2005, doi: 10.2174/1381612013397898.

[51] C. Carella *et al.*, "Serum thyrotropin receptor antibodies concentrations in patients with Graves' disease before, at the end of methimazole treatment, and after drug withdrawal: Evidence that the activity of thyrotropin receptor antibody and/or thyroid response modify during," *Thyroid*, vol. 16, no. 3, pp. 295-302, 2006, doi: 10.1089/thy.2006.16.295.

[52] P. Laurberg, "Remission of Graves' disease during anti-thyroid drug therapy. Time to reconsider the mechanism?," *European Journal of Endocrinology*. 2006, doi: 10.1530/eje.1.02295.

[53] P. Laurberg, G. Wallin, L. Tallstedt, M. Abraham-Nordling, G. Lundell, and O. Törring, "TSH-receptor autoimmunity in Graves' disease after therapy with anti-thyroid drugs, surgery, or radioiodine: A 5-year prospective randomized study," *Eur. J. Endocrinol.*, vol. 158, no. 1, pp. 69-75, 2008, doi: 10.1530/EJE-07-0450.

[54] N. B. Tütüncü, T. Tütüncü, A. Özgen, and T. Erbas, "Long-term outcome of Graves' disease patients treated in a region with iodine deficiency: Relapse rate increases in years with thionamides," *J. Natl. Med. Assoc.*, vol. 98, no. 6, pp. 926-930, 2006.

[55] E. Fröhlich and R. Wahl, "Thyroid autoimmunity: Role of anti-thyroid antibodies in thyroid and extra-thyroidal diseases," *Front. Immunol.*, vol. 8, no. MAY, pp. 521(1-16), 2017, doi: 10.3389/fimmu.2017.00521.

[56] V. Fatourechi, D. D. F. Ahmed, and K. M. Schwartz, "Thyroid acropachy: Report of 40 patients treated at a single institution in a 26-year period," *J. Clin. Endocrinol. Metab.*, vol. 87, no. 12, pp. 5435-5441, 2002, doi: 10.1210/jc.2002-020746.

[57] R. S. Bahn, "Graves' ophthalmopathy," *New England Journal of Medicine*, vol. 362, no. 8. 2010, doi: 10.1056/NEJMra0905750.

[58] V. Michelangeli, C. Poon, J. Taft, H. Newnham, D. Topliss, and P. Colman, "The prognostic value of thyrotropin receptor antibody measurement in the early stages of treatment of Graves' disease with anti-thyroid drugs," *Thyroid*, vol. 8, no. 2, pp. 119-124, 1998, doi: 10.1089/thy.1998.8.119.

[59] T. Männistö, P. Mendola, U. Reddy, and S. K. Laughon, "Neonatal outcomes and birth weight in pregnancies complicated by maternal thyroid disease," *Am. J. Epidemiol.*, vol. 178, no. 5, pp. 731-740, 2013, doi: 10.1093/aje/kwt031.

[60] S. L. Samuels, S. M. Namoc, and A. J. Bauer, "Neonatal Thyrotoxicosis," *Clinics in Perinatology*, vol. 45, no. 1. pp. 31-40, 2018, doi: 10.1016/j.clp.2017.10.001.

[61] N. Hamada *et al.*, "Persistent high TRAb values during pregnancy predict increased risk of neonatal hyperthyroidism following radioiodine therapy for refractory hyperthyroidism," *Endocrine Journal*, vol. 58, no. 1. pp. 55-58, 2011, doi: 10.1507/endocrj.K10E-123.

[62] H. Umar, N. Muallima, J. M. F. Adam, and H. Sanusi, "Hashimoto's thyroiditis following Graves' disease.," *Acta Med. Indones.*, vol. 42, no. 1, pp. 31-35, 2010.

[63] C. W. Schardt, S. M. McLachlan, J. Matheson, and B. R. Smith, "An enzyme-linked immunoassay for thyroid microsomal antibodies," *J. Immunol. Methods*, vol. 55, no. 2, pp. 155-168, 1982, doi: 10.1016/0022-1759(82)90028-X.

[64] A. E. Ohwovoriole, T. J. Wilkin, L. Scott-Morgan, P. Johnston, and W. Mould, "Improved elisa for thyroid microsomal auto-antibodies: Comparison with haemagglutination and immunofluorescent techniques," *Int. Arch. Allergy Immunol.*, vol. 86, no. 2, pp. 183-189, 1988, doi: 10.1159/000234569.

[65] C. Massart, R. Sapin, J. Gibassier, A. Agin, and M. D'Herbomez, "Intermethod variability in TSH-receptor antibody measurement: Implication for the diagnosis of graves disease and for the follow-up of graves ophthalmopathy," *Clin. Chem.*, vol. 55, no. 1, pp. 183-186, 2009, doi: 10.1373/clinchem.2008.115162.

[66] K. Zöphel *et al.*, "TSH receptor antibody (TRAb) assays based on the human monoclonal autoantibody M22 are more sensitive than bovine TSH based assays," *Horm. Metab. Res.*, vol. 42, no. 1, pp. 65-69, 2010, doi: 10.1055/s-0029-1241196.

[67] R. Tozzoli, M. Bagnasco, D. Giavarina, and N. Bizzaro, "TSH receptor autoantibody immunoassay in patients with Graves' disease: Improvement of diagnostic accuracy over different generations of methods. Systematic review and meta-analysis," *Autoimmun. Rev.*, vol. 12, no. 2, pp. 107-113, 2012, doi: 10.1016/j.autrev.2012.07.003.

[68] J. I. Lee *et al.*, "Diagnostic value of a chimeric TSH receptor (Mc4)-based bioassay for graves' disease," *Korean J. Intern. Med.*, vol. 26, no. 2, pp. 179-186, 2011, doi: 10.3904/kjim.2011.26.2.179.

[69] C. Giuliani *et al.*, "A TSHR-LH/CGR chimera that measures functional thyroid-stimulating autoantibodies (TSAb) can predict remission or recurrence in Graves' patients undergoing anti-thyroid drug (ATD) treatment," *J. Clin. Endocrinol. Metab.*, vol. 97, no. 7, 2012, doi: 10.1210/jc.2011-2897.

[70] S. D. Lytton, Y. Li, P. D. Olivo, L. D. Kohn, and G. J. Kahaly, "Novel chimeric thyroid-stimulating hormone-receptor bioassay for thyroid-stimulating immunoglobulin," *Clin. Exp. Immunol.*, vol. 162, no. 3, pp. 438-446, 2010, doi: 10.1111/j.1365-2249.2010.04266.x.

[71] K. Kamijo, H. Murayama, T. Uzu, K. Togashi, and G. J. Kahaly, "A novel bioreporter assay for thyrotropin receptor antibodies using a chimeric thyrotropin receptor (Mc4) is more useful in differentiation of graves' disease from painless thyroiditis than conventional thyrotropin-stimulating antibody assay using porcine," *Thyroid*, vol. 20, no. 8, pp. 851-856, 2010, doi: 10.1089/thy.2010.0059.

[72] S. L. La'ulu, P. R. Slev, and W. L. Roberts, "Performance characteristics of

5 automated thyroglobulin autoantibody and thyroid peroxidase autoantibody assays," *Clin. Chim. Acta*, vol. 376, no. 1-2, pp. 88-95, 2007, doi: 10.1016/j.cca.2006.07.018.

[73] F. D'Aurizio, R. Tozzoli, D. Villalta, G. Pesce, and M. Bagnasco, "Immunoassay of thyroid peroxidase autoantibodies: Diagnostic performance in automated third generation methods. A multicentre evaluation," *Clin. Chem. Lab. Med.*, vol. 53, no. 3, pp. 415-421, 2015, doi: 10.1515/cclm-2014-0545.

Chapter 7

Deiodinase Enzymes and Their Activities in Graves' Hyperthyroidism

Ildikó Molnár

Abstract

The origin of hyperthyroidism in Graves' Disease was displayed demonstrating the complexity of the processes. The role of stimulating TSH receptor antibodies is the one factor for the production of increased thyroidal T_3 and T_4. The T_3 and T_4 formation in colloid-embedded thyroglobulin and the activities of thyroidal deiodinases [type 1 (DIO1) and type 2 (DIO2)] play a crucial role in that. The findings of different authors were summarized with respect to highlighting the role of tissue-specific deiodinase activities. Apart from the results of experimental studies, the clinical results were brought to the front. The role of tissue-specific type 2 deiodinase activity was demonstrated according to thyroid function, the presence of autoantibodies against thyroid peroxidase (TPO), thyroglobulin (Tg) and TSH receptor. Autoantibodies against human eye muscle membrane and cytosol antigens had influencing effects on tissue-specific DIO2 activities, and the antieye muscle antibody immunoglobulin isotypes were associated with eye muscle enlargements. Antithyroid drug (ATD) therapy demonstrated relevant effects on tissue-specific DIO2 activities, which were manifested in the alterations of thyroid hormone levels. An asymptomatically appearance of autoantibodies against peptides corresponding to amino acid sequence of DIO2 was detected associating with thyroid hormone and anti-TPO, anti-Tg and TSH receptor antibody levels during the therapy.

Keywords: hyperthyroidism, Graves' Disease, type 1 and type 2 deiodinases, ophthalmopathy, autoantibodies

1. Introduction

Graves' hyperthyroidism is characterized by increased thyroid hormone levels (T_4 and T_3) with the supprimation of TSH levels, diffuse enlargement of thyroid glands and associated symptoms with orbitopathy or/and dermopathy [1, 2]. The course of disease is characterized by duality. The main autoimmune processes are manifested in thyrotoxicosis with a lymphocytic infiltration and diffuse thyroid enlargement, which can be associated with orbitopathy in 15–25% and pretibial myxedema in 0.5–4.5% [3]. The autoimmune processes are associated with the development of autoantibodies against different antigens, such as thyroid antigens [TSH receptor, thyroid peroxidase (TPO) enzyme and thyroglobulin (Tg)] and IGF-1 receptor, as well as against extraocular muscle membrane and cytosol antigens, and intracellular particles (flavoprotein subunit of mitochondrial succinate dehydrogenase, sarcalumenin, calsequestrin, collagen XII)] in thyroid-associated

IntechOpen

ophthalmopathy [4–7]. The increased production of proinflammatory cytokines (IL-1, IL-6, TNFα), chemokines and costimulatory ligands on fibroblasts and adipocytes lead to inflammatory and infiltrating processes, and glycosaminoglycan (GAG) accumulation resulting in local tissue enlargements [8, 9]. In orbitopathy, the local infiltrating processes are responsible for the proptosis and sometimes the damage of nervi optici that can reach vision loss in the final stage. TSH receptor stimulating antibodies are kept to be the causative factors for hyperthyroidism. Autoantibodies against IGF-1 nearby receptor are involved in the edematous-infiltrative processes [10]. Antibodies against thyroid peroxidase (TPO) and thyroglobulin (Tg) are the relevant thyroid autoantibodies in Graves' Disease [11]. The binding of IgG and IgA autoantibodies to human extraocular muscle was different: IgG types bound endomysially, while IgA types bound to muscle fibers [12].

Deiodinase enzymes, DIO1, DIO2 and DIO3 are responsible for the conversion of T_4 to active T_3 hormone, the maintenance of the local T_3 levels and the inactivation of T_4 and T_3 hormones [13, 14]. Deiodinase enzymes show tissue-specific expression, which limits their functions. Many drugs, iodine and selenium supply, proinflammatory cytokines and autoantibodies can influence DIO activities [15, 16]. The increased T_4 levels are connected to the acceleration of the physiological degradation of DIO2 enzyme [17]. The common localization of DIO2 enzyme between thyroid and eye muscle tissues suggests that its autoantigenic role can be important in Graves' ophthalmopathy [18, 19]. 5′-deiodinase enzymes (DIO1 and DIO2) play a crucial role in thyroid hormone synthesis. TPO enzyme plays a role in the iodination of tyrosyl residues and their coupling to T_3 and T_4 in the colloid-embedded Tg with the interaction of hydrogen peroxide (H_2O_2) at the apical plasma membrane of thyrocytes [20]. The schematically illustrated process of thyroid hormone synthesis is exhibited in **Figure 1** highlighting the role of DIO1 and DIO2 activities.

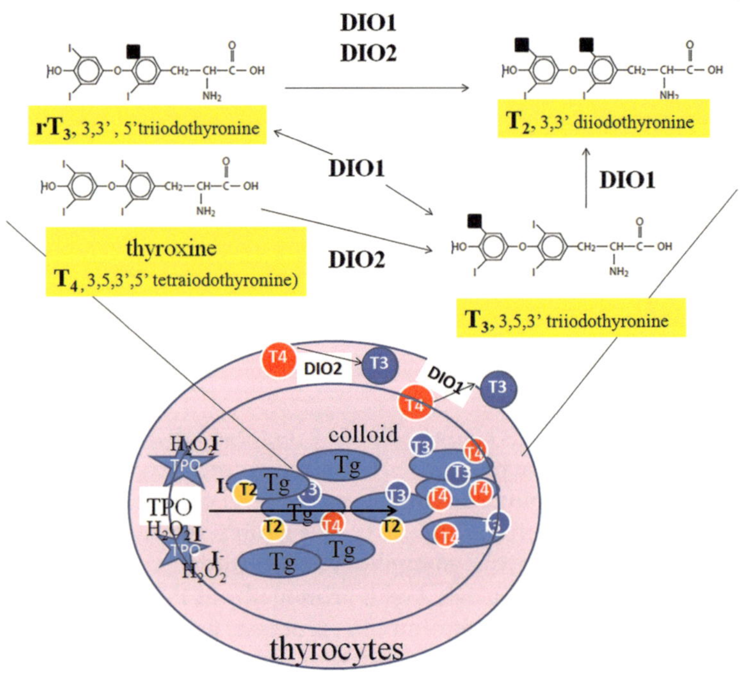

Figure 1.
Schematic illustration of thyroid hormone synthesis and thyroidal deiodinase activities (DIO1 and DIO2). DIO1: Type 1 deiodinase; DIO2: Type 2 deiodinase; Tg: Thyroglobulin; TPO: Thyroid peroxidase; T2, T3 and T4: Iodothyronines with 2, 3 and 4 iodides.

This review emphasizes the role of deiodinases in the hyperthyroidism of Graves' Disease with respect to the thyroid functional stages and the relationship with antithyroid autoantibodies and autoantibodies against extraocular muscle and peptides corresponding to amino acid sequence of DIO2, as well as with the antithyroid drug (ATD) therapies.

2. Three types of deiodinase enzymes are involved in thyroid hormone activation and inactivation

Three types of deiodinase enzymes (DIO1, DIO2, DIO3) are responsible for the activation and inactivation of thyroxine (T_4) and triiodothyronine (T_3) thyroid hormones [21]. Deiodinase enzymes demonstrate tissue-specific localization. DIO1 enzyme is expressed in the liver, kidney and thyroid parenchymal cells localized in the plasma membrane [22]. Its active center is found in the cytosol. T_4 plays as a prohormone for the active T_3 hormone. T_4 has four iodine bindings at the 3,3′, 5 and 5′ positions. DIO1 enzyme is able to cleave iodine from 5 (inner ring deiodination, step of T_4 inactivation) or 5′ position (outer ring deiodination, step of active T_3 hormone production). The dual effect of DIO1 enzyme plays a crucial role in the excessive thyroid hormone production, called hyperthyroidism. DIO2 enzyme is a widespread 5′-deiodinase expressed in thyroid, skeletal muscle and adipose tissues, hypothalamus, pituitary, skin, osteoblast, astroglia, retina, cochlea, placenta and endothelial cells localized in the endoplasmic reticulum [23]. Its active center is found in the cytosol. DIO1 expression can be induced transcriptionally by T_3 and TSH receptor stimulating antibodies. Fasting and chronic illnesses decrease DIO1 activity. The inhibitory effect on thyroidal DIO1 and DIO2 activities was demonstrated *in vitro* in the presence of proinflammatory cytokines (IL-1, IL-6 and TNFα) [24]. The inhibitory rate was higher on DIO2 than on DIO1 activities. The inhibitory degree was dose-dependent. Thyroidal DIO1 activity is responsible for only 6% of the daily T_3 production [25]. Propylthiouracil (PTU) inhibits its activity. DIO2 plays a crucial role in the maintenance of intracellular T_3 levels via 5′-deiodination, converting T_4 to T_3. Its increased activity is partly present in hyperthyroidism; however, its activity is decreased in nonthyroidal illness [26]. DIO2 is a posttranslationally T_4-dependent enzyme, which accelerates its proteasomal degradation. DIO2 enzyme is involved in the feedback mechanism of hypothalamic–pituitary-thyroid axis [27]. The normal development and regeneration of skeletal muscle requires DIO2 activity [28].

DIO3 is an enzyme located in the plasma membrane. It has both extra- and intracellular activity [29]. DIO3 plays a crucial role in fetal development and tissue-repair. It is expressed in placenta, uterus, neurons, skin, alveolar cells, glial cells, urothelium, gastrointestinal tract, hypothalamus and skeletal muscle [30]. DIO3 inactivates T_3 through inner ring 5-deiodination. Its increased activity is responsible for the consumptive hypothyroidism observated in hepatic hemangiomas [31]. Nether DIO2 nor DIO3 are PTU sensitive enzymes. Hypothyroidism is connected to an increase in DIO1 and DIO2 activities, but DIO3 activities are decreased [22]. Hyperthyroidism is connected to an increase in both thyroidal DIO1 and DIO2, but to a decrease in extrathyroidal DIO2 activities. Iopodic acid, the contrast material with high iodine content decreases the activities of all deiodinase enzymes. The alterations in T_4 and T_3 levels according to thyroid function have a different effect on the deiodinase enzyme activities in the living cells vs. sonicated cells [23]. No protein synthesis can happen in sonicated cells. Therefore, the sonicated cell content could be regarded as a deiodinase enzyme solution.

3. The role of DIO1 and DIO2 deiodinase enzymes in thyroid hormone production of Graves' hyperthyroidims

Hyperthyroidism is characterized by increased serum FT_4 and FT_3 levels, which can be associated with Graves' Disease, toxic goiter, destruction-induced thyrotoxicosis and subacute thyroiditis. Thyroid follicular cells possess both DIO1 and DIO2 enzymes, but not DIO3 enzyme. The amount of produced FT_4 and FT_3, and the ratio of FT_3 to FT_4 can help with the diagnosis [32]. Serum FT_3 levels are predominant and are better formed than FT_4 in hyperthyroidism connected to Graves' Disease or toxic goiter [33]. In Graves' hyperthyroidism, the increase in the daily production of T_3 and T_4 was 7-fold and 3.5-fold, respectively. Laurberg and coworkers demonstrated that the major source of excess T_3 derived from increased thyroidal DIO1 and DIO2 activities (in a ratio of 3 to 1). This is in contrast to what is found in euthyroidism, where 20% of T_3 came from thyroidal production and 80% from extrathyroidal deiodination [25]. In hyperthyroidism, a large part of T_3 levels was produced by the thyroid (in 57–77%) by way of converting T_4 to T_3 with decreased peripheral deiodination. The extrathyroidal DIO2 activities were decreased in hyperthyroidism with the exception of the thyroidal one due to the increased thyroidal formation of T_4 and T_3. Maia and coworkers supported that thyroidal DIO1 activity is responsible for 67% of T_3 production in hyperthyroidism [22]. In HEK 293 cells, which transiently expressed DIO1 and DIO2 enzymes, the effect of 2–20-200 pM T_4 was studied on these cells modeling hypo-, eu- and hyperthyroid states. DIO1 activity was continuous, but DIO2 activity was decreased by the concentration of 200 pM T_4. Salvatore and coworkers emphasized the greater role of DIO2 enzyme in the excess T_3 in Graves' hyperthyroidism [34]. Ito and coworkers suggested that thyroidal DIO1 and specifically, DIO2 could be contributed to the higher ratio of FT_3 to FT_4 in Graves' hyperthyroidism [35]. The lower ratio of T_3 to T_4 can help us with the diagnosis of destruction-induced thyrotoxicosis and subacute thyroiditis [36]. Values less than of 20 confirm the above mentioned diseases, while the values above 20 are connected to Graves' hyperthyroidism. Weetman and coworkers made the DIO1 and DIO2 activities responsible for the syndrome of low T_4 with increased T_3 levels during PTU treatment [37]. Thyroidal DIO1 activity is mainly regulated by cAMP at pretranslational levels, similarly to TSH receptor stimulating antibody-induced cAMP. Thyroglobulin and iodine contents of thyroid can influence the generation of T_4 and T_3 through the rate of hydrolysis from the colloid-embedded thyroglobulin. This condition can contribute to the alterations in the production of thyroid hormones. Very few reports could be found, which explained in detail the thyroid hormone production connecting to the formation of the coupling mechanism alone or together with deiodinase conversion. Iodide alone inhibited both thyroidal deiodinase activities rapidly decreasing the circulating T_3 by 50% and T_4 by 70% [33]. Ipodate is also a potent inhibitor for DIO1 and DIO2 enzymes due to its iodine content of 64%. Ipodate with PTU resulted in a profound decrease in serum T_3. In untreated Graves' hyperthyroidism, the T_3 content of Tg was 2-fold of what was found in euthyroidism [38]. In hyperthyroidism, local DIO2 activity is required for the intrapituitary production of T_3, which is responsible for the acute decrease in TSH levels [39].

4. *In vitro* model for the measurement of tissue-specific DIO2 activities

In our study, homogenized (supernatant of 100 000 x g separated by centrifugations) thyroidal, skeletal and eye muscle tissue fractions, called cytosol fractions were applied for the measurements of deiodinase enzyme activities [40]. Thyroid tissues were obtained from the removal of euthyroid goiter; the removal of skeletal muscle during accident surgery and the removal of extraocular muscle during strabismus surgery. All tissue fractions contained DIO2 enzyme, the activity of which was measured in the presence of patient sera with Graves' Disease with respect to the different thyroid hormonal stages. The DIO2 content of cytosol fractions was proofed before the study using guinea pig sera immunized with TCSS and LVFR peptides. Both peptides were corresponding to amino acid sequences of human DIO2 (GenBank AAD45494–1) and contained the selenocysteine at position 133 in the active center of the enzyme: *LVVNFGSATCPPFTSQLPAFRKLVEEFSS.* TCSS peptide (aa 132–152): T**CC**PP**TF**SQLPAFRKLVEEFSS was synthesized with double cysteins replaced at position 133, as well as amino acids reserved at positions 136 and 137. LVFR peptide (aa 124–144): LVVNFGSAT**C**PPFTSQLPAFR was 100% identical to the original amino acid sequence. The bindings of immunized sera to cytosol fractions and to tissue sections were investigated with enzyme-linked immunosorbent assay (ELISA) and immunohistochemistry, respectively. Immunized sera against TCSS peptide resulted in more intensive positive bindings to the cytosol fractions and gave positive reactions to tissue sections.

The patient sera of hyper-, eu- and hypothyroid Graves' Disease were added to thyroidal, skeletal and eye muscle cytosol fractions, which contained DIO2 enzyme activities. The study could be considered as an *in vitro* model, in which the patient sera included the actual hormonal and autoantibody parameters. The effects of these parameters were measured on DIO2 activities. The results, after evaluating them with respect to the parameters, may contribute to gaining useful data for the course and treatment of disease. Thyroidal DIO1 activities were inhibited by 2 μM PTU. The sample mixture contained 12.5 μg protein per cytosol fraction. Radioiodine labeled T_4 (^{125}I-T_4) 1 kB/50 μl was the substrate in reducing condition [20 mM dithiothreitol (DDT)]. The results were extrapolated at 1 pmol/T_4 of patient serum. DIO2 enzyme activity was expressed as pmol of T_4 converted per mg/min of protein. The whole protocol is described in detail in our previous paper [41].

5. Recent research with tissue-specific DIO2 activities in Graves' hyperthyroidims

5.1 Measurement and evaluation of DIO2 enzyme activities: DIO2 enzyme activities were measured after adding patient sera with Graves' ophthalmopathy to thyroidal, skeletal and eye muscle cytosol fractions, all containing DIO2 enzymes. The results were then evaluated according to thyroid functional stages

Fifty-two patients with Graves' Disease, of whom 37 had ophthalmopathy, were investigated [42]. The difference in the disease duration, the ratio of FT_3 to FT_4 and the serum levels of TSH receptor antibodies was significant between the Graves' patients with and without ophthalmopathy. The difference in DIO2 activities was relevant and constant among thyroidal, skeletal and eye muscle cytosol fractions in hyper-, eu- and hypothyroidism in Graves' ophthalmopathy. The effect of increased serum FT_4 levels was 1.9 times greater on eye muscle DIO2 than thyroidal DIO2 activity. The findings demonstrated that, the tissue-specific DIO2 activities also play a crucial role in the T_3 content of peripheral tissues in hyperthyroidism. The skeletal muscle and thyroidal DIO2 activities were lower by 27% and 47%, respectively in hyperthyroidism, as well as were lower by 27% and 87%, respectively in hypothyroidism compared to eye muscle DIO2 activity. DIO2 activities of all cytosol fractions were 6.3 times lower in hyperthyroidism and 3.5 times greater in hypothyroidism compared to those in euthyroidism (**Figure 2**). In hyperthyroidism, the thyroidal DIO2 activity was better inhibited than that of peripheral tissues. In hypothyroidism, increased thyroidal DIO2 activity could be found together with increased peripheral tissue DIO2 activities.

The effects of FT_3 hyperthyroidism were identical on DIO2 activities in all cytosol fractions, but their activities were 2 times higher in euthyroidism compared to those found by increased FT_4 levels. No increase in any DIO2 activities could be detected with respect to FT_3 levels in hypothyroidism compared to those in euthyroidism. The decrease in all DIO2 activities was the consequence of the increased FT_4 levels, which demonstrated a substrate-mediated inhibitory effect in hyperthyroidism. Note, however, that the inhibitory effect of proinflammatory cytokines (IL-6, IL-1 and TNFα) and the therapy cannot be excluded in some cases. Our previous study confirmed the role of IL-6 in Graves' ophthalmopathy with active eye signs [43]. The presence of inflammatory orbital events and a longer manifestation of ophthalmopathy were associated with increased serum IL-6 levels. Therefore, the autoimmune features of Graves' Disease can modify DIO2 activities. The increased DIO2 activities in all cytosol fractions in FT_4 hypothyroidism could be explained by the concomitantly increased serum levels of TSH receptor antibodies compared to those in FT_3 hypothyroidism. Nevertheless, serum TSH levels were not suppressed by increased serum FT_4 levels, which could be explained by the pituitary resistance to T_4 [44]. No similar results could be demonstrated for increased T_3 levels. Contrary to FT_4 hypothyroidism, the lack of increased DIO2 activities in FT_3 hypothyroidism support that in this condition the active protein synthesis of DIO2 enzyme is needed for increasing their activities. The partly increased skeletal and eye muscle DIO2 activities in both FT_4 and FT_3 hyperthyroidism excluded a relevant inactivating role of DIO3 in muscle cytosol fractions.

DIO2 activities in all cytosol fractions were significantly lower in Graves' ophthalmopathy with increased serum FT_3 levels keeping the proportional discrepancies constantly among thyroidal, skeletal and eye muscle DIO2 activities. However, Graves' sera without ophthalmopathy resulted in a 5-fold increase in all

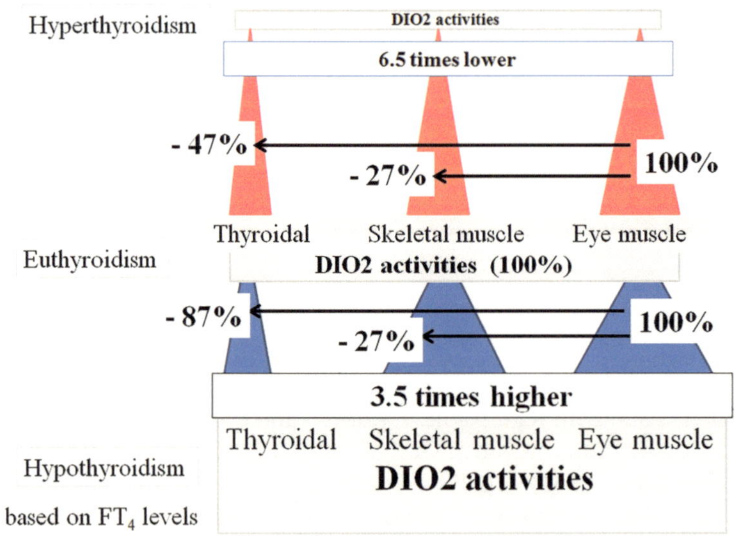

Figure 2.
The effect of patient sera with Graves' Disease on thyroidal, skeletal and eye muscle DIO2 activities with respect to thyroid functional stages based on FT_4 levels. DIO2: Type 2 deiodinase.

DIO2 activities still keeping the proportional discrepancies constant among thyroidal, skeletal and eye muscle DIO2 activities. The elevation in TSH receptor antibody levels did not associated with DIO2 elevation, but it did with TSH suppression and with a lower ratio of FT_3 to FT_4. Note that due to the small number of patients without ophthalmopathy, the conclusions can be limited.

5.2 Effects of antithyroid and antiextraocular muscle autoantibodies on thyroidal, skeletal and eye muscle DIO2 activities

5.2.1 Thyroidal, skeletal and eye muscle DIO2 activities with respect to anti-TPO and TSH receptor autoantibodies in FT_3 hyperthyroid Graves' Disease

The effects of autoantibodies against thyroid peroxidase (TPO) and TSH receptor were investigated on thyroidal, skeletal and eye muscle DIO2 activities in FT_3 hyperthyroid Graves' Disease. A greater number of patients with ophthalmopathy (n = 11) demonstrated anti-TPO antibodies than those without (n = 4) [42]. Anti-TPO antibody positive patients without ophthalmopathy exhibited 5 times greater DIO2 activities in thyroidal and skeletal muscle cytosol fractions, and even 12 times greater in eye muscle cytosol fraction compared to those with ophthalmopathy (**Figure 3**). DIO2 activities were compared between anti-TPO antibody positive and negative patients. The difference in all DIO2 activities were significant between the patients with and without ophthalmopathy in FT_3 hyperthyroid Graves' Disease, as well as between anti-TPO antibody negative and positive patients. DIO2 activities increased 17 times in patients without ophthalmopathy, but decreased by 39% in patients with ophthalmopathy in the presence of anti-TPO antibodies compared to those who were negative for these autoantibodies (**Figure 4**). The alterations could be explained by the greater increased serum FT_4 levels in anti-TPO antibody positive patients with Graves' ophthalmopathy in contrast to the patients without ophthalmopathy. The patients without ophthalmopathy showed reduced FT_4 levels, which were below the normal range, concomitantly with the elevated serum TSH levels. These result are limited by the small patient number of Graves' Disease without ophthalmopathy.

In FT_3 hyperthyroidism, TSH receptor antibody positivity was greater in Graves' ophthalmopathy (n = 11, and 9 out of 11 cases were anti-TPO antibody positive)

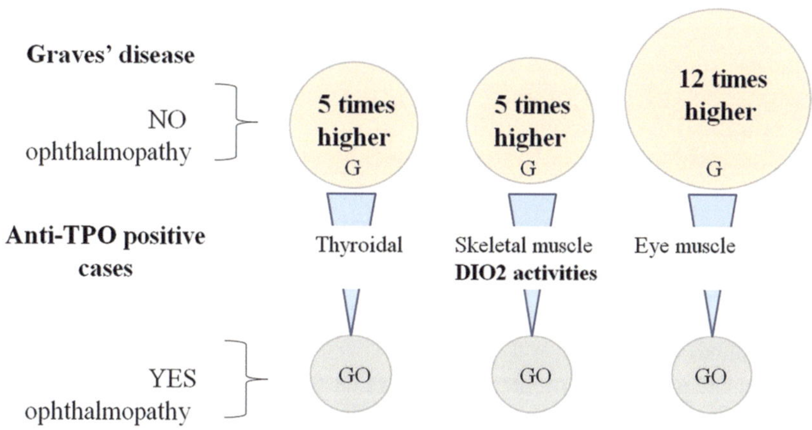

Figure 3.
The effect of patient sera with Graves' Disease on thyroidal, skeletal and eye muscle DIO2 activities in anti-TPO antibody positive patients between with (GO) and without (G) ophthalmopathy. DIO2: Type 2 deiodinase; TPO: Thyroid peroxidase.

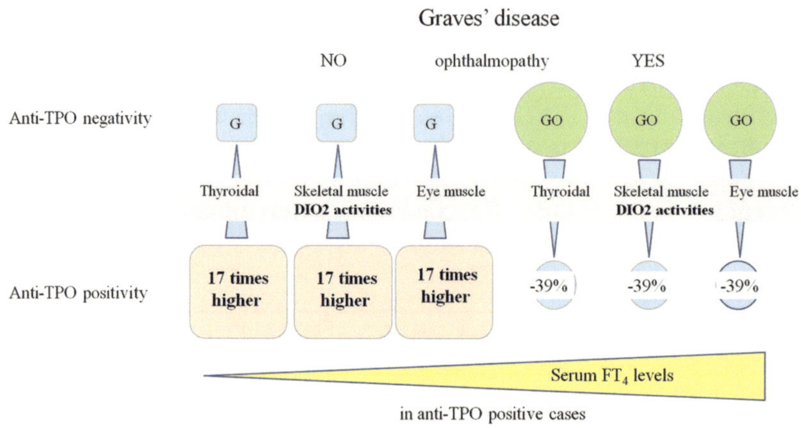

Figure 4.
The effect of patient sera with Graves' Disease on thyroidal, skeletal and eye muscle DIO2 activities between anti-TPO antibody negative and positive patients with (GO) and without (G) ophthalmopathy. DIO2: Type 2 deiodinase; TPO: Thyroid peroxidase.

than in those who had no ophthalmopathy (n = 2) [42]. DIO2 activities were significantly increased in all cytosol fractions (increased by 3.6 times) for TSH receptor antibody positive patients compared to TSH receptor antibody negative patients with Graves' ophthalmopathy, but the opposite was true for patients without ophthalmopathy (**Figure 5**). Surprisingly, in the absence of ophthalmopathy, TSH receptor antibody positive patients demonstrated relevantly decreased DIO2 activities, which were 10 times lower than those found in TSH receptor antibody negative patients in all cytosol fractions, concomitantly with the increased serum TSH levels.

5.2.2 The effects of IgG and IgM isotype antieye muscle cytosol and membrane autoantibodies on eye muscle DIO2 activity in Graves' ophthalmopathy

Next, the effects of antieye muscle cytosol and membrane autoantibodies on eye muscle DIO2 activity were examined in Graves' ophthalmopathy. Before the study, the binding reactivity of sera to human eye muscle membrane and cytosol antigens in tissue sections was controlled. In our previous results using immunohistochemistry and immunoblotting methods, antibodies against TCSS peptide, corresponding to amino acid sequence of DIO2 and eye muscle cytosol or membrane antigens (supernatant or pellet fractions of 100 000 x g, separated by centrifugations) were demonstrated, which gave intensive binding reactions to human thyroid, skeletal and eye muscle tissue sections [40].

The binding of guinea pig sera immunized by TCSS peptide could be inhibited by patient sera added in advance, which sera gave positive reactions to eye muscle tissue sections. Toyoda and coworkers investigated the DIO1 enzyme activity in FRTL-5 rat thyroid cells in the presence of IgG type immunoglobulins derived from untreated hyperthyroid Graves' patients and controls [45]. They demonstrated a relevant increased DIO1 activity, which could be completely abolished by the addition of cycloheximide.

Based on the previously mentioned results we wanted to measure the effects of antieye muscle cytosol and membrane autoantibodies on eye muscle DIO2 activity, as well as to compare DIO2 activity to eye muscle enlargements. The hypothesis was, that antieye muscle autoantibodies may affect DIO2 activity, which can lead to eye muscle enlargement. We investigated the role of antieye muscle antibodies in Graves' Disease [46]. In turn, the appearance of these autoantibodies was not

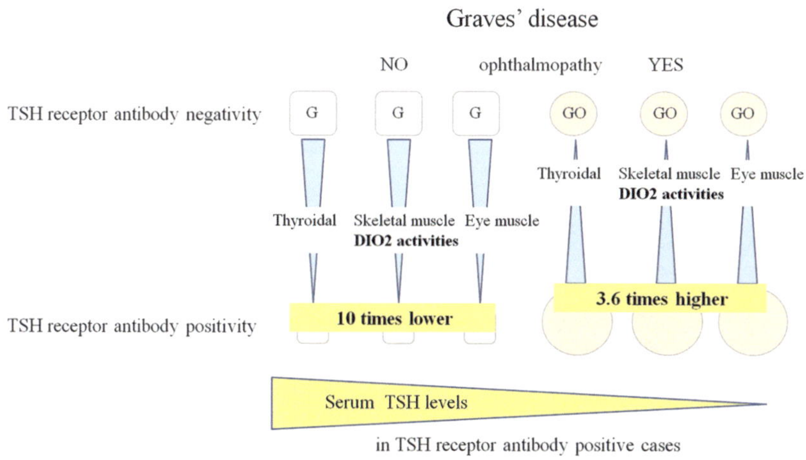

Figure 5.
The effect of patient sera with Graves' Disease on thyroidal, skeletal and eye muscle DIO2 activities between TSH receptor antibody negative and positive patients with (GO) and without (G) ophthalmopathy. DIO2: Type 2 deiodinase.

only connected to ophthalmopathy, but they could also be found in a small part of patients without ophthalmopathy. IgG, IgA and IgM isotype antieye muscle membrane and cytosol autoantibodies were measured with enzyme-linked immunosorbent assay (ELISA) in 32 patients with hyperthyroid Graves' Disease, of whom 20 cases had ophthalmopathy. None of IgA isotype autoantibodies could be detected against membrane and cytosol antigens in any of the patients. A greater number of patients with ophthalmopathy demonstrated IgM (n = 10) and IgG (n = 5) antieye muscle autoantibodies than those without ophthalmopathy, of whom 3 cases had IgG type and 3 cases had IgM type autoantibodies. Surprisingly, the addition of serum containing IgG isotype antieye membrane (EyeM) or cytosol (EyeC) autoantibodies resulted in 6.4 times or 3.9 times increased eye muscle DIO2 activity, respectively compared to those found with IgG negative sera (**Figure 6**). Conversely, the effect of IgM type antieye muscle membrane or cytosol autoantibodies was associated with 3 times or 1.9 times lower eye muscle DIO2 activity, respectively. The presence of IgG type anti-EyeC autoantibodies resulted in 1.5 times greater eye muscle DIO2 activity than anti-EyeM autoantibodies. A similar increase in DIO2 activity could be demonstrated in the presence of IgM type anti-EyeC autoantibodies compared to those with anti-EyeM autoantibodies. In this instance, the increase in eye muscle DIO2 activitiy was 2 times greater. Furthermore, the increase in eye muscle DIO2 activity was 7 times and 5 times higher in the presence of IgG type anti-EyeM and anti-EyeC autoantibodies compared to those in the presence of IgM type anti-EyeM and anti-EyeC autoantibodies, respectively. Eye muscle DIO2 activities strongly correlated with IgG type anti-EyeM and anti-EyeC autoantibody levels. It seems, the autoantibody binding to eye membrane could mediate a signal towards the cytosolic DIO2 enzyme. The findings between eye muscle DIO2 activity and eye muscle enlargement suggest this idea. IgG type anti-EyeM autoantibodies were associated with increased eye muscle enlargement, although the difference was not significant. However, IgM type anti EyeM autoantibodies were associated with a significant decrease in eye muscle enlargement. The fact that IgM type anti-EyeM autoantibodies could play a role in DIO3 activity, could not be excluded. The eye muscle DIO2 activity was more greater in patients with the absence of ophthalmopathy compared to those in the presence of that. Our results suggest that autoantibodies against eye muscle

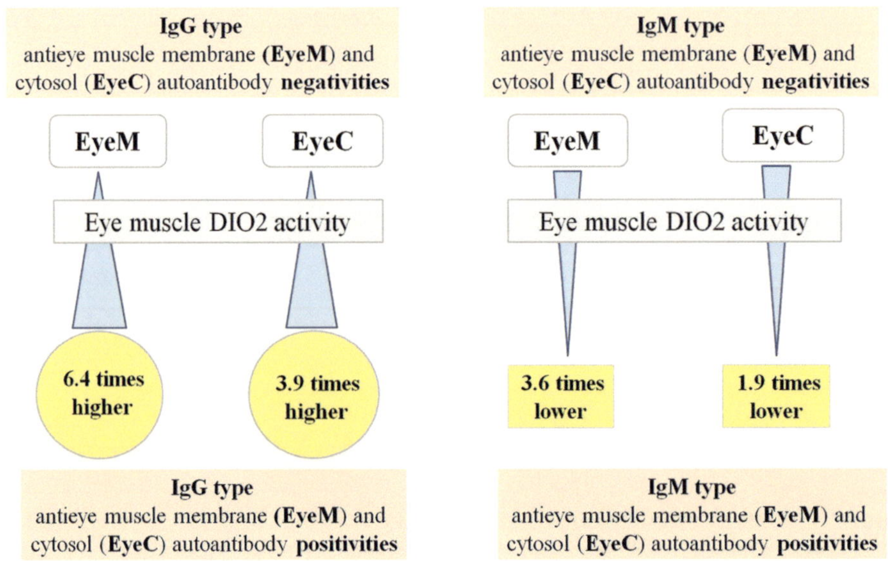

Figure 6.
The effect of patient sera containing IgG and IgM type antieye muscle membrane (EyeM) and cytosol (EyeC) autoantibodies on eye muscle DIO2 activity in Graves' ophthalmopathy. DIO2: Type 2 deiodinase.

antigens have a role in the development of ophthalmopathy through the eye muscle enlargements. The limitation of this study was the small patient number containing IgM isotype anti-EyeM and IgG isotype anti-EyeC antibodies. Another limitation could be the measurement method of the eye muscle enlargements, which was done using ultrasound in the absence of CT or MRI possibilities.

5.3 The effect of antithyroid drugs on tissue-specific DIO2 activities, as well as their role in the induction of autoantibodies against DIO2 peptides

5.3.1 The effect of antithyroid drugs on thyroidal, skeletal and eye muscle DIO2 activities

Antithyroid drugs (ATD) are used very often in the therapy of Graves' hyperthyroidism. Methimazole (MMI) and propylthiouracil (PTU) are the medicines used to block the synthesis of thyroid hormones in Hungary. ATDs are thioamide derivates with the binding reaction to DIO1 enzyme forming an intermediary selenyl-iodide-DIO1 enzyme complex (presumably the same is true for DIO2 also). In addition, they inhibit the activity of TPO enzyme due to the impairment of H_2O_2 generation and the coupling of iodotyrosines. MMI may be a selective DIO1 blocker and inhibits thyroidal H_2O_2 generation. However, MMI has no remarkable effect on DIO2 activity. PTU is a very strong inhibitor for DIO1 activity. None of the patients were treated with PTU in the tissue-specific DIO2 activity study.

The difference in thyroidal DIO2 activities was significant between those with and without ophthalmopathy in FT_3 hyperthyroidism who did not undergo MMI therapy [42]. MMI therapy was associated with a greater increase in thyroidal, skeletal and eye muscle DIO2 activities in both patients without and with ophthalmopathy (the increase was 17 times and 4 times higher, respectively) compared to the increases in patients who were not treated with MMI. MMI therapy was associated with greater TSH levels and greater ratio of FT_3 to FT_4 in patients without ophthalmopathy, and greater TSH receptor antibody levels in patients with ophthalmopathy (**Figure 7**).

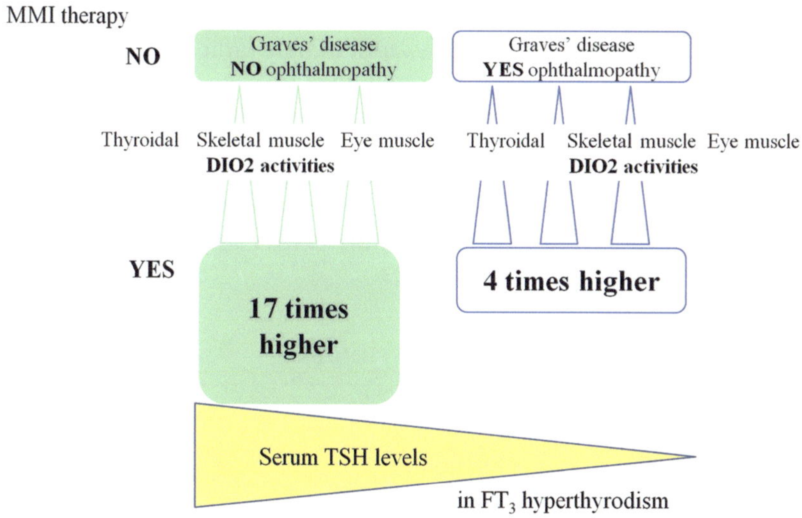

Figure 7.
The effect of patient sera who were treated with methimazole (MMI) on thyroidal, skeletal and eye muscle DIO2 activities in hyperthyroid Graves' Disease with and without ophthalmopathy. DIO2: Type 2 deiodinase.

5.3.2 Occurrence of antibodies against peptides corresponding to amino acid sequence of DIO2 during antithyroid drug therapy and the efficacy of therapy

In another study, the occurrence of autoantibodies against DIO2 peptides, such as TCSS (cyspeptide) and LVFR (hompeptide) peptides were investigated in 78 patients with hyperthyroid Graves' Disease [47]. The relationships were examinated among ATD therapies, antibodies against TPO, thyroglobulin (Tg) and TSH receptor, as well as thyroid hormone levels. The appearance of autoantibodies against cys-, hompeptide or both peptides could be detected in 24, 4 or 9 cases, respectively, in Graves' Disease. The appearance of these autoantibodies was not associated with the clinical signs of urticaria or ANCA-associated vasculitis. These anticys- and antihompeptide antibodies could be demonstrated in 12 and 3 cases in hyperthyroidism, and in 10 and 1 cases in euthyroidism. A significant difference was found in the occurrence of anticyspeptide antibodies between PTU (n = 3 out of 3 cases) and MMI (n = 13 out of 42 cases) therapies. The frequency of antipeptide antibodies was smaller in Graves' ophthalmopathy (9 cases for anticyspeptide antibodies and 1 for antihompeptide antibodies). The exact mechanism is not clear, but ATDs are thioamide drugs with the binding feature to DIO and TPO enzymes blocking the T_4 conversion to T_3, and the iodination with the phenolic coupling of iodothyrosine residues. Their higher binding features are connected to their greater reactivity with free radicals. Not only the asymptomatic occurrence of autoantibodies against cys- and/or hompeptide was surprising in hyperthyroid Graves' Disease, but also their strong relationship with decreasing anti-TPO and increasing TSH receptor antibody levels (**Figure 8**). In hyperthyroidism, two antipeptide antibodies possessed distinct features with relation to the occurrence of anti-TPO, anti-Tg and TSH receptor antibody levels, as well as to the thyroid hormone levels and the ratio of FT_3 to FT_4. Antibodies against cyspeptide were rather stimulating: Positive correlation could be demonstrated between anticyspeptide antibodies and serum FT_4 levels; the ratio of FT_3 to FT_4 was increased when those antibodies were present compared to when they were absent. In Graves' ophthalmopathy, the serum FT_4 and FT_3 levels were lower in the presence of antibodies against cyspeptide compared to when those antibodies were absent. The ratio of FT_3 to FT_4 was increased in patients without ophthalmopathy compared to those when it was present (**Figure 9**). Antibodies against hompeptide and both peptides were rather inhibiting: anti-TPO and anti-Htg antibodies levels were reduced in their presences compared to when they were absent. In hyperthyroid Graves' ophthalmopathy, antibodies against both peptides were associated with reduced antibody levels against TPO and Tg, but with increased TSH receptor antibody levels, particularly when the clinical activity score (CAS) was above 4. In FT_4 hyperthyroidism, MMI treated Graves' patients without ophthalmopathy, demonstrated significantly increased FT_3 to FT_4 ratio with the occurrence of anticyspeptide autoantibodies.

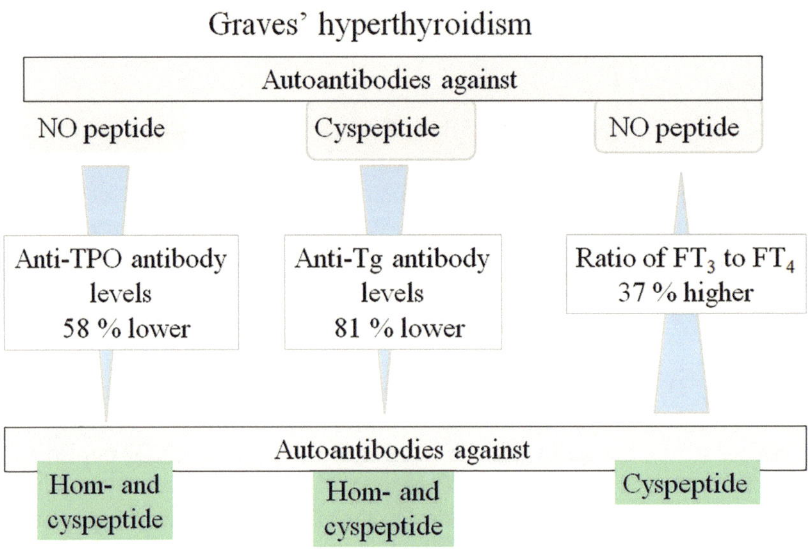

Figure 8.
The effect of patient sera containing autoantibodies against peptides (hom – and/or cyspeptide) corresponding to amino acid sequence of DIO2 on the levels of anti-TPO and anti-Tg autoantibodies, as well as on the ratio of FT_3 to FT_4 in hyperthyroid Graves' Disease. DIO2: Type 2 deiodinase; TPO: Thyroid peroxidase; Tg: Thyroglobulin.

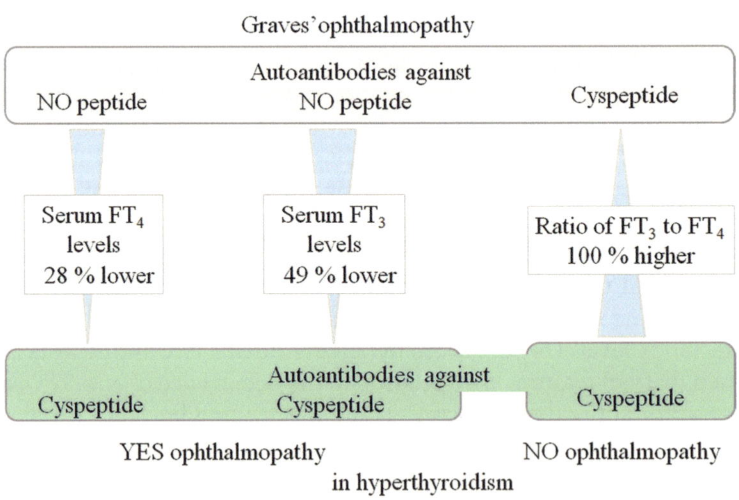

Figure 9.
The effect of patient sera containing autoantibodies against cyspeptide corresponding to amino acid sequence of DIO2 on serum FT_4 and FT_3 levels, as well as on the ratio of FT_3 to FT_4 in hyperthyroid Graves' ophthalmopathy and between the presence and absence of ophthalmopathy. DIO2: Type 2 deiodinase.

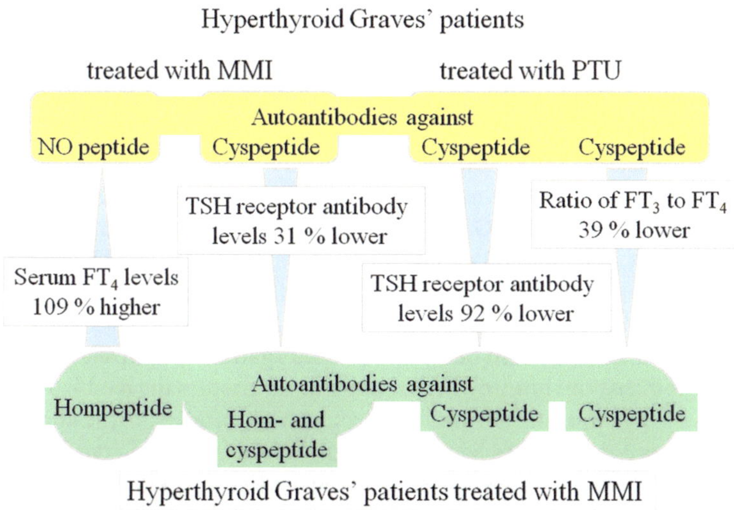

Figure 10.
The effect of patient sera containing autoantibodies against peptides (hom- and/or cyspeptide) corresponding to DIO2 amino acid sequence on serum FT_4 and TSH receptor antibody levels, as well as on the ratio of FT_3 to FT_4 in hyperthyroid Graves' Disease treated with methimazole (MMI) and propylthiouracil (PTU). DIO2: Type 2 deiodinase.

The results in thyroid hormone levels supported that the presence of antipeptide antibodies before the treatment and their absence during the treatment with MMI may contribute to the worsening of orbital processes in hyperthyroid Graves' ophthalmopathy. Antibodies against DIO2 peptides may influence the therapeutic efficacy during the treatment (**Figure 10**). In MMI treatment, the presence of antibodies against hompeptide only was connected to increased serum FT_4 levels, but when autoantibodies against both hom- and cyspeptide were present, it resulted in a relevant decrease in TSH receptor antibody levels. MMI treatment demonstrated lower TSH receptor antibody levels and lower ratio of FT_3 to FT_4 in the appearance of anticyspeptide autoantibodies compared to those treated with PTU. The exact role of antipeptide antibodies and their relationship with antithyroid autoantibodies, as well as the possibility of the occurrence of autoantibodies against other amino acid sequence of the whole DIO2 protein need futher investigations.

6. Conclusions

In hyperthyroid Graves' Disease the thyroid hormone excess is dominantly T_3. The thyroidal production of T_3 and T_4 excess can derive from the thyroidal T_4 and T_3 formation in the colloid-embedded Tg mediated by thyroidal TPO, and the additional production of T_3 due to deiodinase enzymes mediated conversion from T_4 resulting in the ratio of 3 to 1 for DIO1 and DIO2 activities in the cytosol, respectively. The results using *in vitro* model for the study of tissue-specific DIO2 activities confirmed the dominance of thyroidal DIO1 activity, but the thyroidal DIO2 activity seemed to be more reduced compared to skeletal and eye muscle DIO2 activities. The degree of DIO2 activities was tissue-specific, but the extent of their decreases in hyperthyroidism and increases in hypothyroidism was identical. The findings highlighted that the increase in tissue-specific DIO2 activity needed an active protein synthesis only in FT_3, but not in FT_4 hypothyroidism. The appearance of anti-TPO, TSH receptor, and antieye muscle membrane and cytosol autoantibodies modified the tissue-specific DIO2 activities, which manifested in both increased and decreased serum TSH levels and sometimes in eye muscle enlargements. Besides the effect of ATDs on tissue-specific DIO2 activities, autoantibodies against peptides corresponding to amino acid sequences of DIO2 also appeared asymptomatically in Graves' Disease. Furthermore, they were also detectable before ATD therapy, and the therapy increased their occurrences. The antipeptide autoantibodies were associated with alterations in serum FT_4 and FT_3 levels, as well as in the levels of autoantibodies against TPO, Tg and TSH receptor. In Graves' ophthalmopathy, the tissue-specific DIO2 activities were much more reduced and they were connected to a lack of appearance of antipeptide autoantibodies. The occurrence of anticyspeptide autoantibodies was associated with lower serum FT_4 and FT_3 levels compared to those in patients who were negative for these autoantibodies. Although, autoantibodies could be demonstrated against eye muscle cytosol antigens, which inhibited the binding of antipeptide antibodies derived from guinea pig immunization to eye muscle in immunohistochemical studies, these antieye muscle and antipeptide autoantibodies had no pathognomonic role in Graves' ophthalmopathy. These findings above explain why the duality of features causes a greater complexity of hyperthyroidism in Graves' Disease.

Conflict of interest

The author declares no conflict of interest.

Author details

Ildikó Molnár
EndoMed Debrecen Kft, Debrecen, Hungary

*Address all correspondence to: molilendomed@gmail.com

References

[1] Prabhakar BS, Bahn RS, Smith TJ: Current perspective on the pathogenesis of Graves' disease and ophthalmopathy. Endocrine Reviews, 2003;24:802-835.

[2] Kahaly GJ, Bartalena L, Hegedüs L, Leenhardt L, Poppe K, Pearce SH: 2018 European thyroid association guideline for the management of Graves' hyperthyroidism. European Thyroid Journal, 2018;7:167-186.

[3] Schwartz KM, Fatourechi V, Ahmed DDF, Pond GR: Dermopathy of Graves' disease (Pretibial myxedema): Long-term outcome. Journal of Clinical Endocrinology and Metabolism, 2002;76:438-446.

[4] Jyonouchi SC, Valyasevi RW, Harteneck DA, Dutton CM, Bahn RS: Interleukin-6 stimulates thyrotropin receptor expression in human orbital preadipocyte fibroblasts from patients with Graves' ophthalmopathy. Thyroid, 2001;11:929-934.

[5] Gunji K, De Bellis A, Kubota S, Swanson J, Wengrowicz S, Cochran B, Ackrell BAC, Salvi M, Bellastella A, Bizzarro A, Sinisi AA, Wall JR: Serum antibodies against the flavoprotein subunit of succinate dehydrogenase are sensitive markers of eye muscle autoimmunity in patients with Graves' hyperthyroidism. Journal of Clinical Endocrinology and Metabolism,1999;84:1255-1262.

[6] De Bellis A, Sansone D, Coronella C, Conte M, Iorio S, Perrino S, Battaglia M, Bellastella G, Wall JR, Bellastella A, Bizzarro A: Serum antibodies to collagen XIII: a further good marker of active Graves' ophthalmopathy. Clinical Endocrinology, 2005;62:24-29.

[7] Smith TJ, Tsai CC, Shih MJ, Tsui S, Chen B, Han R, Naik V, King CS, Press C, Kamat S, Goldberg RA, Phipps RP, Douglas RS, Gianoukakis AG: Unique attributes of orbital fibroblasts and global alterations in IGF-1 receptor signaling could explain thyroid-associated ophthalmopathy. Thyroid, 2008;18:983-988.

[8] Siddiqi A, Monson JP, Wood DF, Besser GM, Burrin JM: Serum cytokines in thyrotoxicosis. Journal of Clinical Endocrinology and Metabolism, 1999;84:435-439.

[9] Rotondi M, Chiovato L, Romagnani S, Serio M, Romagnani P: Role of chemokines in endocrine autoimmune diseases. Endocrin Reviews 2007; 28:492-520.

[10] Łacheta D, Miśkiewicz P, Gluszko A, Nowicka G, Struga M, Kantor I, Poślednik KB, Mirza S, Szczepański MJ: Immunological aspects of Graves' ophthalmopathy. BioMed Research International, 2019; Article ID 7453260. DOI: 10.1155/2019/7453260.

[11] Bresson D, Cerutti M, Devauchelle G, Pugnière M, Roquet F, Bès C, Bossard C, Chardèst T, Péraldi-Roux S: Localization of the discontinous immunodominant region recognized by human anti-thyroperoxidase autoantibodies in autoimmune thyroid diseases. Journal of Biological Chemistry, 2003;278: 9560-9569.

[12] Molnár I, Kaczur V, Boros A, Krajczár G, Balázs C: IgA autoantibodies against human eye muscle antigen detected by western blotting and immunohistochemical methods in Graves' disease. Journal of Endocrinological Investigation, 1995;18:408-414.

[13] Bianco AC, Kim BW: Deiodinases: implications of the local control of thyroid hormone action. Journal of Clinical Investigation, 2006;116:2571-2579.

[14] Salvatore D: Deiodinases: keeping the thyroid hormone supply in balance. Journal of Endocrinology, 2011;209:259-260.

[15] St. Germain DL, Galton VA, Hernandez A: Minireview: Defining the roles of the iodothyronine deiodinases: Current concepts and challenges. Endocrinology, 2009;150:1097-1107.

[16] Bianco AC, de Conceição RR: The deiodinase trio and thyroid hormone signaling. Methods in Molecular Biology, 2018;1801:67-83.

[17] Steinsapir J, Bianco AC, Buettner C, Harney J, Larsen PR: Substrate-induced down-regulation of human type 2 diodinase (hD2) is mediated through proteasomal degradation and requires interaction with the enzyme's active center. Endocrinology, 2000;141:1127-1135.

[18] Khoo TK, Bahn RS: Pathogenesis of Graves' ophthalmopathy: The role of autoantibodies. Thyroid, 2007;17:1013-1018.

[19] Salvatore D, Simonidea WS, Dentice M, Zavacki AM, Larsen PR: Thyroid hormones and skeletal muscle – new insights and potential implications. Nature Reviews Endocrinology, 2014;10:206-214.

[20] Carvalho DP, Dupuy C: Thyroid hormone biosynthesis and release. Molecular and Cellular Endocrinology, 2017;458:6-15.

[21] Larsen PR, Zavacki AM: Role of iodothyronine deiodinases in the physiology and pathophysiology of thyroid hormone action. European Thyroid Journal, 2012;1:232-242.

[22] Maia AL, Goemann IM, Meyer ELS, Wajner SM: Deiodinases: the balance of thyroid hormone. Type 1 iodothyronine deiodinase in human physiology and disease. Journal of Endocrinology, 2011;209:283-297.

[23] Maia AL, Kim BW, Huang SA, Harney JW, Larsen PR: Type 2 iodothyronine deiodinase is the major source of plasma T3 in euthyroid humans. Journal of Clinical Investigation, 2005;115:2524-2533.

[24] Molnár I, Balázs C, Szegedi G, Sipka S: Inhibition of type 2, 5′-deiodinase by tumor necrosis factor alpha, interleukin-6 and interferron gamma in human thyroid tissue. Immunology Letters, 2002;80:3-7.

[25] Laurberg P, Vestergaard H, Nielsen S, Christensen SE, Seefeldt T, Helleberg K, Pedersen KM: Sources of circulating 3,5,3′-triiodothyronine in hyperthyroidism estimated after blocking of type 1 and type 2 iodothyronine deiodinases. Journal of Clinical Endocrinology and Metabolism, 2007;92:2149-2156.

[26] de Vries EM, Fliers E, Boelen A: The molecular basis of the non-thyroidal illness syndrome. Journal of Endocrinology, 2015;225:R67-R81.

[27] Christoffolete MA, Ribeiro R, Sinfru P, Fekete C, da Silva WS, Gordon DF, Huang SA, Crescenzi A, Harney JW, Ridgeay EC, Larsen PR, Lechan RM, Bianco AC: Atypical expression of type 2 iodothyronine deiodinase in thyrotrophs explains the thyroxine-mediated pituitary thyrotropin feedback mechanism. Endocrinology, 2006;147:1735-1743.

[28] Dentice M, Marsili A, Ambrosio R, Guardiola O, SibilioA, Palk JH, Minchiotti G, DePinho RA, Fenzi G, Larsen PR, Salvatore D: The FoxO3/type 2 deiodinase pathway is required for normal mouse myogenesis and muscle regeneration. Journal of Clinical Investigation, 2010;120:4021-4030.

[29] Dentice M, Salvatore D: Deiodinases: The balance of thyroid hormone. Local impact of thyroid hormone inactivation. Journal of Endocrinology, 2011; 209: 273-282.

[30] Larsen PR: Type 2 iodothyronine deiodinase in human skeletal muscle: New insights into its physiological role and regulation. Journal of Clinical Endocrinology and Metabolism, 2000;94:1893-1895.

[31] Luongo C, Trivisano L, Alfano F, Salvatore D: Type 3 deiodinase and consumptive hypothyroidism: a common mechanism for a rare disease. Frontiers in Endocrinology, 2013;4:1-7. DOI:10.3389/fendo.2013.00115.

[32] Sriphrapradang C, Bhasipol A: Differentiating Graves' disease from subacute thyroiditis using ratio of serum free triiodothyronine to free thyroxine. Annals of Medicine and Surgery, 2016;10:69-72.

[33] Larsen PR, Abuid J: Triiodothyronine and thyroxine in hyperthyroidism. Comparison of the acute changes during therapy with antithyroid agents. Journal of Clinical Investigation, 1974;54:201-208.

[34] Salvatore D, Tu H, Harney JW, Larsen PR: Type 2 iodothyronine deiodinase is highly expressed in human thyroid. Journal of Clinical Investigation, 1996;98: 962-968.

[35] Ito M, Toyoda N, Nomura E, Takamura Y, Amino N, Iwasaka T, Takamatsu J, Míyauchi A, Nishikawa M: Type 1 and type 2 iodothyronine deiodinases in the thyroid gland of patients with 3,5,3′-triiodothyronine-predominant Graves' disease. European Journal of Endocrinology, 2011;164:95-100.

[36] Amino N, Yabu Y, Miki T, Morimoto S, Kumahara Y, Mori H, Iwatani Y, Nishi K, Nakatani K, Miyai K: Serum ratio of triiodothyronine to thyroxine, and thyroxine-binding globulin and calcitonin concentrations in Graves' disease and destruction-induced thyrotoxicosis. Journal of Clinical Endocrinology and Metabolism, 1981;53:113-116.

[37] Weetman AP, Shepherdley CA, Mansell P, Ubhi CS, Visser TJ: Thyroid over-expression of type 1 and type 2 deiodinase may account for the syndrome of low thyroxine and increasing triiodothyronine during propylthiouracil treatment. European Journal of Endocrinology, 2003;149:443-447.

[38] Laurberg P: Thyroxine and 3, 5, 5′- triiodothyronine content of thyroglobulin in thyroid needle aspirates in hyperthyroidism and hypothyroidism. Journal of Clinical Endocrinology and Metabolism, 1987;64:969-974.

[39] Larsen PR, Dick TE, Markovitz BP, Kaplan MM, Gard TG: Inhibition of intrapituitary thyroxine to 3, 5, 3′-triiodothyronine conversion prevents the acute suppression of thyrotropin release by thyroxine in hypothyroid rats. Journal of Clinical Investigation, 1979;64:117-128.

[40] Molnár I, Szombathy Z, Kovács I, Szentmiklósi JA: Immunohistochemical studies using immunized guinea pig sera with features of anti-human thyroid, eye and skeletal antibody and Graves' sera. Journal of Clinical Immunology, 2007;27: 172-180.

[41] Molnár I, Czirják L: Euthyroid sick syndrome and inhibitory effect of sera on the activity of thyroid 5′-deiodinase in systemic sclerosis. Clinical and Experimental Rheumatology, 2000;18:719-724.

[42] Molnár I, Szentmiklósi AJ, Somogyiné-Vári É: Hyperthyroidism in

patients with Graves' ophthalmopathy, and thyroidal, skeletal and eye muscle specific type 2 deiodinase enzyme activities. Experimental Clinical Endocrinology and Diabetes, 2017;125:514-521.

[43] Molnár I, Balázs C: High circulating IL-6 level in Graves' ophthalmopathy. Autoimmunity, 1997;25:91-96.

[44] Schneider MJ, Fiering SN, Pallud SE, Parlow AF, St. Germain DL, Galton VA: Targeted disruption of the type 2 selenodeiodinase gene (DIO2) results in a phenotype of pituitary resistance to T_4. Molecular Endocrinology, 2001;15:2137-2148.

[45] Toyoda N, Nishikawa M, Horimoto M, Yoshikawa N, Mori Y, Yoshimura M, Masaki H, Tanaka K, Inada M: Graves' immunoglobulin G stimulates iodothyronine 5′-deiodinating activity in FRTL-5 rat thyroid cells. Journal of Clinical Endocrinology and Metabolism, 1990;70:1506-1511.

[46] Molnár I, Somogyiné-Vári É: Anti-eye muscle IgG and IgM antibodies are associated with eye muscle type 2 deiodinase activities in hyperthyroid Graves' ophthalmopathy. Journal of Clinical and Cellular Immunology, 2016;7:1-5.

[47] Molnár I, Szentmiklósi AJ, Gesztelyi R, Somogyiné-Vári É: Effect of antithyroid drugs on the occurrence of antibodies against type 2 deiodinase (DIO2), which are involved in hyperthyroid Graves' disease influencing the therapeutic efficacy. Clinical and Experimental Medicine, 2019;19:245-254.

Section 3

Therapy for Graves' Disease

Chapter 8

Treatment of Graves' Disease in Adults

Mauricio Alvarez Andrade and Lorena Pabón Duarte

Abstract

Graves' Disease is an autoimmune disease, with a genetic susceptibility, activated by environmental factors like stress, iodine excess, infections, pregnancy and smoking. It is caused by thyroid stimulating immunoglobulin (TSI) or thyroid stimulating antibody (TSAb) and is the most common cause of hyperthyroidism with an incidence of 21 per 100,000 per year. Treatment of Graves' Disease includes antithyroid drugs such as methimazole and propylthiouracil, radioactive iodine therapy and thyroidectomy. Methimazole, an antithyroid drug that belongs to the thioamides class, is usually the first line of treatment due to lower risk of hepatotoxicity compared to propylthiouracil. Radioactive iodine therapy is reserved for those patients who do not respond to antithyroid drugs or have contraindication or adverse effects generated by antithyroid drugs, and thyroid surgery is an option in people with thyroid nodular disease with suspected malignancy or large goiters such as predictors of poor response to antithyroid drugs and radioactive iodine therapy. Multiple factors influence the management of patients with Graves' Disease including patient and physician preferences, access to medical services and patients features such as age, complications and comorbidities.

Keywords: Hyperthyroidism, Graves' Disease, antithyroid agents, methimazole, propylthiouracil, thyroidectomy

1. Introduction

Graves' Disease is the most common cause of hyperthyroidism with an incidence of 21 per 100,000 per year [1], with a F:M ratio ranging from 3 to 5:1 [2–4]. The usual age of presentation ranges from 20 to 50 years old.

Graves' Disease is an autoimmune disease, with a genetic susceptibility, activated by environmental factors like stress, iodine excess, infections, pregnancy and smoking. It is caused by thyroid stimulating immunoglobulin (TSI) or thyroid stimulating antibody (TSAb). TSI stimulate follicular thyroid cells by binding to the thyroid stimulating hormone (TSH) receptor on the thyroid cell membrane to produce the thyroid hormone synthesis and liberation as well as gland growth, with consequent hyperthyroidism and bocio [1, 5].

Graves' Disease produces varied symptoms such as sweating, insomnia, weight loss, anxiety, muscle weakness, loss of libido. Clinical signs include tachycardia, systolic hypertension, heart failure, atrial fibrillation, tremors, hyperkinesia, hyperreflexia, hot skin, palmar erythema, onycholysis, alopecia, goiter and impaired mental status. Among the most characteristic signs of the disease are thyroid orbitopathy and the infrequent pretibial myxedema. Orbitopathy is characterized by proptosis, palpebral retraction, chemosis, and periorbital edema [1, 5].

Treatment of Graves' Disease includes antithyroid drugs such as methimazole and propylthiuracil, radioactive iodine therapy and thyroidectomy. Methimazole, an antithyroid drug that belongs to thionamides class, usually is the first line of treatment due to lower risk of hepatotoxicity compared to propylthiuracil. Radioactive iodine therapy is reserved for those patients who do not respond to antithyroid drugs or have contraindication or adverse effects generated by antithyroid drugs, and thyroid surgery is an option in people with thyroid nodular disease with suspected malignancy or large goiters such as predictors of poor response to antithyroid drugs and radioactive iodine therapy [5–9].

Multiple factors influence the management of patients with Graves' Disease including patient and physician preferences, access to medical services and patients features such as age, complications and comorbidities.

2. Antithyroid drugs

2.1 Methimazole

Methimazole, an antithyroid drug that belongs to the thionamide class, with few exceptions is usually the first line of treatment due to the lower risk of hepatotoxicity compared to propylthiuracil [10, 11].

The mechanism of action of methimazole is to block the production of thyroid hormone by interfering with the iodination of tyrosine residues of thyroglobulin by inhibiting the enzyme thyroid peroxidase and then the synthesis of thyroxine and triiodothyronine. Furthermore, methimazole inhibits iodine oxidation and the binding of iodotyrosyl residues [10, 11].

The route of administration of methimazole is oral. The starting dose depends on the severity of the disease, in most cases it varies between 20 to 40 mg per day, with titration every 4 to 8 weeks and variable maintenance doses and a maximum dose of 60 to 80 mg. does not require dose adjustment except in patients with severe hepatic impairment [10, 11]. The recommended starting dose in mild cases is 15 mg per day and moderate to severe cases 30 mg per day.

Although methimazole has a half-life of less than 6 hours, the half-life has been shown to be greater than 6 hours in follicular cells [12, 13], and the effectiveness of administering it in a single daily dose in usual doses is effective [14–17].

In patients with thyroid storm, higher doses are required, with a starting dose of 60 to 80 mg per day with the dose divided every 4 to .8 hours, with a maximum dose of 120 mg [18].

Serious adverse effects of methimazole include agranulocytosis, hepatotoxicity, and teratogenicity. Agranulocytosis usually occurs in the first months of treatment but can occur at any time during treatment, it is characterized by an absolute granulocyte count less than 500 per ml, fever and sore throat, so it should be indicated to the patient attend the emergency room in case of these symptoms. Treatment consists of stopping methimazole if the granulocyte count is less than 1000 per ml and antibiotic treatment. Agranulocytosis due to methimazole predicts the risk of agranulocytosis due to propylthiuracil, therefore the use of propylthiuracil should also be avoided in these patients. Methimazole hepatotoxicity can occur at any dose, is characterized by cholestasis and slowly recovers after discontinuation of the drug [19–21].

The teratogenicity of methimazole occurs by free crossing the placenta, especially in the first trimester, the effects include aplasia cutis, umbilical malformations, facial dysmorphism, esophageal and choanal atresia as well as craniofacial malformations. For this reason, the use of propylthiuracil in the first trimester of pregnancy is preferred [19–21].

2.2 Propylthiuracil

Propylthiuracil is an antithyroid drug that is frequently used as a second treatment option in hyperthyroidism after methimazole due to an increased risk of hepatotoxicity, as well as in patients with a contraindication to methimazole or radioactive iodine therapy. Propylthiuracil is preferred as the first line of treatment in patients with thyroid storm because of its greater effect in theory, by inhibiting the peripheral conversion of t4 to t3 by inhibiting thyroid deiodinase. Propylthiuracil is also preferred in the first trimester of pregnancy because of the toxicity of methimazole [20, 21].

The mechanism of action of propylthiuracil is inhibition of thyroid peroxidase, which oxidizes iodine and incorporates it into the tyrosine molecule, preventing the formation of diiodotyrosine and monoiodothyronine. Unlike methimazole, it has a peripheral effect by inhibiting the conversion of T4 to T3 by inhibition of deiodinase [19, 20].

The route of administration is oral. The presentation is tablet of 50 mg. The initial dose depends on the severity with the usual starting dose 300 mg daily divided every 8 hours, with titration of the dose up to a maximum dose of 600 to 900 mg daily. The usual maintenance dose is 100 to 150 mg per day. In patients with thyroid storm the usual dose is 500 to 1000 mg daily divided every 4 hours [19–21].

Hepatic injury is one of the most worrisome adverse effects of the use of propylthiuracil, it occurs frequently in the first 6 months of treatment, however it can occur at any time, the symptoms are specific and the initial diagnosis is made by elevation of liver function markers. Due to the high risk of hepatotoxicity in pregnancy, methimazole is preferred in the second and third trimester of pregnancy [19–21].

Less frequently, propylthiuracil has been associated with ANCA-associated vasculitis that can cause glomerulonephritis, alveolar hemorrhage, central nervous system compromise, and leukocytoclastic vasculitis, may improve with drug withdrawal or require additional immunosuppressive treatment [19–21].

Agranulocytosis can occur in up to 0.5% of patients, especially in the first 3 months of treatment, the symptoms as in methimazole agranulocytosis are sore throat and fever and the patient should be advised of attend the emergency department in case of presenting these symptoms. Other adverse effects are hypersensitivity, hypothyroidism, and potential teratogenicity. Less frequently, multiple adverse effects have been described, including dermatological manifestations, interstitial nephritis, neuritis, paresthesia, headache, vertigo, lymphadenopathy, splenomegaly, aplastic anemia, fever, and lupus-like [19–21].

3. Initial treatment and relapse risk factors

Antithyroid drugs are the initial treatment for hyperthyroidism due to Graves' Disease, with the exception of patients who have contraindications. Methimazole is preferred as the first line of treatment due to a lower risk of liver toxicity and propylthiuracil as the second line of treatment, with the exceptions previously described [20, 21]. The relapse rate after initial antithyroid drug treatment based on a meta-analysis with more than 1000 patients is 52% [22].

There are factors that predict a higher remission rate with antithyroid drugs, some studies have identified factors such as female gender, not smoking, absence of orbitopathy, duration of treatment, pharmacological hypothyroidism, higher levels of TSH during treatment, more than 3 months of discontinuation of antithyroid drugs and lower levels of FT4 and FT3, antimitochondrial antibody level and factors associated with a higher relapse rate such as antithyroid use for more than 24 months [23–25], Scores such as GREAT have also been created that give a higher relapse risk score to people under 40 years of age, with greater ft4 level, higher levels of Thyrotropin-binding Inhibitory Immunoglobulin (TBII), greater degree of goiter and HLA polymorphisms [26].

After 12 to 18 months of antithyroid treatment, the patient should be reassessed and depending on the risk factors for relapse as well as the TRBII titers, continuing treatment with antithyroid drugs for an additional 12 months or taking the patient to therapy may be considered. Ablative with iodine 131 or surgery, depending on the age, comorbidities and desire of the patient, taking into account risks and benefits of each therapy. In selected patients, one option is to continue treatment with antithyroid drugs. In patients seeking pregnancy or pregnancy who are being treated with methimazole, it is recommended to switch to propylthiuracil during the first trimester of pregnancy [27].

The use of combined therapy with methimazole and levothyroxine has been evaluated in some studies, however it has been found that it does not increase the rate of remission of the disease with the probability of increasing adverse effects [28, 29], with the exception of one study which demonstrated a probable benefit in bone mineralization with the use of combination therapy [30].

3.1 Beta blockers

Beta-blockers are an adjuvant to antithyroid drugs, radioactive iodine, or surgery. They have been used for more than 20 years to modify the severity of general symptoms due to excess thyroid hormones by blocking the hyperadrenergic effects. The effects of the different beta-blockers depend on their selectivity for B1 receptors, membrane stabilizing activity, sympathomimetic activity, and lipid solubility [31–33].

Some beta-blockers such as propranolol have effects on the metabolism of thyroid hormones by decreasing the conversion of T4 to T3, decreasing the levels of active hormone T3, this effect is not typical of all beta-blockers and has been associated with the stabilization activity of membrane [31–33].

When comparing treatment with propranolol and metoprolol, it has been shown that both are equally effective in controlling the symptoms and signs of thyrotoxicosis, however propranolol produces a decrease in T3 and an increase in reverse rT3 by the mechanism previously described, findings that are not known. Found in patients treated with metoprolol [31–33].

In conclusion, beta-blockers are effective in treating the metabolic and hyperadrenergic symptoms of hyperthyroid states and in the case of Graves' Disease they are an adjuvant treatment to antithyroid drugs and ablative therapies [31–33].

3.2 Iodine 131 (I131) therapy

Ablative treatment with radioiodine or thyroidectomy result in better cure rates and overcome the risk of non-compliance with thionamides, but both treatments incur the need for permanent levothyroxine therapy [34].

The mechanism of action of I131 is physiological, it is taken up by the thyroid gland and incorporated into thyroid hormone, releasing beta particles that cause ionizing damage and tissue necrosis, this results in ablation of functional thyroid tissue. On average, it takes between 6 to 18 weeks before an euthyroid or hypothyroid state is achieved following I131 treatment. After a single dose of radioiodine, around 15–25% of patients remain hyperthyroid and require additional treatment [35].

Iodine therapy represents a cost-effective treatment option for Graves' Disease. In the United States is the preferred therapy, whereas in Europe, Australia and most of Asia, it is reserved as second line for patients who relapse after initial thionamide treatment [34, 36]. The recent National Institute for Health and Care Excellence (NICE) guidelines recommends that radioiodine should now be the first line treatment for Graves' Disease in the UK because of its superior cost-effectiveness and efficacy of radioiodine compared to thionamides [34].

Previous studies have reported factors related to success of radioiodine therapy (RIT) including: gender (lower remission rates in males), more severe hyperthyroidism, thyroid size, serum TSH receptor antibody titers and thyroid uptake on radionuclide scans [36]. A recent study included 336 patients aged 22–75 years who were diagnosed with Graves' Disease and treated with iodine therapy, which 220 (65.5%) were smokers. In regards of the treatment, 115 (52.2%) of patients received single RIT and 105 (47.8%) received second dose of RAI due to recurrent hyperthyroidism. In non-smokers (n = 116, 34.5%), 91 (78.6%) received single activity of RAI, while 25 (21.4%) required second RIT due to recurrent hyperthyroidism [36].

Potential complications of I131 therapy include: worsening of Graves' ophthalmopathy (15–20% of patients) and development of a radiation thyroiditis (1% of patients), which appears within 2 weeks after I131 therapy and can be associated with neck tenderness and swelling. The risk of exacerbation or new occurrence of Graves' eye disease can be mitigated by glucocorticoid prophylaxis [35, 36].

Regarding outcomes of radioiodine therapy, data from 101 patients in an Australian 10 year cohort reported remission following a single dose of I131 in 73 patients (79.3%), 64 patients became hypothyroid (87.6%) and 9 patients (12.3%) remained euthyroid. Individuals who did not achieve remission with a single dose were more likely to have higher TSH receptor antibody titers at diagnosis. The median time from I131 administration to hypothyroidism was 4 months. There was no difference in technetium uptake, I131 administered activity, duration of medical therapy, pre-treatment free thyroxine or duration of disease [35].

The safety of radioiodine with respect to long-term mortality risk has been subject of debate; observational studies from the United States, Sweden, UK and Finland reported increased all-cause mortality compared to the background general population in patients who received radioiodine therapy for hyperthyroidism, attributable to cardiovascular disorders, and in some cases, mortality increased with higher radioiodine doses. Along cancer mortality, there are reports of increased, similar or decreased cancer mortality risk in radioiodine-treated patients with hyperthyroidism. The increased mortality was seen in younger versus older patients, and in patients with toxic nodules compared to Graves' Disease. Mortality cancer risk was dose dependent, and it attributable to upper gastroesophageal, respiratory tract or breast tumors, suggesting that the malignancies were a consequence of internal exposure to radioactivity in iodide accumulating organs. A critical appraisal of these and other treatment-related mortality studies in hyperthyroidism is therefore necessary to ascertain the safety of the proposed NICE approach [34].

There are several studies that compare mortality in radioiodine versus thionamide treated patients. Some showed excess cancer deaths in thionamide but not radioiodine-treated patients, and others showed reduced mortality in association with radioiodine but only after it led to hypothyroidism, implying survival advantages of hyperthyroidism control [34].

3.3 Surgery

Thyroidectomy is the oldest form of Graves' treatment and has been found to be as effective as ATDs and radioiodine in normalizing serum thyroid hormone levels within 6 weeks of therapy. A meta-analysis that included 8 studies and a total of 1402 patients with hyperthyroidism has shown that thyroidectomy has the lowest relapse rate (10%) when compared with RAI (15%) and ATD (52%) as well as another meta-analysis which showed a 100% cure rate among patients who underwent total thyroidectomy [37].

Indications for thyroidectomy include large goiters, goiters causing airway obstruction/ dysphagia, moderate to severe ophthalmopathy (because radioiodine may worsen ophthalmopathy), pregnant or breastfeeding women (If the patient is unable to tolerate propylthiuracil or methimazole after the first trimester, persistent hyperthyroidism after radioablation and ATD therapy, or a nodule with abnormal cytology on fine needle aspiration (FNA) [37].

Regards of mortality outcomes in radioiodine versus thyroidectomy cohorts. A 1982 Mayo clinic study showed no difference of mortality in radioiodine versus surgically treated women with hyperthyroidism, but two studies from Finland and Sweden have shown an increase in all-cause mortality and cardiovascular mortality in radioiodine treated patients compared to thyroidectomy patients; differences in cancer related mortality were not observed between the two groups in these cohort. Excess cardiovascular morbidity was not seen in radioiodine or in surgically who developed hypothyroidism, suggesting that the survival advantages of surgery over radioiodine therapy may be related to the superior hyperthyroidism control achieved with thyroidectomy [34].

Preparing for surgery [37]:

- Thyrotoxic patients should be rendered euthyroidic before undergoing surgery, some believe that there is a risk of hemodynamic instability if thyroid function is not controlled

- Beta blockers should be used up to and after surgery until thyroid function levels are within the normal limits

- Antithyroid drug therapy is used up until the day of surgery

- According to ATA guidelines, preoperative potassium iodide (KI), saturated solution of potassium iodide (SSKI), or Lugol solution should be used, this treatment has been shown to decrease thyroid blood flow, vascularity, and intraoperative blood loss. Although, there have also been other studies that show no change in outcomes when using these products.

- Calcium and vitamin D levels should be measured prior to surgery to establish a baseline level

- Serum calcium and albumin levels should be measured in the postoperative setting

- Parathyroid hormone is tested postoperatively after thyroidectomy to screen for transient and later permanent hypoparathyroidism

- Postoperative hypocalcemia can be avoided by pretreating with calcium carbonate 1 g for 3 weeks prior the procedure

- All patients should take 1 g calcium carbonate TID for 2 weeks until the levels of calcium and parathyroid hormone (PTH) are measured again

Total thyroidectomy is preferred to subtotal thyroidectomy. Total thyroidectomy versus subtotal thyroidectomy is a balance between risk of recurrence of hyperthyroidism and incidence of hypothyroidism [37].

One randomized trial of total thyroidectomy vs. subtotal thyroidectomy followed 191 patients over a span of 5 years. Total thyroidectomy had a recurrence of 0% versus 4.7% in patients undergoing subtotal thyroidectomy. It was also found that transient hypoparathyroidism occurred in 12.6% of total thyroidectomy and permanent hypoparathyroidism in 0.5% patients. In the subtotal thyroidectomy cohort, 6.8% had transient hypoparathyroidism and 0% had permanent hypoparathyroidism [38].

A systematic review and meta-analysis of total vs. subtotal thyroidectomy for Graves' Disease, found that the odds ratio (OR) of transient and permanent hypoparathyroidism favors subtotal thyroidectomy, the OR of the recurrence of hyperthyroidism favors total thyroidectomy. Permanent recurrent laryngeal nerve injury was found to be equivalent between the 2 operations [39].

3.4 Thyroid storm

Thyroid storm is a life-threatening complication of severe disease with a high risk of mortality. Once thyroid storm is recognized, the patient should be managed in an appropriate location such as an Acute Medical Unit, high-dependency area or intensive care unit [40, 41].

Thyroid storm has multiple aims: supportive care, inhibition of new hormone synthesis, inhibition of thyroid hormone release, peripheral β-adrenergic receptor blockade, preventing peripheral conversion of T4 to T3 and identifying and treating precipitating factors [41].

General supportive care includes intravenous resuscitation, electrolyte replacement and nutritional support. Fluid losses could result from the combination of fever, diaphoresis, vomiting, and diarrhea. Normal saline can be given for replacement [40, 41]. Antipyretics can be administered to relieve pyrexia, but salicylates should be avoided as they are associated with displacement of thyroid hormone binding from thyroid binding globulin [40].

Thionamides inhibit synthesis of thyroid hormones. Iodine (lugol solution, potassium iodide can be given to stop thyroid hormone release. Iodine-containing solution should not be given to patients with iodine overload, iodine-induced hyperthyroidism, or those with amiodarone-induced thyrotoxicosis. In these situations, an alternative such as lithium or potassium perchlorate may be used instead [41].

Conversion of T4 to T3 is blocked by PTU, propranolol, and glucocorticoid. For PTU and propranolol, this effect is not quantitatively significant. Therefore, glucocorticoids like hydrocortisone or dexamethasone are essential in treatment [41].

Peripheral β-adrenergic receptor blockade is made by using propranolol. It can be given intravenous in slow 1–2 mg boluses, which may be repeated every 10–15 min until the desired effect is achieved. Orally, propranolol therapy usually begins at 20–120 mg per dose, or 160–320 mg/day [41].

Propranolol could be used for the management for secondary atrial fibrillation. Alternatively, esmolol, with a shorter acting effect could also be used. Intravenous calcium channel blockers may be considered if β-blockers are contraindicated, other alternatives are digoxin and amiodarone [41].

The incidence of thromboembolism in thyrotoxic patients is considerable. In view of the hypercoagulable state and increased incidence of mitral valve prolapse in thyrotoxicosis-related atrial fibrillation, anticoagulant should be started [41].

In the case of acute heart failure, which is associated with a high cardiac output state, initial management is with loop diuretics. Vasodilators such as nitrates should be avoided as thyrotoxicosis is associated with vasodilatation and systemic vascular resistance [41].

4. Future therapies

Although antithyroid drugs, radioactive iodine and surgery have been the treatment options in the las few decades, in recent years treatment options based on immunobiology such as biologics, small molecules and peptide immunomodulation have been investigated. These treatments are in different stages of development and are aimed at immunomodulation of B lymphocytes such as rituximab, iscalimab and belimumab, blocking of immunoglobulin recycling, signaling of TSH receptors as antagonists of TSH receptor, immune tolerance as immunomodulatory TSH receptor peptides, with the benefit of a lower risk of toxicity and since they are targeted treatments, a lower risk of immunosuppression and the hope of higher rates of remission [42].

5. Conclusions

Graves' Disease is the most common cause of hyperthyroidism. Treatment options are still antithyroid drugs, radioactive iodine and surgery. Antithyroid drugs continue to be the first line of treatment, except for patients with contraindications or intolerance, radioactive iodine therapy has gained more force in some management guidelines such as the NICE 2019 guidelines. Surgical ablation is still an option in a smaller proportion of patients with particular conditions. New treatment options with biological and immunomodulatory therapy are under development and in the future may be a treatment option with a lower risk of toxicity and perhaps higher rates of cure.

Author details

Mauricio Alvarez Andrade[1*] and Lorena Pabón Duarte[2]

1 Keralty, Bogotá, Colombia

2 Fundación Cardioinfantil, Bogotá, Colombia

*Address all correspondence to: mauricioalvarez613@gmail.com

References

[1] Hussain YS, Hookham JC, Allahabadia A, Balasubramanian SP. Epidemiology, management and outcomes of Graves' disease-real life data. Endocrine. 2017 Jun;56(3):568-578.

[2] McGrogan A, Seaman HE, Wright JW, de Vries CS. The incidence of autoimmune thyroid disease: a systematic review of the literature. Clin. Endocrinol. (Oxf). 2008;69(5):687-696. doi: 10.1111/j.1365-2265.2008.03338.x.

[3] Cooper GS, Stroehla BC. The epidemiology of autoimmune diseases. Autoimmun. Rev. 2003;2(3):119-125. doi: 10.1016/S1568-9972(03)00006-5.

[4] Nystrom HF, Jansson S, Berg G. Incidence rate and clinical features of hyperthyroidism in a long-term iodine sufficient area of Sweden (Gothenburg) 2003-2005. Clin. Endocrinol. (Oxf). 2013;78(5):768-776. doi: 10.1111/cen.12060.

[5] Antonelli A, Fallahi P, Elia G, Ragusa F, Paparo SR, Ruffilli I, Patrizio A, Gonnella D, Giusti C, Virili C, Centanni M, Shoenfeld Y, Ferrari SM. Graves' disease: Clinical manifestations, immune pathogenesis (cytokines and chemokines) and therapy. Best Pract Res Clin Endocrinol Metab. 2020 Jan;34(1):101388. doi: 10.1016/j.beem.2020.101388. Epub 2020 Feb 4. PMID: 32059832.

[6] Benker G, Vitti P, Kahaly G, Raue F, Tegler L, Hirche H, Reinwein D. Response to methimazole in Graves' disease. The European Multicenter Study Group. Clin Endocrinol (Oxf). 1995 Sep;43(3):257-63. doi: 10.1111/j.1365-2265.1995.tb02030.x. PMID: 7586593.

[7] Raber W, Kmen E, Waldhäusl W, Vierhapper H. Medical therapy of Graves' disease: effect on remission rates of methimazole alone and in combination with triiodothyronine. Eur J Endocrinol. 2000 Feb;142(2):117-24. doi: 10.1530/eje.0.1420117. PMID: 10664518.

[8] Huang H, Shi Y, Liang B, Cai H, Cai Q, Lin R. Optimal iodine supplementation during antithyroid drug therapy for Graves' disease is associated with lower recurrence rates than iodine restriction. Clin Endocrinol (Oxf). 2018 Mar;88(3):473-478. doi: 10.1111/cen.13543. Epub 2018 Jan 23. PMID: 29288501.

[9] Park S, Song E, Oh HS, Kim M, Jeon MJ, Kim WG, Kim TY, Shong YK, Kim DM, Kim WB. When should antithyroid drug therapy to reduce the relapse rate of hyperthyroidism in Graves' disease be discontinued? Endocrine. 2019 Aug;65(2):348-356. doi: 10.1007/s12020-019-01987-w. Epub 2019 Jun 24. PMID: 31236779.

[10] LiverTox: Clinical and Research Information on Drug-Induced Liver Injury [Internet]. Bethesda (MD): National Institute of Diabetes and Digestive and Kidney Diseases; 2012–. Antithyroid Agents. 2014 Feb 16. PMID: 31643916.

[11] Jansson R, Lindström B, Dahlberg PA. Pharmacokinetic properties and bioavailability of methimazole. Clin Pharmacokinet. 1985 Sep-Oct;10(5):443-50.

[12] Jansson R, Dahlberg PA, Johansson H, Lindström B. Intrathyroidal concentrations of methimazole in patients with graves' disease. J Clin Endocrinol Metab. (1983) 57:129-32. doi: 10.1210/jcem-57-1-129 43.

[13] Liu L, Lu H, Liu Y, Liu C, Xun C. Predicting relapse of Graves' disease following treatment with antithyroid drugs. Exp Ther Med. 2016

Apr;11(4):1453-1458. doi: 10.3892/etm.2016.3058. Epub 2016 Feb 9. PMID: 27073464; PMCID: PMC4812122.

[14] Shiroozu A, Okamura K, Ikenoue H, Sato K, Nakashima T, Yoshinari M, et al. Treatment of hyperthyroidism with a small single daily dose of methimazole. J Clin Endocrinol Metab. (1986) 63:125-8. doi: 10.1210/jcem-63-1-125 Frontiers in Endocrinology | www.frontiersin.org 10 May 2020 | Volume 11 | Article 286 Abbara et al. Endocrine Response to Anti-thyroid Drugs 38.

[15] Macfarlane IA, Davies D, Longson D, Shalet SM, Beardwell CG. Single daily dose short term carbimazole therapy for hyperthyroid graves' disease. Clin Endocrinol. (1983) 18:557-61. doi: 10.1111/j.1365-2265.1983. tb00593.x 39.

[16] . Gupta SK, Mithal A, Godbole MM. Single daily dose of carbimazole in the treatment of hyperthyroidism. Natl Med J India. (1992) 5:214-6

[17] Mashio Y, Beniko M, Matsuda A, Koizumi S, Matsuya K, Mizumoto H, et al. Treatment of hyperthyroidism with a small single daily dose of methimazole. Endocr J. (1997) 44:553-8. doi: 10.1507/endocrj.44.553.

[18] Idrose AM. Acute and emergency care for thyrotoxicosis and thyroid storm. Acute Med Surg. 2015 May 12;2(3):147-157. doi: 10.1002/ams2.104. PMID: 29123713; PMCID: PMC5667251.

[19] Abbara A, Clarke SA, Brewster R, Simonnard A, Eng PC, Phylactou M, Papadopoulou D, Izzi-Engbeaya C, Sam AH, Wernig F, Jonauskyte E, Comninos AN, Meeran K, Kelsey TW, Dhillo WS. Pharmacodynamic Response to Anti-thyroid Drugs in Graves' Hyperthyroidism. Front Endocrinol (Lausanne). 2020 May 12;11:286. doi: 10.3389/fendo.2020.00286. PMID: 32477269; PMCID: PMC7236601.

[20] Nicholas W, Fischer R, Stevenson R, Bass J. Single daily dose of methimazole compared to every 8 hours propylthiouracil in the treatment of hyperthyroidism. South Med J. 9:973– 6. doi: 10.1097/00007611-199509000-00018

[21] Nakamura H, Noh JY, Itoh K, Fukata S, Miyauchi A, Hamada N, et al. Comparison of methimazole and propylthiouracil in patients with hyperthyroidism caused by graves' disease. J Clin Endocrinol Metab. (2007) 92:2157-62. doi: 10.1210/jc. 2006-2135

[22] Sundaresh V, Brito JP, Wang Z, Prokop LJ, Stan MN, Murad MH, Bahn RS. Comparative effectiveness of therapies for Graves' hyperthyroidism: a systematic review and network meta-analysis. J Clin Endocrinol Metab. 2013 Sep;98(9):3671-7. doi: 10.1210/jc.2013-1954. Epub 2013 Jul 3. PMID: 23824415; PMCID: PMC3763977.

[23] Panagiotis A, Fotini A, Polyzos SA, Katergari S, Karathanasi E, Zouli C, et al. Predictors of long-term remission in patients with graves' disease: a single center experience. Endocrine. (2013) 44:448-53. doi: 10.1007/s12020-013-9895-0 48.

[24] Edmonds CJ, Tellez M. Treatment of Graves' disease by carbimazole: high dose with thyroxine compared to titration dose. Eur J Endocrinol. 1994 Aug;131(2):120-4.

[25] Hwang SM, Kim MS, Lee DY. Predictive factors for early response to methimazole in children and adolescents with Graves disease: a single-institute study between 1993 and 2013. Ann Pediatr Endocrinol Metab. 2016 Jun;21(2):70-4. doi: 10.6065/apem.2016.21.2.70. Epub 2016 Jun 30. PMID: 27462582; PMCID: PMC4960017.

[26] Vos XG, Endert E, Zwinderman AH, Tijssen JGP, Wiersinga WM. Predicting the risk of recurrence before the start of

antithyroid drug therapy in patients with graves' hyperthyroidism. J Clin Endocrinol Metab. (2016) 101:1381– 9. doi: 10.1210/jc.2015-3644

[27] Kahaly GJ, Bartalena L, Hegedüs L, Leenhardt L, Poppe K, Pearce SH. 2018 European Thyroid Association Guideline for the Management of Graves' Hyperthyroidism. Eur Thyroid J. 2018 Aug;7(4):167-186. doi: 10.1159/000490384. Epub 2018 Jul 25. PMID: 30283735; PMCID: PMC6140607.

[28] Rittmaster RS, Abbott EC, Douglas R, Givner ML, Lehmann L, Reddy S, Salisbury SR, Shlossberg AH, Tan MH, York SE. Effect of methimazole, with or without L-thyroxine, on remission rates in Graves' disease. J Clin Endocrinol Metab. 1998 Mar;83(3):814-8. doi: 10.1210/jcem.83.3.4613. PMID: 9506733.

[29] A. Lucas, I. Salinas, F. Rius, E. Pizarro, M.L. Granada, M. Foz, A. SanmartÍ, Medical Therapy of Graves' Disease: Does Thyroxine Prevent Recurrence of Hyperthyroidism? The Journal of Clinical Endocrinology & Metabolism, Volume 82, Issue 8, 1 August 1997, Pages 2410-2413

[30] Fan Yang, Tingting Yu, Xiaolan Jiang et al. Coupling methimazole with L-thyroxine on bone of older patients with Graves' disease. Int J Clin Exp Med 2016;9(9):18458-18464

[31] Geffner DL, Hershman JM. Beta-adrenergic blockade for the treatment of hyperthyroidism. Am J Med. 1992 Jul;93(1):61-8. doi: 10.1016/0002-9343(92)90681-z. PMID: 1352658.

[32] Wiersinga WM. Propranolol and thyroid hormone metabolism. Thyroid. 1991 Summer;1(3):273-7. doi: 10.1089/thy.1991.1.273. PMID: 1688102.

[33] Murchison LE, How J, Bewsher PD. Comparison of propranolol and metoprolol in the management of hyperthyroidism. Br J Clin Pharmacol. 1979 Dec;8(6):581-7. doi: 10.1111/j.1365-2125.1979.tb01048.x. PMID: 391258; PMCID: PMC1429912.

[34] Okosieme OE, Taylor PN, Dayan CM. Should radioiodine now be first line treatment for Graves' disease? Thyroid Res. 2020 Mar 9;13:3. doi: 10.1186/s13044-020-00077-8. PMID: 32165924; PMCID: PMC7061474.

[35] Fanning E, Inder WJ, Mackenzie E. Radioiodine treatment for graves' disease: a 10-year Australian cohort study. BMC Endocr Disord. 2018 Dec 12;18(1):94. doi: 10.1186/s12902-018-0322-7. PMID: 30541519; PMCID: PMC6292026.

[36] Plazinska MT, Sawicka-Gutaj N, Czarnywojtek A, Wolinski K, Kobylecka M, Karlińska M, Prasek K, Zgorzalewicz-Stachowiak M, Borowska M, Gut P, Ruchala M, Krolicki L. Radioiodine therapy and Graves' disease - Myths and reality. PLoS One. 2020 Jan 13;15(1):e0226495. doi: 10.1371/journal.pone.0226495. PMID: 31929534; PMCID: PMC6957158.

[37] Smithson M, Asban A, Miller J, Chen H. Considerations for Thyroidectomy as Treatment for Graves Disease. Clinical Medicine Insights: Endocrinology and Diabetes Volume 12: 1-5. DOI 10.1177/1179551419844523.

[38] Barczynski M, Konturek A, Hubalewska-Dydejczyk A, Golkowski F, Nowak W. Randomized clinical trial of bilateral subtotal thyroidectomy versus total thyroidectomy for Graves' disease with a 5-year follow-up. Br J Surg. 2012;99:515-522.

[39] Feroci F, Rettori M, Borrelli A, et al. A systematic review and meta-analysis of total thyroidectomy versus bilateral subtotal thyroidectomy for Graves' disease. Surgery. 2014;155:529-540

[40] Carroll R, Matfin G. Endocrine and metabolic emergencies: thyroid storm. Ther Adv Endocrinol Metab (2010) 1(3) 139145

[41] Idrose A. Acute and emergency care for thyrotoxicosis and thyroid storm. Acute Medicine & Surgery 2015; 2: 147-157

[42] Laura C Lane, Tim D Cheetham, Petros Perros, Simon H S Pearce, New Therapeutic Horizons for Graves' Hyperthyroidism, *Endocrine Reviews*, Volume 41, Issue 6, December 2020, bnaa022,

Chapter 9

Radioiodine for Graves' Disease Therapy

Aisyah Elliyanti

Abstract

Radioiodine-131 (RAI) is an isotope of the chemical element iodine and is commonly used for hyperthyroidism, including Graves' Disease. It is given orally, and its concentration in the thyroid gland. The RAI transport involves a natrium iodide symporter (NIS) role that brings two cations sodium (Na+) and one anion of iodide (I-) across the membrane. The process is facilitated by the enzyme Na+/K+ ATPase. RAI is a beta (β) and gamma (γ) particles emitter. β particle is used for therapy and γ particle for imaging (theranostic). β particle inhibits cell growth by inducing cell death through apoptosis or necrosis of some of the sufficient thyroid cells. The aim of RAI therapy in Graves' Disease is to control hyperthyroidism and render the patient hypothyroidism. It is easier to manage patients with hypothyroidism with levothyroxine and fewer complications. This review will focus on RAI's therapeutic approach in Graves' Disease, including patient preparation, selecting activity dose, adverse events, contraindication, controversies issues such as malignancy and fertility, the follow-up to ensuring the patient remains euthyroid or need a replacement therapy if they become hypothyroidism. RAI therapy is safe as definitive therapy and cost-effective for Graves' Disease therapy.

Keywords: hyperthyroidism, hypothyroidism, malignancy, pregnancy, replacement therapy

1. Introduction

Graves' Disease is an autoimmune disorder that affects the thyroid gland, and it causes 50–80% of hyperthyroid cases and is associated with a firm diffuse goiter [1–3]. Its etiology is not entirely understood. The disease occurs in patients with having a genetic history and combination with environmental factors and lifestyles. Graves' Disease (GD) is characterized by elevated thyroid-stimulating receptor antibodies with increased thyroid hormone production [4–6]. GD can also affect other organs, including the eyes and skin. The annual incidence rate has been estimated at 14–50 cases per 100,000 persons. The peak incidence is between 30–50 years. Even though the disease may affect every age, the incidence is higher in women than men, with a 6:1 ratio [2, 5].

Graves' Disease treatments depend on the presentation. The treatment consists of symptomatic therapy and reduction of thyroid hormone synthesis. The symptomatic therapy, such as a beta-adrenergic blocker, is given for patients with tachycardia, a history of cardiovascular disease, and elderly patients [2, 6]. Therapies for reducing thyroid hormone synthesis are antithyroid drugs (ATDs), radioactive iodine (RAI), and thyroidectomy [2, 3, 6–8]. All three options have advantages and disadvantages. There is no consensus on which one is the best choice, and it is one of the more debatable issues. The treatment choice is likely to be influenced by local availability, treatment cost, patient's preferences, and socio-economy that caused vary from country to country.

Antithyroid drugs are widely used in Europe and most of Asia as first-line therapy. However, RAI is used by most physicians in the United States of America. [3, 6–8]. Hertz and Roberts were used radioiodine I-130 for the first time on March 31, 1941, for hyperthyroidism treatment [9, 10]. Its radiation was delivered rapidly to the thyroid cells over a day or two. Since the Atomic Energy Commission was allowed to supply the fission products for peaceful medical use in August 1946, I-130 was replaced by I-131 because I-131 was much cheaper [9]. RAI is used for therapy and imaging (theranostic). It is a beta (β) and gamma (γ) emitter with a half-life of 8.05 days. A β particle has a peak energy of 0.606 MeV, with a maximum range of ~3 mm in the tissue used for therapy. The peak of γ particle is 0.364 MeV is used for imaging [4, 11, 12]. The longer physical half-life of RAI ensures long-term irradiation of the target tissues, becoming a potential advantage.

RAI therapy aims to treat hyperthyroidism by destroying sufficient thyroid cells to reach either euthyroid or hypothyroid conditions. Radioactive iodine is safe as definitive therapy, cure rates ~80–90%, and cost-effective, rarely or minor side-effects. [4, 6, 7, 11–14]. The choice of therapy depends on the patient's preference. The choice of therapy should take into account local availability and cost-effectiveness. In practical terms, RAI is administrated as an outpatient visit, and it is an advantage. RAI is recommended for optimal treatment of Graves' Disease by the American Thyroid Association (ATA) and American Association of Clinical Endocrinologists (AACE) guidelines for the management of thyrotoxicosis 2011 and ATA 2016 [3, 6, 15]. The recent guidelines of the United Kingdom (UK) National Institute for Health and Care Excellence (NICE) recommend that radioiodine should now be the first-line treatment for Graves' Disease in the UK [7].

2. Transport radioiodine

RAI is administrated in a capsule or liquid. Once it is ingested, it is quickly absorbed into the bloodstream in the gastrointestinal (GI) tract. It is taken up by

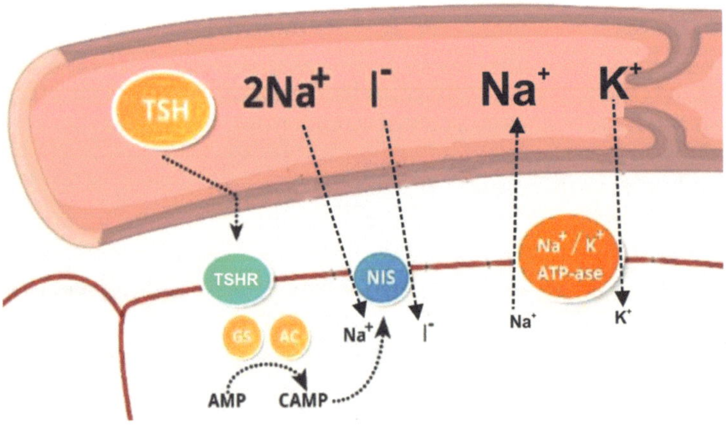

Figure 1.
Natrium iodide symporter brings two cations of sodium (Na^+) and one anion of iodide (I^-) cross the epithelial thyroid cells' at the basolateral membrane. The process is facilitated by the enzyme Na+/K+ ATPase.

thyroid cells through active transport, which is the same natural iodine process. The transport involves a natrium iodide symporter (NIS) role that brings two cations sodium (Na^+) and one anion of iodide (I^-). The process is facilitated by an enzyme Na+/K+ ATPase, as shown in **Figure 1**. NIS is a transmembrane glycoprotein that contains 13 membrane-spanning segments and three N-linked carbohydrates. It resides in the basolateral membrane of epithelial thyroid cells [16–20]. Besides the thyroid cell, NIS is expressed by extra-thyroid tissues [20]. NIS expression increased RAI uptake for diagnostic and therapy in thyroid extra-thyroid organ.

3. The mechanism action of RAI

β particle of RAI inhibits cell growth by inducing cell death through apoptosis or necrosis. Cell responses to radiation are influenced by various factors that lead to different responses between cells. The amount of RAI radiation received by cells is affected by the capture and accumulation of RAI and its biological half-life, which correlates with the effects. Cell responses to radiation are influenced by the cell's sensitivity and the complexity of the cells' micro-environments [21, 22]. Due to the small therapeutic range of β particles within the tissues, naturally, no β particles escape from the thyroid. So, the remaining non-target tissue (i.e., parathyroid glands) still safe even though high activity RAI dose is given to the patients. [4, 11, 23].

A β particle of RAI has a low Linear Energy Transfer (LET) value (0.2 KeV/μm). It causes cell death, direct and indirect. The decay of radioisotopes in the cell (self-dose) cause DNA damage through direct breakage of molecular bonds. The formation of free radicals or the decay of radioisotopes in adjacent cells (cross-fire) indirectly causes cell death, as shown in **Figure 2**. The condition leads to a reduction of thyroid function and diminished thyroid size [24, 25].

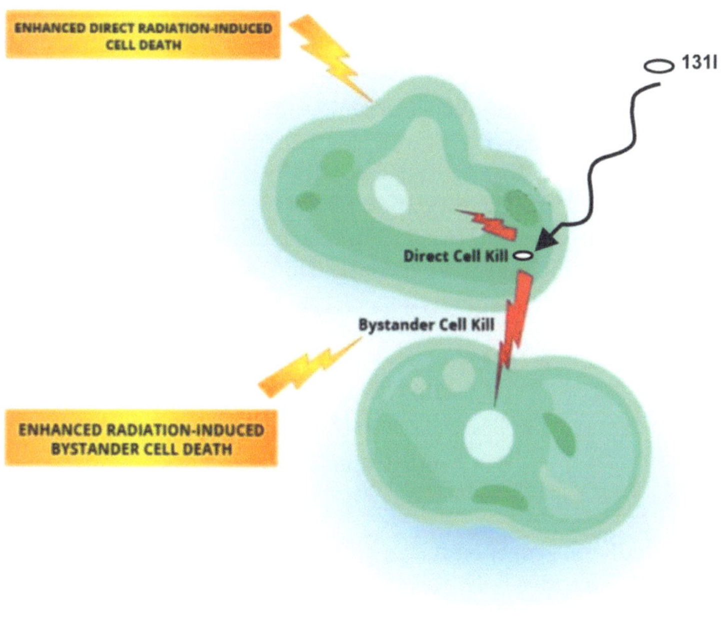

Figure 2.
RAI radiation damages a DNA directly (lethal and sub-lethal) or indirectly from adjacent cell radiation (cross-fire/bystander).

4. Treatment protocol

Many studies reported various approaches to RAI therapy published by different institutions. It remains a matter of debate when choosing the treatment protocols, whether a calculated dose that considers radioiodine uptake (RAIU) and thyroid volume measurements versus a fixed-dose, or a high dose versus a low dose, or whether short term versus long term medical management. RAI administrates as low as reasonably achievable (ALARA) dose that is an essential principle for radiation treatment [23, 25].

5. Radioiodine dose

RAI therapy is well established for the definitive treatment of GD. However, Its approach remains controversial due to differing treatment control goals. It is between hyperthyroidism versus avoidance of hypothyroidism. Various methods of RAI doses have been used to deliver adequate radiation to the thyroid gland. Radiation dose to the thyroid depends on the RAI uptake, thyroid volume, and biologic half-life of the RAI. Actually, RAI activity dose measured based an amount of the radiation delivered to the thyroid gland rather than administered activity, but few publications confirm this unequivocally [23]. Three approaches for determining the administered RAI activity doses. 1. Based on the calculation of thyroid volume and the RAI uptake 24 hours. 2. Based on thyroid volume, RAI uptake, effective half-life. 3. Fixed activity dose [4, 11].

In calculation approaches, the thyroid volume, RAI uptake, and effective half-life are factors determine the activity dose. It is recommended a delivered activity of RAI about 3–8 MBq (80–220 μCi) per gram of thyroid mass, with absorbed radiation dose 100–150 Gy to restore a euthyroid status, whereas the total ablation dose is in the range 200–300 Gy [12, 14, 23]. Naturally, the normal thyroid mass is about 20 grams. Ultrasound, x-ray/MRI studies, and scintigraphy thyroid can be used to evaluate thyroid volume. However, ultrasonography is superior to all of these techniques because of its relatively low cost, wide availability, ease of technically.

The RAI uptake should be appropriately prepared to ensure its real thyroid uptake. The patient should be advised to avoid meals for at least 2 hours before and 2 hours after the oral administration of RAI for the test. The thyroid uptake can also be measure by intravenous administration of Tc-99 m pertechnetate. The pertechnetate is trapped but not be organification by the thyroid. The measurement usually after 20 minutes of the injection [6, 11, 23]. GD uptakes usually high unless the patient has a history of iodine intake recently. However, the calculated dose versus fixed-dose effectiveness is an equally successful outcome [6, 26]. Radioactive iodine uptake (RAIU) can be calculated using formula (1) [12].

$$\text{RIAU}(\%) = \frac{\text{thyroid counts}(cpm)}{\text{Administrated counts}(cpm)} x\,100. \quad (1)$$

An effective half-life is needed for an accurate absorbed dose calculation to the thyroid [6, 11]. Effective half-life is the combination of the physical half-life (constant for a particular nucleus) and the biological half-life (varies from patient to patient). A radionuclide in a living tissue decays in two ways, physical decay and biological elimination from the body is called biological half-life. The effective half-life of RAI in the thyroid can be determined by measuring its uptake at several different periods following RAI administration. It may vary from 1.2 to 7.5 days in hyperthyroidism (i.e., the variation factor is 6.25). The effective half-life calculation is cumbersome. It has a lot of calculations and assumptions that may have a human error. Effective half-life calculation will increase the accuracy of RAI activity dose [11]. However, the outcome has not been shown to be better, so the method is rarely used [6].

Fixed-dose of RAI activities is a simple protocol and convenient to use. It can be administered as a single dose and be repeated as necessary, with a range of 185–740 MBq (5- 20 mCi). The administration dose is given based on validated clinical parameters and an estimated thyroid size by palpation or measurement by ultrasonography or scintigraphy [26, 23, 25].

The majority of patients cure with a single RAI dose [11, 13]. Many physicians prefer a single high RAI dose, which leads to hypothyroidism. Cure rate high dose reach 85% - 94.4%, and 66–74% for low dose [4, 11, 14]. A single high dose or ablative dose concept is preferred by a physician today. It can avoid patients' frequent visits and laboratory testing for hypothyroid onset detection. It decreases the risk of persistent or recurrent hyperthyroidism [23]. A low dose is administered to achieve a euthyroid state to avoid hypothyroidism. 50%–90% of patients become hypothyroidism within 3–12 months [13]. Around 14% of hyperthyroid patients required second therapy. Persistence hyperthyroidism showed 7.3% after received 555 MBq (15 mCi) RAI [12, 13].

On the other hand, the low activity dose is generally not recommended because many patients need RAI retreatment. Furthermore, most patients will become hypothyroid after RAI [4, 23, 25]. Finally, therapy aims to control hyperthyroidism and render the patient to be hypothyroidism. The therapy outcome can be accomplished equally by administering a fixed RAI activity dose or calculating the activity based on the thyroid RAIU and size.

6. Patient preparation

Certain evaluations for adequate treatment include the treatment history such as ATDs, food or medication containing iodine that blocked radioiodine uptake that needs to discontinue before the treatment, and the duration of their period as shown in **Table 1**.

Pharmaceutical	Withdrawal duration
ATDs (propylthiouracil, methimazole carbimazole)	7–14 days before therapy 7 days after therapy
Thyroid hormones • Triiodothyronine • Thyroxine	 10–14 days 3–4 weeks
Lugol solution	2–3 weeks
Vitamins containing iodine	7–10 days
Amiodarone	3–6 months
Intravenous radiographic contrast agents • Water soluble • Lipophilic	 6–8 weeks 1–6 months

Table 1.
Pharmaceuticals containing iodine block of RAI uptake [4, 6, 11, 23, 25].

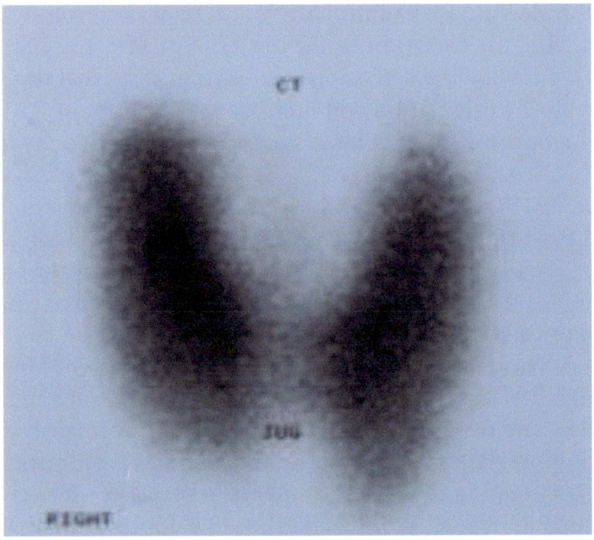

Figure 3.
Scintigraphy thyroid showed enlargement of both thyroid lobes, with high diffuse uptake of a Tc-99 m pertechnetate.

The patient should also be advised to avoid meals for at least 2 hours before and 2 hours after the oral administration of RAI. Large meals can slow the absorption of RAI. Laboratory results, including free T4, free T3, Thyroid-stimulating hormone (TSH). Thyroid scintigraphy is used to assess the potential variability distribution of RAI in the thyroid gland. Graves' Disease scintigraphy pattern is a diffuse high uptake at the thyroid gland. It can differentiate between Graves' Disease with toxic adenoma and toxic multinodular goiter, as shown in **Figure 3**. Ultrasonography assessment may be useful if patients have a contraindication for the scintigraphy, such as during breastfeeding and pregnancy [6]. The choice of testing depends on cost, local availability, and expertise. RAIU measurements are not required when fixed activities are used. Thyroid ultrasonography can be used to determine thyroid volume. Pregnancy test for child-bearing females within 72 hours before the RAI administration, and when pregnancy is excluded, the test can be omitted.

For patients with ophthalmopathy, RAI can exacerbate existing Graves' ophthalmopathy (GO) [11, 12, 23]. Smokers, high serum triiodothyronine pre-treatment, posttherapy hypothyroidism, and thyroid-stimulating receptor antibody are also associated with an increased risk of developing or worsening ophthalmopathy [23]. Steroids prevent the risk of RAI-induced ophthalmopathy without influence the outcome of therapy. Mild and active ophthalmopathy pre-exists patients with high-risk factors associated with development or worsening of ophthalmopathy should receive steroid prophylaxis [25, 27, 28].

RAI therapy may need to be repeated. Patients also need a long-term follow- up because of the likelihood of eventual hypothyroidism and very uncommon side effects. Written information must be provided, and the patient should obtain written informed consent before therapy.

7. Contraindication

Absolute contraindications of RAI are in pregnancy and during breastfeeding and in patients who cannot comply with radiation safety regulations. Relative contraindications are uncontrolled hyperthyroidism and active thyroid orbitopathy (especially in smokers) [4, 6, 12, 25]. RAI is not contraindicated in large goiters, even if partially retrosternal or intrathoracic [25]. A higher cure rate reaches up to 96%, even for thyroid size of more than 40 gram [12].

8. Adverse effects

Some patients, especially those who have large thyroid mass, may notice a transient swelling of goiter for approximately one week after therapy, salivary gland discomfort, or dyspnoea. Nausea that could develop into vomiting depends on the amount of administered activity for RAI. Antiemetic treatment can reduce the symptom. The effects are infrequent when the patients received <1.1 103 MBq (<30 mCi). Those effects are usually observed on a high dose >3.7 103 MBq (> 100 mCi) of RAI [29].

RAI treatment can cause a transient exacerbation of hyperthyroidism. The β- adrenergic blocker should be considered in symptomatic and asymptomatic patients who have hyperthyroidism risk (i.e., elderly patients and patients with comorbidities) [6]. Even though it is rare, the radiation can induce thyroiditis and thyroid hormone release into the circulation leading to thyroid storm precipitation [4, 6, 12]. The condition is more likely occurring in patients with a large thyroid mass and who received higher RAI activities. Elderly patients and patients with significant pre-existing heart disease, severe systemic illness, or debility may benefit from pre-treatment with ATDs. However, ATDs should be withdrawn for one week before RAI therapy and resumed a week afterward [4, 6, 23, 25].

The aim of RAI therapy in GD is to control hyperthyroidism and render hypothyroidism. It is easier to manage hypothyroidism with levothyroxine and fewer complications compared to treat hyperthyroidism with ATDs in the long term, leading to undesirable therapy effects [30]. The number of mortality reduced in hyperthyroid patients who become hypothyroidism after RAI therapy. The condition is implying the survival advantages of hyperthyroidism control. The risk of mortality of patients with hyperthyroidism, whether caused by cardiovascular or cancer, appears to be driven by thyroid hormone excess [4, 31].

9. Malignancy

The challenge of RAI's late effect is concern developing the risk of malignancy after RAI treatment. Based on multi-center trials, there was no association of any clinical malignancy of RAI for the therapy. [7, 9, 11, 13, 23, 29, 31]. The malignancy is associate with a small risk of pre-existing or coexisting thyroid cancer in patients with toxic nodular goiter. Graves' Disease was not related to cancer development after RAI therapy [23].

10. Pregnancy

Conception should be delayed after six months of the therapy. The same period applies for males to allow irradiated spermatozoa and complete ovarian recovery for patients without undergone gonadal function and thyroid hormone under control [12]. Child-bearing women have no evidence of decreased fertility after received RAI treatment and no adverse outcome on subsequent pregnancies [32]. The incidence of intrauterine growth restriction, neonatal gender, and premature birth did not significantly differ between patients who received RAI therapy and antithyroid drugs (ATDs). However, a higher abortion rate was found in Graves' Disease patients who received RAI and ATDs [33].

Furthermore, patients with intractable Graves' Disease and too high thyroid-stimulating receptor antibody who want to pregnant soon should not receive radioiodine therapy to avoid developing fetal or neonatal hyperthyroidism [34]. RAI exposures in the first ten weeks of pregnancy do not affect fetal growth, but after ten weeks, the exposures can affect the growth [35]. Studies reported have no evidence of genetic damage and congenital anomaly, miscarriage, and preterm birth in patients who received RAI with the general population [7, 11, 13, 25, 36–38].

11. Follow-ups

Long-term follow-up after RAI therapy is needed. The likelihood of eventual hypothyroidism can occur within 2–3 months after therapy or even decades later, with a small, ongoing annual incidence. Lifelong thyroid hormone supplementation would then become necessary and should be started when thyroid-stimulating hormone elevation is detected and should have as its goal a euthyroid, symptom-free state [23]. Transient hypothyroidism is reported in 3–20% of cases. It does not invariably lead to permanent hypothyroidism, but thyroid hormone supplementation is generally recommended.

12. Conclusions

RAI therapy is safe as definitive therapy and cost-effective for Graves' Disease definitive treatment. The treatment has to be individualized. Patients should fully understand the treatment procedures to reach the desired outcome and handle the risks and adverse effects. Three approaches for determining the administered RAI activity doses. 1. Based on the calculation of thyroid volume and the RAI uptake 24 hours. 2. Based on thyroid volume, RAI uptake, effective half-life. 3. Fixed activity dose. However, the effectiveness is an equally successful outcome between them. RAI treatment aims in GD is to control hyperthyroid rather than avoidance of hypothyroidism. Hypothyroidism can occur within the first three months after RAI therapy or even decades later. Lifelong follow-up is needed to ensure recurrence of disease, and hypothyroidism is detected. Thyroid hormone supplementation would then become necessary and should be started when thyroid-stimulating hormone elevation is detected. Long-term studies show that radiation does not induce genetic damage or malignancy. However, conception should be delayed at least for six months after the therapy. So, the physician needs to provide written information for the patients to avoid miss interpretation.

Conflict of interest

The authors declare no conflict of interest.

Author details

Aisyah Elliyanti[1,2*]

1 Department of Medical Physics, Faculty of Medicine, Universitas Andalas, Padang, Indonesia

2 Nuclear Medicine Division of Radiology Department, Dr. M. Djamil Hospital, Padang, Indonesia

*Address all correspondence to: aelliyanti@med.unand.ac.id

References

[1] Chen YK, Lin CL, Chang YJ, Cheng FTF, Peng CL, et al. Cancer Risk in Patients with Graves' Disease: A Nationwide Cohort Study. Thyroid.2013;32(7):879-884

[2] Pokhrel B, Bhusal K. Graves Disease. [Updated 2020 Jul 21]. In: StatPearls [Internet]. Treasure Island (FL): StatPearls Publishing; 2020. Available from: https://www.ncbi.nlm.nih.gov/books/NBK448195/

[3] Karyampudi A, Hamide A, Halanaik D, Sahoo JP, Kamalanathan S. Radioiodine therapy in patients with Graves' disease and the effects of prior carbimazole therapy. Indian J Endocrinol Metab. 2014;18(5):688-693

[4] Mumtaz M, Lin LS, Hui KC, Mohd Khir AS. Radioiodine I-131 for the therapy of graves' disease. Malays J Med Sci. 2009;16(1):25-33.

[5] Campi, Irene & Salvi, Mario. Graves' Disease. 2018;doi: 10.1016/B978-0-12-801238-3.98495-2.

[6] Ross DS, Burch HB, Cooper DS, Greenlee MC, Laurberg P, Maia AL, Rivkees SA, Samuels M, Sosa JA, Stan MN, Walter MA. 2016 American Thyroid Association Guidelines for Diagnosis and Management of Hyperthyroidism and Other Causes of Thyrotoxicosis. Thyroid. 2016;26(10):1343-1421. doi: 10.1089/thy.2016.0229.

[7] Okosieme OE, Taylor PN, Dayan CM. Should radioiodine now be first line treatment for Graves' disease?. Thyroid Res. 2020;13:3. doi:10.1186/s13044-020-00077-8

[8] Kornelius E, Yang YS, Huang CN, Wang YH, Lo SC, Lai YR, Chiou JY. The trends of hyperthyroidism treatment in Taiwan: A nationwide population-based study. Endocr Pract. 2018;24(6):573-579. doi: 10.4158/EP-2017-0266.

[9] Bonnema SJ, Hegedüs L. Radioiodine therapy in benign thyroid diseases: effects, side effects, and factors affecting therapeutic outcome. Endocr Rev. 2012;33(6):920-980. doi: 10.1210/er.2012-1030.

[10] Slonimsky E, Tulchinsky M. Radiotheragnostics Paradigm for Radioactive Iodine (Iodide) Management of Differentiated Thyroid Cancer. Current Pharmaceutical Design. 2020;26:3812.doi: 10.2174/1381612826666200605121054

[11] Wazir M. Radioactive iodine therapy for hyperthyroidism: Physics, treatment protocols and radiation protection in Handbook of Hyperthyroidsm.2009

[12] Stokkel, M. & Handkiewicz-Junak, Daria & Lassmann, Michael & Dietlein, Markus & Luster, Markus. EANM procedure guidelines for therapy of benign thyroid disease. European journal of nuclear medicine and molecular imaging. 2010;37. 2218-28. doi :10.1007/s00259-010-1536-8.

[13] Al-Kaabi JM, Hussein SS, Bukheit CS, Woodhouse NJ, Elshafie OT, Bererhi H. Radioactive iodine in the treatment of Graves' disease. Saudi Med J. 2002;23(9):1049-1053.

[14] Radhi HT, Jamal HF, Sarwani AA, Jamal AJ, Al Alawi MF. Efficacy of a single fixed 131I dose of Radioactive iodine for the treatment of hyperthyroidism. Clin. Invest. 2019; 9(4): 111-120

[15] Bahn RS, Burch HB, Cooper DS, Garber JR, Greenlee MC, Klein I, et al. Hyperthyroidism and other causes of thyrotoxicosis: Management guidelines of the American Thyroid Association and American Association of Clinical Endocrinologists. Endocr Pract. 2011;17:456-520.

[16] Ravera S, Reyna-Neyra A, Ferrandino G, Amzel LM, Carrasco N. The Sodium/Iodide Symporter (NIS): Molecular Physiology and Preclinical and Clinical Applications. Annu Rev Physiol. 2017;79:261-289. doi: 10.1146/annurev-physiol-022516-034125.

[17] Elliyanti A, Rusnita D, Afriani N, Susanto YD, Susilo VY, Setiyowati S, et al. Analysis natrium iodide symporter expression in breast cancer subtypes for radioiodine therapy response. Nucl Med Mol Imaging. 2020;54(1):35-42.

[18] Darrouzet E, Lindenthal S, Marcellin D, Pellequer JL, Pourcher T. The sodium/iodide symporter: state of art of its molecular characterization. Biochim Biophys Acta. 1838;2013:244-253.

[19] Elliyanti A, Susilo VY, Setiyowati S, Rao PV. An Iodine Treatments Effect on Cell Proliferation Rates of Breast Cancer Cell Lines; In Vitro Study. Open Access Maced J Med Sci. 2020;8(B):1064-1070.

[20] Micali S, Bulotta S, Puppin C, Territo A, Navarra M, et al. Sodium iodide symporter (NIS) in extrathyroidal malignancies: focus on breast and urological cancer. BMC Cancer. 2014;14:303.

[21] Kogai T, Brent GA. The Sodium Iodide Symporter (NIS): Regulation and Approaches to Targeting for cancer Therapeutics. Pharmacology&Therape utics.2012;135:355-370

[22] Kim HW, Kim JE, Hwang MH, Jeon YH, Lee SW, Lee J, Zeon SK, Ahn BC. Enhancement of natural killer cell cytotoxicity by sodium/iodide symporter gene-mediated radioiodine pretreatment in breast cancer cells. PLoS One. 2013;8(8):e70194. doi: 10.1371/journal.pone.0070194.

[23] Silberstein EB, Alavi A, Balon HR, Clarke SE, Divgi C, Gelfand MJ, Goldsmith SJ, Jadvar H, Marcus CS, Martin WH, Parker JA, Royal HD, Sarkar SD, Stabin M, Waxman AD. The SNMMI practice guideline for therapy of thyroid disease with 131I 3.0. J Nucl Med. 2012 ;53(10):1633-1651. doi: 10.2967/jnumed.112.105148.

[24] Hingorani M, Spitzweg C, Vassaux G, Newbold K, Melcher A, Pandha H, Vile R, Harrington K. The biology of the sodium iodide symporter and its potential for targeted gene delivery. Curr Cancer Drug Targets. 2010;10(2):242-67. doi: 10.2174/156800910791054194.

[25] Kahaly G, J, Bartalena L, Hegedüs L, Leenhardt L, Poppe K, Pearce S, H: 2018 European Thyroid Association Guideline for the Management of Graves' Hyperthyroidism. Eur Thyroid J 2018;7:167-186. doi: 10.1159/000490384

[26] de Rooij A, Vandenbroucke JP, Smit JW, et al. Clinical outcomes after estimated versus calculated activity of radioiodine for the treatment of hyperthyroidism: systematic review and meta-analysis. 2009. In: Database of Abstracts of Reviews of Effects (DARE): Quality-assessed Reviews [Internet]. York (UK): Centre for Reviews and Dissemination (UK); 1995-.https://www.ncbi.nlm.nih.gov/books/NBK78254/

[27] Vannucchi G, Covelli D, Campi I, Currò N, Dazzi D, Rodari M, Pepe G, Chiti A, Guastella C, Lazzaroni E, Salvi M. Prevention of Orbitopathy by Oral or Intravenous Steroid Prophylaxis in Short Duration Graves' Disease Patients Undergoing Radioiodine Ablation: A Prospective Randomized Control Trial Study. Thyroid. 2019 ;29(12):1828-1833. doi: 10.1089/thy.2019.0150.

[28] Shiber S, Stiebel-Kalish H, Shimon I, Grossman A, Robenshtok E. Glucocorticoid regimens for prevention of Graves' ophthalmopathy progression following radioiodine treatment:

systematic review and meta-analysis. Thyroid. 2014 ;24(10):1515-1523. doi: 10.1089/thy.2014.0218.

[29] Tulchinsky M, Brill AB. Spotlight on the Association of Radioactive Iodine Treatment With Cancer Mortality in Patients With Hyperthyroidism is Keeping the Highest Risk From Antithyroid Drugs in the Blind Spot. Clin Nucl Med. 2019;44(10):789-791. doi: 10.1097/RLU.0000000000002792.

[30] Chen DY, Jing J, Schneider PF, et al. Comparison of the long- term efficacy of low dose 131I versus antithyroid drugs in the treatment of hyperthyroidism. Nucl Med Commun.2009; 30: 160-168

[31] Ron E, Doody MM, Becker DV, et al. Cancer mortality following treatment for adult hyperthyroidism. Cooperative Thyrotoxicosis Therapy Follow-up Study Group. JAMA. 1998;280(4):347-355. doi: 10.1001/jama.280.4.347.

[32] Vini L, Hyer S, Al-Saadi A, Pratt B, Harmer C. Prognosis for fertility and ovarian function after treatment with radioiodine for thyroid cancer. Postgrad Med J. 2002;78(916):92-93. doi:10.1136/pmj.78.916.92

[33] Zhang LH, Li JY, Tian Q, et al. Follow-up and evaluation of the pregnancy outcome in women of reproductive age with Graves' disease after 131Iodine treatment. J Radiat Res. 2016;57(6):702-708. doi:10.1093/jrr/rrw049

[34] Hamada N, Momotani N, Ishikawa N, Yoshimura Noh J, Okamoto Y, Konishi T, Ito K, Ito K. Persistent high TRAb values during pregnancy predict increased risk of neonatal hyperthyroidism following radioiodine therapy for refractory hyperthyroidism. Endocr J. 2011;58(1):55-58. doi: 10.1507/endocrj.k10e-123.

[35] Tran P, Desimone S, Barrett M, Bachrach B. I-131 treatment of graves' disease in an unsuspected first trimester pregnancy; the potential for adverse effects on the fetus and a review of the current guidelines for pregnancy screening. Int J Pediatr Endocrinol. 2010;2010:858359. doi: 10.1155/2010/858359.

[36] Brandão Carmen Dolores G., Miranda Angélica E., Corrêa Nilson Duarte, Sieiro Netto Lino, Corbo Rossana, Vaisman Mario. Radioiodine therapy and subsequent pregnancy. Arq Bras Endocrinol Metab. 2007; 51(4): 534-540.

[37] Dottorini ME, Lomuscio G, Mazzucchelli L, Vignati A, Colombo L. Assessment of female fertility and carcinogenesis after iodine-131 therapy for differentiated thyroid carcinoma. J Nucl Med. 1995;36(1):21-27.

[38] Balenovic A, Vlasic M, Sonicki Z, Bodor, Kusic Z. Pregnancy Outcome after Treatment with Radioiodine for Differentiated Thyroid Carcinoma, Coll. Antropol. 2006; 30 : 743-748

Chapter 10

RAI Therapy for Graves' Hyperthyroidism

Ioannis Iakovou, Evanthia Giannoula, Paraskevi Exadaktylou and Nikitas Papadopoulos

Abstract

Graves' Disease is the most common cause of hyperthyroidism. It has multiple manifestations and it requires appropriate diagnostic and therapeutic management. Once it has been established that the patient is hyperthyroid and the cause is GD, the patient and physician must choose between three effective and relatively safe initial treatment options: antithyroid drugs (ATDs), radioiodine (RAI) therapy, or thyroidectomy. RAI has been used to treat hyperthyroidism for more than seven decades. It is well tolerated and complications are rare, except for those related to orbitopathy. Most patients are effectively treated with one therapeutic dose of I-131. The patient usually notes symptomatic improvement within 3 weeks of therapy. However, the full therapeutic effect takes 3 to 6 months because stored hormone must first be released. Radioiodine therapy may not initially be effective in up to 10% of patients. They require repeat treatment, usually with a higher administered dose.

Keywords: RAI, hyperthyroidism, therapy, Graves' Disease, Nuclear Medicine, theranostics, guidelines

1. Introduction

Thyrotoxicosis is a very common clinical syndrome caused by an excess of thyroid hormones in the serum. It results in a generalized acceleration of metabolic processes. Occasionally, thyrotoxicosis may be due to other causes. Graves' Disease is the commonest cause of hyperthyroidism, typically presenting in patients between 40–60 years. It is characterized by the presence of thyroid stimulating hormone receptor antibodies (TRAbs) but pathogenesis is not completely understood [1]. The thyroid stimulating hormone receptor (TSHR) is a transmembrane G-protein-coupled receptor (GPCR) and when it is activated by thyroid stimulating hormone (TSH) it stimulates thyroid hormone production [2]. TRAbs mimic the action of TSH leading to hyperthyroidism. Although autoimmune mechanisms are responsible for the syndrome of GD, management has been largely directed toward controlling the hyperthyroidism. Three therapeutic methods are available: (1) antithyroid drug therapy (ATD), (2) surgery, and (3) radioiodine treatment (RAI) and have proved to be effective, safe and cost-effective. They can be the first-line treatment for hyperthyroidism not only due to Graves' Disease, but also due to toxic adenoma, and toxic multinodular goiter [3]. Nowadays research has turned its focus on the potential use of immunotherapy in GD [4, 5]. It is remarkable that the

IntechOpen

selection of the right therapy for each patient still poses a challenge to the clinician as there is no single best therapy for all patients [6].

Radioactive iodine (I-131), has been commonly used for the treatment of both benign and malignant thyroid conditions since the 1940s. In the early days of nuclear medicine, endocrinologists were attracted to the field by the potential of radioiodine for diagnosis and therapy. Today thyroid diagnosis and therapy continue to have an important role in the practice of nuclear medicine. The story of radioiodine started in 1935 at the Massachusetts Institute of Technology in cooperation with the Thyroid Unit of the Massachussetts General Hospital. Diagnostic thyroid studies were performed for the first time in 1937 using iodine-128. In 1938, not more than one year later, I-130 and I-131 were discovered, followed by the first treatment of benign thyroid disease in. Hertz and Roberts were the first to do so on March 31, 1941; Hamilton and John Lawrence, began on October 12, 1941. In 1946 the Oak Ridge National Laboratory produced I-131 for routine use and from this time on I-131 treatment is increasingly performed not only in benign thyroid disease but also in differential thyroid cancer (DTC) [7].

Nuclear medicine involves the administration of radiopharmaceuticals to patients for diagnostic and therapeutic purposes. The theranostic approach is an established tool for specific molecular targeting, both for diagnostics and therapy. Most radiopharmaceuticals are a combination of radioactive molecule, a radionuclide, that permits external detection and a biologically active molecule or drug that acts as a carrier and determines localization and biodistribution. For a few radiotracers (e.g., radioiodine), the radioactive atoms themselves confer the desired localization properties [8]. RAI in GD includes the systemic administration of 131-I for selective irradiation of hyperfunctioning thyroid gland. The efficacy and safety of this treatment and the advantages over thyroid surgery and ATDs have been documented and are widely accepted. Several guidelines, protocols and recommendations have been released by various scientific societies including the European Association of Nuclear Medicine (EANM), and the American Society of Nuclear Medicine Molecular Imaging (SNMMI), European Thyroid Association (ETA) and American Thyroid Association (ATA) whose procedural guidelines are updated in last decade and will be discussed in this chapter.

2. Physical and radiobiological properties of (radio)iodine

Physicians responsible for treating thyroid disorders should have an understanding of the clinical pathophysiology and natural history of the disease processes. They also should be familiar with iodine uptake and metabolism. Iodine is a micronutrient of crucial importance for the health and well-being of all individuals. It is mostly obtained from food sources. Thyroid gland plays the central role in the metabolism of iodine. When iodine enters the bloodstream it is then taken up by thyroid follicular cells through an active transport system the sodium iodide symporter (NIS) which is located at the basolateral membrane of the follicular cell [9]. Then, peroxidase promotes iodine to bound to thyroglobulin (Tg) and in particular to tyrosine which is then iodinated. The latter leads to the formation of 3-monoiodotyrosine (MIT) and 3,5-diiodotyrosine (DIT) which are coupled afterwards leading to the formation of thyroid hormones. Two molecules of DIT form thyroxine (T4) hormone and when one MIT and one DIT molecule couple they form Triiodothyronine (T3) hormone. Thyroid hormones remain stored in the thyroid cells in a thick fluid that is called colloid. Colloid can store a 3 month supply of thyroid hormones. Thyroid stimulating hormone (TSH) regulates thyroid hormone production. In particular it stimulates NIS expression which then activates follicular cells through TSH receptor (TSH-R). The uptake and metabolism of the radioactive iodine (I-123 and I-131) does not differ from nutritional iodine uptake in the normal or hyperfunctional gland.

I-131used for the treatment of thyroid disorders has a physical half life of 8.4 days and undergoes beta-minus decay emitting a principle primary gamma photon of 364 kiloelectron volts (keV) (81% abundance). The 364-keV photons are not optimal for gamma cameras. The detection sensitivity for I-131 (i.e. the amount of photons detected by the gamma camera) is poor. Approximately half of the photons penetrate a 3/8-inch crystal without being detected. Other higher energy I-131 emissions will pass though the collimators holes leading to image degradation. Beta-minus decay also results to emission of beta particles of 0.606 megaelectron volt (MeV) (89% abundance) which are responsible for the therapy outcome but cannot be used for imaging. The I-131 high-energy beta emissions and long physical half-life of gamma emissions result in a high radiation dose to the patient, particularly to the thyroid. Thyroid gland which is the target organ of RAI treatment receives ultimately a high radiation dose ~0.01Gy/μCi, and this defines the maximum applicable administered dose [10]. Radiobiological effects of radioiodine on tissues are direct (radiation deposit within DNA) or indirect. Indirect effects produce free radicals that in turn react with critical macromolecules. The cellular effect of the ionizing radiation leads to genetic damage, mutations, or cell death. The DNA damage from radiation is mediated via a combination of direct effects, through breakage of molecular bonds, or indirectly through the formation of free radicals. This leads to a decrease in thyroid function and/or reduction in thyroid size. There are neither good measures of individual radiosensitivity nor ideal methods of predicting the clinical response to RAI therapy [11].

3. Treatment choices for Graves' hyperthyroidism

Patients with overt Graves' hyperthyroidism should be treated with any of the following modalities: RAI therapy, ATDs, or thyroidectomy. Once the diagnosis has been made, the treating physician and patient should discuss each of the treatment options, including the logistics, benefits, expected speed of recovery, drawbacks, potential side effects, and costs. This sets the stage for the physician to make recommendations based on best clinical judgment and allows the final decision to incorporate the personal values and preferences of the patient. The treatment selection should also take into account the local availability and the associated costs. Whenever surgery is selected as treatment one should consider the use of expert high-volume thyroid surgeons with on average lower risk of complications; lack of that expertise should be considered against the known risk of alternative choices. Long-term continuous treatment of hyperthyroidism with ATDs may be considered in selected cases [12]. Despite the use of these three treatments for decades, selection of the optimal therapy for GD still poses a challenge for both the physician and the patient.

3.1 Thyroidectomy

Thyroidectomy, in particular subtotal thyroidectomy, is the oldest way of treating hyperthyroidism [13]. A Swiss surgeon, Theodor Kocher (1841–1917) won the Nobel Prize for Medicine and Physiology in 1909 after performing the first successful surgeries for GD [14]. Nowadays, thyroidectomy is the least preferable therapeutic selection for GD worldwide [15]. However, in some circumstances it is regarded as the most preferable treatment option. In particular, it is indicated for women who are planning a pregnancy in less than 6 months (provided they are rendered euthyroid with ATD), in patients with large goiters (≥80 g) or with compressive symptoms, in cases of coexisting hyperparathyroidism which will lead to a surgery and when thyroid cancer is suspected. Also, surgery is preferred in patients with moderate to severe active Graves orbitopathy (GO), in cases of large thyroid nodules that are additionally cold (has lower radiopharmaceutical uptake than the surrounding thyroid tissue) on scintigraphy, when TRAb values are very high or radioiodine uptake is low. Thyroidectomy should not be considered in patients with comorbid conditions such as cardiopulmonary disease and end-stage malignancy. Lack of access to a high-volume thyroid surgeon may also, directs against the choice of surgery. During pregnancy it can be considered as an emergency treatment of hyperthyroidism, when rapid control of the latter is crucial and ATD therapy cannot be used, but it is followed by a higher rate of complications such as hypoparathyroidism and recurrent laryngeal nerve (RLN) injury [12].

Thyroidectomy can be associated with postoperative complications, such as hypocalcemia, wound infection, hematoma, recurrent laryngeal nerve (RLN) injury, and Horner's syndrome. Those complications are dependent on surgeon's experience and skills as well as on removal approaches and the type and extent of the disease, having a great impact on patient's quality of life. Studies have shown that surgeons experience and post surgery complications are inversely proportional. In rare cases, after subtotal thyroidectomy recurrence of GD may be present [16].

3.2 Antithyroid drugs

ATD represent the predominant therapy in Europe, Asia, and as a bridge therapy in the USA [17]. The thionamides, propylthiouracil (PTU), carbimazole (CBZ), and the active metabolite of the latter, methimazole (MMI) by inhibiting thyroid peroxidase enzymes they cause a decrease in thyroid hormone production. Moreover studies have shown that they have an immunosuppressive effect resulting in reduction of TSH-RAb levels, intercellular adhesion molecule-1 (ICAM-1) and soluble IL-2 receptor (sIL-2R) [18]. ATD are indicated especially in younger patients and in cases when a short term treatment is needed prior to RAI or surgery. Moreover, patients with mild disease (small size of goiter, negative or low TRAb values), of old age with comorbidities who are at high risk of postoperative complications or patients with a history of head and neck irradiation or surgery, are candidates for ATD therapy. In pregnancy ATD are the first line therapy for GD. Also ATD are indicated, in cases of people receiving care in nursing facilities and therefore radiation safety precautions cannot be preserved, in patients with moderate to severe active Graves' orbitopathy (GO) and in those who need more rapid biochemical disease control. Finally, ATD should be considered when there is lack of access to an experienced thyroid surgeon [12]. Adverse events of antithyroid medication range from milder adverse events such ascutaneous eruptions, gastrointestinal disorders and arthralgias to more serious complications as agranulocytosis, frank polyarthritis and hepatotoxicity. Adverse events of methimazole seem to be dose related (40 mg/day or more) while such thing has not been associated pylthiouracil doses [19].

3.3 RAI therapy

RAI treatment is a very effective therapy of GD. Accordintg to the NICE guidance, which is prepared for the National Health Service in England, it is used as first line treatment and in cases of hyperthyroidism recurrence post ATD therapy. The aim of this therapy is to radiate thyroid cells rendering the patient eu/hypothyroid. Although for many years it has been the most preferable treatment in USA, currently there is a tendency toward ATD therapy [20]. RAI treatment is performed after failure of ATD therapy to control hyperthyroidism or when the latter is contraindicated. Also RAI is preferred in patients with commodities who are at high risk of surgical complications, or in those with a history of prior surgery or irradiation of the head and neck. RAI treatment is the therapy of choice when there is no access to an experienced thyroid surgeon and in patients with periodic thyrotoxic hypokalemic paralysis, right heart failure pulmonary hypertension, or congestive heart failure [12]. RAI treatment is contraindicated when there is suspicion of thyroid cancer, in women who are pregnant or are breastfeeding and in those who cannot follow radiation safety rules. As RAI treatment has a risk of worsening Graves orbitopathy it is contraindicated in case of moderate to severe orbitopathy [12].

4. Patient preparation for RAI therapy

A close collaboration between, endocrinology and nuclear medicine, departments is required for the management of patients with thyroid disease who are candidates for RAI therapy. The determination of the activity, as well as the administration of radioiodine are responsibilities of the nuclear medicine physician. According to the EANM guidelines for the treatment of benign thyroid disease prior to any intervention a detailed medical history is needed including previous therapies for hyperthyroidism and especially any potential intake of iodine-containing medication (such as amiodarone and contrast media) or food [21]. The medical history should include medical conditions, surgeries, allergies and medications (especially those who may interfere with radioiodine uptake). Nuclear medicine physician should provide oral and written information about RAI therapy procedure, possible side effects, risk of recurrence and possible retreatment as well as radiation safety precautions post RAI therapy [14, 22] and rule out any possibility of pregnancy prior treatment. It is mandatory for female patients of childbearing age to undergo a pregnancy test 3 days prior to radioiodine administration and provide written signed declaration stating that they are not pregnant. Serum pregnancy test is preferable than urine test as it is more sensitive [23]. If previous hysterectomy has been reported or the patient is in postmenopausal state then the test can be omitted. Patients of both sexes should avoid conception 6 months post RAI therapy. RAI therapy is contraindicated in breastfeeding and it should be administrated 6 weeks to 3 months after lactation is disrupted [21]. To increase radioiodine uptake (RAIU), iodine restriction for 1 to 2 weeks and ATD withdrawal 3–7 days before RAI administration are also recommended.

Serum levels of TSH, FT3, FT4, TPO and TSI should be measured prior RAI therapy. Thyroid volume is assessed by ultrasonography (US) and in cases of a large goiter magnetic resonance imaging (MRI) is performed in order to estimate possible extension in the mediastinum. Computed Tomography (CT) is not preferred as the contrast media impair with the radioiodine uptake. Thyroid scintigraphy with ^{99m}Tc pertechnetate ($^{99m}TcO4$) and radioiodine is also mandatory to provide metabolic information of the organ. Radioactive iodine thyroid uptake (RAIU) at 4-6 h and

24 h post administration must be measured. RAIU increases gradually over 24 h but in some patients it can be increased rapidly reaching maximum values at 4 to 12 h and return to normal after 24 h. In some nuclear medicine departments a fixed dose of radioiodine is used, therefore RAIU calculation is not needed.

For nodules >1–1,5 cm, with suspicious findings in US (hypoechoic nodules solid or cystic with hypoechoic solid component, with irregular shape, calcifications and presence of invasion in adjacent structures) which appear in scintigraphy as "cold' or with a decreased uptake, fine needle aspiration (FNA) biopsy is recommended [24].

Patients with GD may present with ophthalmopathy. An experienced ophthalmologist should estimate the severity of the disease as RAI therapy has been associated with exacerbation of the ophthalmopathy. Corticosteroid therapy should be considered [12]. Studies have shown a possible correlation between Grave's ophthalmopathy (GO) progression post RAI therapy in smokers. Cessation of smoking is recommended. RAI therapy in cases of active moderate-to-severe ophthalmopathy is contraindicated [25].

As transient elevation of thyroid hormones due to actinic thyroiditis may present, ATD therapy should be discontinued approximately one week before and be resumed 3–7 days post RAI therapy [18]. B-adrenergic blockade should be administered in cases of patients who are at a higher risk of complications due to hyperthyroidism.

4.1 Patients' information for RAI therapy

Patients should be properly and adequately educated concerning the procedures they will undergo, the precautions they should take, the outcomes and possible adverse events of RAI therapy. Fulfilling these needs requires a collaborative approach among patients and health care professionals. Patients should receive both written and verbal information. More modern approaches such as mobile health (mHealth) could also be helpful [26]. Except for the pre- and posttreatment use of thyroid specific medication, risk of recurrent disease and subsequent retreatment(s), early and late side effects, health care professionals should prepare the patients regarding radiation protection initiatives to reduce radiation doses to family members and general population, according to national rules. Unlike thyroid cancer patients, those who receive RAI therapy to treat benign thyroid diseases do not need hospitalization.

RAI capsule is administered on an outpatient basis, in authorized Nuclear Medicine Departments. After RAI administration the patient is advised to avoid eating or drinking anything for 2 h, to allow time for the iodine to be absorbed. After this time patients should eat as normal and drink plenty of fluids.

For a few weeks after the treatment patient's thyroid gland will be radioactive. The amount of radioactivity is gradually decreasing. During this period, which is estimated for each patient individually, they are advised to avoid or restrict to minimum radiation exposure to their environment. Patients are guided to reduce the radiation exposure to other people by limiting the amount of time they spend with them and by keeping more than three meters away from them. They must not share a bed with anyone or sleep within 2 meters of anyone, even if there is a wall between beds. For 1–1 ½ months after RAI treatment, patients should not spend more than a few minutes each day within arm's reach of any children or pregnant women. Of course, they also need to limit close and prolonged contact with any other people, and stay away from crowded places such as cinemas, theaters, public transport as well as their work place, where they may be close to the same person for a prolonged period of time.

Although, most of the radioactivity is concentrated in thyroid gland, for a few days after RAI treatment, some of the radioiodine is excreted by urine and sweat. Around 90% of administered radioiodine activity is excreted mainly through the kidneys. Thus, patients with renal insufficiency may retain radioiodine activity over a long period, thereby leading to more intense internal exposure to radiation than that observed in normal ones [27]. Drinking plenty of fluids and emptying bladder frequently can help minimize bladder and adjacent tissues' exposure. Patients are advised to take care with personal hygiene in the first few days after treatment. They are instructed to always flush the toilet after use and always wash their hands. They are also guided to use their own towels and face cloth. Their clothes do not need to be washed separately unless they experience any incontinence [28, 29].

5. Radiation dosimetry and dose calculation

The aim of RAI therapy in GD is to cure hyperthyroidism. This is achieved by radiating and therefore destroying thyroid cells. The outcome is the patient to return to an euthyroid state or to become hypothyroid. RAI therapy is very effective, even in cases of possible retreatments, with a cure rate ~ 100%. Individualized dose of radioiodine for rendering a patient euthyroid is not feasible [30]. While several studies have been conducted, regarding the association between the optimal dose of radioiodine, thyroid's volume (based on ultrasound) and radioiodine turnover [31], there is lack of consensus for the proper dose regimen. The majority is in favor of rendering the patient hypothyroid [20] applying high radioiodine doses [32] to avoid the possibility of treatment's failure or relapse of the disease. Many nuclear departments apply fixed doses [33]. For rendering a patient euthyroid a target dose of ~150 Gy is needed. Higher doses (200–300 Gy) are applied for complete ablation.

The following equation recommended by the EANM, is used to estimate the appropriate radioiodine dose:

$$\mathrm{A}[\mathrm{MBq}] = \frac{F}{\ln 2} \times \frac{\mathrm{M}[\mathrm{g}] \times \mathrm{D}[Gy]}{\int_0^{\infty} RIU(t)\,dt} \tag{1}$$

A: radioiodine activity, F: conversion factor (between coulombs per kilogram and grays), M: mass of the target volume, D: the target dose.

Radioiodine uptake (RIU) is calculated as follows:

$$\mathrm{RIU} = \frac{\textit{Activity in Thyroid Gland}}{\textit{Administered activity}} \times 100\% \tag{2}$$

As it has been mentioned above many nuclear medicine departments apply fixed doses, in a range of 200–800 MBq with the commonest applicable doses of 400–600 MBq. Estimation of the thyroid size is needed (based on ultrasound) [21].

6. RAI therapy outcome

Initially the goal of RAI treatment was to render the patient euthyroid using low doses of I-131. Through the years it has become clear that hypothyroidism is an inevitable and unpredictable progressive outcome of RAI treatment. Nowadays, hypothyroidism is the desired result of RAI treatment and it has been described by many authors as the elimination of hyperthyroidism [34]. RAI treatment fails when persistent hyperthyroidism occurs. In the majority of the patients thyroid hormones return to normal levels while clinical symptoms are reduced 4–8 weeks post therapy. More than 80% of the patients become hypothyroid 16 weeks post RAI therapy. Hypothyroidism, in rare cases can be transient and the patient may return to a euthyroid state or remainhyperthyroid. The latter is often associated with no decrease of thyroid size [12]. The desired outcome of RAI treatment is dependent on multivariable factors such as thyroid size, dose regimens, compensation of hyperthyroidism, iodine intake (diet or iodine containing medicine) and the timing of the withdrawal of ATDs.

When low dose regimes are preferred, then the possibilities of treatment failure increase and ATD continuance and/or RAI retreatment are needed. Unfortunately, the field of RAI dose regimen still remains vast and things become more complicated when a fixed dose is compared to an individualized one. Many authors suggest that a calculated dose of radioiodine has no advantage over a fixed dose, while others recommend individual dose showing correlation between the success of therapy and the radiation dose actually absorbed by the thyroid [35]. Other factors that influence treatment outcome have been studied as well. In their retrospective cohort study, Aung et al. found that RAI treatment failure was more frequent in patients with high levels, of thyroid hormone or TRABs and in those who received ATD after RAI treatment. There were no correlation found among RAI treatment failure and other parameters such as age, sex or smoking. Moreover approximately 7% of the patients developed GO and 13.3% of them required surgery. There seemed to be a correlation between high thyroid hormone levels and orbitopathy whereas high TRAB levels had no effect in the development of orbitopathy [36].

Despite more than 75 years' experience with RAI treatment of GD, it is not always feasible to predict the efficacy of the treatment or the factors that will eventually affect it. The "GREAT" score, a predictive model consisting of clinical and biochemical variables has been introduced as a clinical tool that predicts the success of antithyroid drug therapy for Graves' Disease. Calculation of the GREAT 6-point score is as follows: age (<40 or ≥ 40 years: 1 or 0 point, respectively), goiter (not visible to slightly visible or clearly visible: 0 or 2 points), FT4 (<3.1 or ≥ 3.1 ng/dl: 0 or 1 point), and TBII (<6; 6–19.9; >19.9 U/L: 0, 1, or 2 points) resulting in the GREAT score classes of I (0–1 point), II (2–3 points), and III (4–6 points). Higher recurrence rate at the end of follow up is observed in GREAT score class III when compared with class II or class I (16.4%) [37]. However, GREAT score has been suggested for predicting outcome before the start of ATD and to our knowledge there has not been developed yet a clinical tool that can estimate RAI results.

7. Follow-up

Regular review of thyroid function tests in patients who have undergone radioiodine treatment for thyroid disease is essential to assess the efficacy of the treatment and for timely detection of developing hypothyroidism or post treatment immunogenic hyperthyroidism. The first review of thyroid function post RAI therapy should be conducted 1–2 months later by assessing TSH, FT4 and total FT3 values and be repeated every 4–6 weeks for the first 6 months or until the patient becomes hypothyroid and is stable on LT4 treatment [13]. In patients at high risk for endocrine ophthalmopathy or who have received ATD, follow up is recommended at shorter intervals. In cases of RAI treatment for overt hyperthyroidism,

ATD should be initiated 3–5 days post RAI treatment. If RAI retreatment is deemed necessary, it can be conducted 6–12 months later. RAI retreatment is not necessary in cases of post therapy immunogenic hyperthyroidism; ATD administration for a few months is adequate. As it is mentioned above a lifelong testing of thyroid function is necessary, even in patients who have returned to an euthyroid state post RAI treatment.

8. Adverse events

Actinic thyroiditis is the result of radioiodine therapy. As radioiodine is accumulated by thyroid cells the emitted betta particles cause cellular necrosis and stored thyroid hormones are released into the circulation causing a transient exacerbation of hyperthyroidism. This effect is greater in radioiodine therapy of a toxic nodular goiter as the levels of stored thyroid hormones are bigger [38]. This transient elevation of thyroid hormones can be asymptomatic or it can lead to atrial fibrillation, heart failure and rarely to thyroid storm with a possible fatal outcome. The latter demands admission to an intensive care unit and administration of ATDs and steroids (intravenously) as well as b-blockers [16].

Hypothyroidism is another side effect of radioiodine therapy and according to the ATA guidelines, it is the main goal of the therapy [12]. This outcome is more common in GD rather than in toxic goiter or in solitary hyperfuctionong nodules [16]. It requires lifelong follow up and LT4 treatment. In cases of failure to accomplish a hypothyroid state post radioiodine treatment, an increase in cardiovascular and cerebrovascular deaths has been noted [12].

Actinic thyroiditis is accompanied by thyroid pain and swelling which is prevalent the first week post therapy. In a few patients this can lead to dyspnea while the majority is asymptomatic. In cases of a large goiter with signs of tracheal compression, corticosteroids before radioiodine therapy should be considered. Sialadenitis, xerostomia or altered taste are adverse effects seen in patients with differentiated thyroid cancer who receive radioiodine therapy, however in patients with GD no permanent damage has been reported.

Ionizing radiation has been associated with increased incidence of leukemia and many solid cancers [39]. An increase in the incidence of thyroid carcinoma in children after Chernobyl accident has been reported [40]. Many studies have evaluated the possible correlation between radioiodine therapy in GD and the risk of malignancy. In a multicenter retrospective cohort study taken place in USA and UK, known as Cooperative Thyrotoxicosis Therapy Follow-up Study Group, 35,593 hyperthyroid patients were included and evaluation of cancer mortality among those patients and especially in those who received radioiodine treatment, was made. The results showed no significant increase in cancer mortality and this was due to the fact that mean doses of radiation among organs except for the thyroid were < 200 mGy. It has to be mentioned that the study cannot provide any information for the children population as themean age of the patients was 46 years [41]. Kitahara et al. [42] extended the previous study and found that radioiodine therapy of GD was correlated with a dose dependent increase in the incidence of all solid tumors and especially of breast cancer, while Greenspan et al., [43] challenged those previous results. Ameta analysis by Hieu et al., [44] found no increase in cancer risk post radioiodine therapy in benign thyroid disorders except perhaps for the thyroid, kidney and the stomach cancer, which the authors estimate that it should be investigated with further studies. The latter has also been challenged by Salvatori et al., [45] as the main reason for increased incidence of cancer in hyperthyroid patients is not radioiodine therapy but hyperthyroidism itself. Thyroid hormones through $\alpha\nu\beta3$, a membrane receptor which is overexpressed in tumor cells, play a crucial role in cancer cell proliferation, angiogenesis and metastasis.

9. Conclusion

Thyrotoxicosis is a very common clinical syndrome caused by an excess of thyroid hormones in the serum. Graves' Disease is the commonest cause of hyperthyroidism. Graves' Disease is the commonest cause of hyperthyroidism. It has multiple manifestations and it requires appropriate diagnostic and therapeutic management. There are three effective treatment options: RAI therapy, ATDs, or thyroidectomy. RAI treatment has been used to treat thyroid disorders, both malignant and benign, for many decades and in many cases it is preferred first- line treatment. In Graves' Disease radioiodine radiates and therefore destroys the follicle cells of the hyperfunctioning thyroid gland providing a definite therapy of hyperthyroidism as well as improving patient's quality of life. It is well tolerated with rare complications except for those related to orbitopathy.

Conflict of interest

The authors declare no conflict of interest.

Author details

Ioannis Iakovou[1*], Evanthia Giannoula[1], Paraskevi Exadaktylou[2] and Nikitas Papadopoulos[3]

1 Second Academic Nuclear Medicine Department, Aristotle University of Thessaloniki, University General Hospital AHEPA, Thessaloniki, Greece

2 Third Academic Nuclear Medicine Department, Aristotle University of Thessaloniki, General Hospital Papageorgiou, Thessaloniki, Greece

3 General Hospital "Georgios Gennimatas", Thessaloniki, Greece

*Address all correspondence to: iiakovou@auth.gr; iiakovou@icloud.com

References

[1] Hussain YS, Hookham JC, Allahabadia A, Balasubramanian SP. Epidemiology, management and outcomes of Graves' disease-real life data. Endocrine. 2017; 56(3):568-578. DOI:10.1007/s12020-017-1306-5

[2] Davies TF, Yin X, Latif R. The genetics of the thyroid stimulating hormone receptor: history and relevance. Thyroid. 2010 Jul;20(7): 727-36. DOI: 10.1089/thy.2010.1638

[3] Sundaresh V, Brito JP, Thapa P, Bahn RS, Stan MN. Comparative Effectiveness of Treatment Choices for Graves' Hyperthyroidism: A Historical Cohort Study. Thyroid. 2017 Apr;27(4):497-505. doi: 10.1089/thy.2016.0343. Epub 2017 Feb 6. PMID: 28049375; PMCID: PMC5385429.

[4] Brancatella A,Viola N, Brogioni S, Montanelli L, Sardella C, Vitti P, Marcocci C, Lupi I., Latrofa F. Graves' Disease Induced by Immune Checkpoint Inhibitors: A Case Report and Review of the Literature. Eur Thyroid J. 2019 Jul;8(4):192-195. DOI: 10.1159/000501824

[5] Pearce SHS, Dayan C, Wraith DC, Barrell K, Olive N, Jansson L, Walker-Smith T, Carnegie C, Martin KF, Boelaert K, Gilbert J, Higham CE, Muller I, Murray RD, Perros P, Razvi S, Vaidya B, Wernig F, Kahaly GJ. Antigen-Specific Immunotherapy with Thyrotropin Receptor Peptides in Graves' Hyperthyroidism: A Phase I Study. Thyroid. 2019 Jul;29(7):1003-1011. DOI: 10.1089/thy.2019.0036

[6] Sundaresh V, Brito JP, Thapa P, Bahn RS, Stan MN. Comparative Effectiveness of Treatment Choices for Graves' Hyperthyroidism: A Historical Cohort Study. Thyroid. 2017 Apr;27(4):497-505. DOI: 10.1089/thy.2016.0343

[7] Sawin CT, Becker DV. Radioiodine and the treatment of hyperthyroidism: the early history. Thyroid. 1997 Apr;7(2):163-76. doi: 10.1089/thy.1997.7.163. PMID: 9133679.

[8] Yordanova A, Eppard E, Kürpig S, et al. Theranostics in nuclear medicine practice. *Onco Targets Ther*. 2017;10:4821-4828. Published 2017 Oct 3. doi:10.2147/OTT.S140671

[9] Ahad F, Ganie SA. Iodine, Iodine metabolism and Iodine deficiency disorders revisited. Indian J EndocrinolMetab. 2010;14(1):13-17. PMCID: PMC3063534 PMID: 21448409

[10] Ziessman HA, O'malley JP, Thrall JH, Fahey FH. Endocrine System. In Ziessman HA, O'malley JP, Thrall JH, Fahey FH (Eds). The Requisites, Nuclear Medicine, 4th edition, Elseviers Saunders, 2014:66-97.

[11] Pouget GP, Lozza C, Deshayes E, Boudousq V, Navarro-Teulon I. Introduction to Radiobiology of Targeted Radionuclide Therapy. Front Med (Lausanne). 2015; 2: 12. DOI: 10.3389/fmed.2015.00012

[12] Ross DS, Burch HB, Cooper DS, Greenlee MC, Laurberg P, Maia AL, Rivkees SA, Samuels M, Sosa JA, Stan MN, Walter MA. 2016 American Thyroid Association Guidelines for Diagnosis and Management of Hyperthyroidism and Other Causes of Thyrotoxicosis. Thyroid. 2016 Oct;26(10):1343-1421. doi: 10.1089/thy.2016.0229. Erratum in: Thyroid. 2017 Nov;27(11):1462. PMID: 27521067.

[13] Rivkees SA, Sklar C, Freemark M. Clinical review 99: The management of Graves' disease in children, with special emphasis on radioiodine treatment. J ClinEndocrinolMetab. 1998 Nov;83(11):3767-76. DOI: 10.1210/jcem.83.11.5239

[14] Alsanea O, Clark OH. Treatment of Graves' disease: the advantages of surgery. Endocrinol Metab Clin North Am. 2000 Jun;29(2):321-37. doi: 10.1016/s0889-8529(05)70134-1. PMID: 10874532.

[15] Bartalena L, Burch HB, Burman KD, Kahaly GJ. A 2013 European survey of clinical practice patterns in the management of Graves' disease. ClinEndocrinol (Oxf). 2016 Jan;84(1):115-20. DOI: 10.1111/cen.12688

[16] Chahardahmasumi E, Salehidoost R, Amini M, Aminorroaya A, Rezvanian H, KachooeiA,Iraj B, Nazem M, Kolahdoozan M. Assessment of the Early and Late Complication after Thyroidectomy. Adv Biomed Res. 2019;8:14. DOI:10.4103/abr.abr_3_19

[17] Emiliano AB, Governale L, Parks M, Cooper DS. Shifts in propylthiouracil and methimazole prescribing practices: antithyroid drug use in the United States from 1991 to 2008. J ClinEndocrinolMetab. 2010 May;95(5):2227-33. DOI: 10.1210/jc.2009-2752

[18] Abraham P., Acharya S. Current and emerging treatment options for Graves' hyperthyroidism. TherClin Risk Manag. 2010 Feb 2;6:29-40. doi: 10.2147/tcrm.s5229

[19] Yu W, Wu N, Li L, Wang J, OuYang H, Shen H. Side effects of PTU and MMIin the treatment of hyperthyroidism: Asystematic review and meta-analysis. EndocrPract. 2020 Feb;26(2):207-217. DOI: 10.4158/EP-2019-0221

[20] Abdi H, Amouzegar A. Management of Graves' Hyperthyroidism: More Than a Century of Progression, Int J EndocrinolMetab. 2020; 18(Suppl):e103943. DOI: 10.5812/ijem.103943

[21] Stokkel MP, HandkiewiczJunak D, Lassmann M, Dietlein M, Luster M. EANM procedure guidelines for therapy of benign thyroid disease. Eur J Nucl Med Mol Imaging. 2010 Nov;37(11):2218-28. DOI: 10.1007/s00259-010-1536-8

[22] Sisson JC, Freitas J, McDougall IR, Dauer LT, Hurley JR, Brierley JD, Edinboro CH, Rosenthal D, Thomas MJ, Wexler JA, Asamoah E, Avram AM., Milas M, Greenlee C. (2011). Radiation safety in the treatment of patients with thyroid diseases by radioiodine 131I : practice recommendations of the American Thyroid Association Thyroid. Apr;21(4):335-46. DOI: 10.1089/thy.2010.0403

[23] Tran P, DeSimone S, Barrett M, Bachrach B. (2010). I-131 Treatment of Graves' Disease in an Unsuspected First Trimester Pregnancy; the Potential for Adverse Effects on the Fetus and a Review of the Current Guidelines for Pregnancy Screening. Int J PediatrEndocrinol. 2010: 858359. DOI: 10.1155/2010/858359

[24] Koike E, Noguchi S, YamashitaH, Murakami T, Ohshima A, Kawamoto H, Yamashita H. Ultrasonographic characteristics of thyroid nodules: prediction of malignancy. Arch Surg. 2001 Mar;136(3):334-7. DOI: 10.1001/archsurg.136.3.334

[25] Kahaly GJ, Bartalena L, HegedüscL, Leenhardtd L, Poppee K, Pearce SH. 2018 European Thyroid Association Guideline for the Management of Graves' Hyperthyroidism. Eur Thyroid J. 2018 Aug;7(4):167-186. DOI: 10.1159/000490384

[26] Giannoula E, Iakovou I, Katsikavelas I, Antoniou P, Raftopoulos V, Chatzipavlidou V, Papadopoulos N, Bamidis P. A Mobile App for Thyroid Cancer Patients Aiming to Enhance Their Quality of Life: Protocol for a

Quasiexperimental Interventional Pilot Study. JMIR Res Protoc. 2020 Mar 13;9(3):e13409. doi: 10.2196/13409. PMID: 32167482; PMCID: PMC7101500.

[27] Holst JP, Burman KD, Atkins F, Umans JG, Jonklaas J. Radioiodine therapy for thyroid cancer and hyperthyroidism in patients with end-stage renal disease on hemodialysis. Thyroid. 2005 Dec;15(12):1321-31. doi: 10.1089/thy.2005.15.1321. PMID: 16405403.

[28] Perros P, Boelaert K, Colley S, Evans C, Evans RM, Gerrard Ba G, Gilbert J, Harrison B, Johnson SJ, Giles TE, Moss L, Lewington V, Newbold K, Taylor J, Thakker RV, Watkinson J, Williams GR; British Thyroid Association. Guidelines for the management of thyroid cancer. Clin Endocrinol (Oxf). 2014 Jul;81 Suppl 1:1-122. doi: 10.1111/cen.12515. PMID: 24989897.

[29] NHS Foundation Trust. Patient Information Radioiodine Treatment. Higher Dose. Available at: https://www.qegateshead.nhs.uk/sites/default/files/users/user15641/IL673%20Radioiodine%20Treatment%20Higher%20Dose.pdf. Accessed January 18, 2121.

[30] Allahabadia A, Daykin J, Holder RL, Sheppard MC, Gough SC, Franklyn JA. Age and gender predict the outcome of treatment for Graves' hyperthyroidism. J ClinEndocrinolMetab. 2000 Mar;85(3):1038-42. DOI: 10.1210/jcem.85.3.6430

[31] Kalinyak JE, McDougall IR. How should the dose of iodine-131 be determined in the treatment of Graves' hyperthyroidism? J ClinEndocrinolMetab. 2003 Mar;88(3):975-7. DOI: 10.1210/jc.2002-021801

[32] Safa AM, Skillern PG. Treatment of hyperthyroidism with a large initial dose of sodium iodide I 131. Arch Intern Med. 1975 May;135(5):673-5. PMID: 1053273.

[33] Mumtaz M, Lin LS, Hui KC, MohdKhir AS. Radioiodine I-131 for the therapy of graves' disease. Malays J Med Sci. 2009 Jan;16(1):25-33. PMID: 22589645; PMCID: PMC3336179

[34] Metso S, Jaatinen P, Huhtala H, Luukkaala T, Oksala H, Salmi J. Long-term follow-up study of radioiodine treatment of hyperthyroidism. ClinEndocrinol (Oxf). 2004 Nov;61(5):641-8. DOI: 10.1111/j.1365-2265.2004.02152.x

[35] Cepková J, Horáček J, Vižďa J, Doležal J. Radioiodine treatment of Graves' disease - dose/response analysis. Acta Medica (Hradec Kralove). 2014;57(2):49-55. doi: 10.14712/18059694.2014.39. PMID: 25257150.

[36] Thuzar-AungT, Zammitt NN, Dover AR, Strachan MWJ, Seckl JR, Gibb FW.Predicting outcomes and complications following radioiodine therapy in Graves' thyrotoxicosis. ClinEndocrinol (Oxf). 2019 Jan;90(1):192-199. DOI: 10.1111/cen.13873

[37] Vos XG, Endert E, Zwinderman AH, Tijssen JG, Wiersinga WM. Predicting the Risk of Recurrence Before the Start of Antithyroid Drug Therapy in Patients With Graves' Hyperthyroidism. J Clin Endocrinol Metab. 2016 Apr;101(4):1381-9. doi: 10.1210/jc.2015-3644. Epub 2016 Feb 10. PMID: 26863422.

[38] Joop-Bonnema S, Hegedüs L. Radioiodine therapy in benign thyroid diseases: effects, side effects, and factors affecting therapeutic outcome. Endocr Rev. 2012 Dec;33(6): 920-80. DOI: 10.1210/er.2012-1030

[39] Gilbert ES.Ionising radiation and cancer risks: what have we learned from epidemiology?Int J Radiat Biol. 2009 Jun;85(6):467-82. DOI: 10.1080/09553000902883836

[40] Farahati J,Demidchik EP, Biko J, Reiners C.Inverse association between age at the time of radiation exposure and extent of disease in cases of radiation-induced childhood thyroid carcinoma in Belarus. Cancer. 2000 Mar 15;88(6):1470-6. DOI: 10.1002/(sici)1097-0142(20000315)88:6<1470::aid-cncr27>3.0.co;2-w

[41] Ron E, Doody MM, Becker DV, Brill AB, Curtis RE, Goldman MB, Harris 3rd BS, Hoffman DA, McConahey WM, Maxon HR, Preston-Martin S, MarshauerME,WongFL,BoiceJD.Cancer mortality following treatment for adult hyperthyroidism. Cooperative Thyrotoxicosis Therapy Follow-up Study Group. JAMA.1998;29;280(4):347-55. DOI: 10.1001/jama.280.4.347

[42] Kitahara CM, Berrington de Gonzalez A, Bouville A, Brill AB, Doody MM, Melo DR, Simon SL, Sosa JA, Tulchinsky M, Villoing D, Preston DL. Association of Radioactive Iodine Treatment With Cancer Mortality in Patients With Hyperthyroidism. JAMA Intern Med.2019 Jul 1;179(8):1034-1042. DOI: 10.1001/jamainternmed.2019.0981

[43] Greenspan BS, Siegel JA, Hassan A, Silberstein EB.There is No Association of Radioactive Iodine Treatment with Cancer Mortality in Patients with Hyperthyroidism. J Nucl Med. 2019 Nov;60(11):1500-1501. DOI: 10.2967/jnumed.119.235929.

[44] Hieu TT, Russell AW, Cuneo R, Clark J, Kron T, Hall P, Doi SAR.Cancer risk after medical exposure to radioactive iodine in benign thyroid diseases: a meta-analysis. EndocrRelat Cancer. 2012 Sep 14;19(5):645-55. DOI: 10.1530/ERC-12-0176

[45] Salvatori M, Treglia G, Perotti G, Giovanella L.Iodine-131 administration and risk of cancer: "appearances can be deceptive".Hormones (Athens). 2013 Apr-Jun;12(2):312-4. doi: 10.14310/horm.2002.1417

Chapter 11

Surgery for Graves' Disease

Kul Ranjan Singh and Anand Kumar Mishra

Abstract

Graves' Disease (GD) is the commonest cause of hyperthyroidism followed by toxic nodular goitre. Patients presenting as goitre with clinical features of hyperthyroidism are to be carefully evaluated with biochemically with thyroid stimulating hormone (TSH), free thyroxine (fT4) and radionuclide scan (Technitium-99/Iodine-123). Those with GD also have raised thyroid receptor stimulating antibody levels. Patients are simultaneously evaluated for eye disease and managed accordingly. Initial treatment is rendering patient euthyroid using anti thyroid drugs (ATD) and if remission does not occur either continue medical therapy or proceed for definitive therapy by radioactive iodine ablation (RAI) or surgery. In last decades there is ample literature preferring surgery as preferred definitive therapy. Surgery in thyroid disease has become safer with development of many intra-operative adjuncts but it should be performed by high volume thyroid surgeon. The procedure of choice is near total or total thyroidectomy as it avoids recurrences. Patients who are not eligible or willing for surgery can be managed with RAI.

Keywords: hyperthyroidism, Graves' Disease, thyroidectomy, radioactive iodine

1. Introduction

Graves' Disease (GD) is the commonest cause of hyperthyroidism world over representing more than 50% of hyperthyroid patients [1]. A woman is 7–10 times more likely to be affected by it [2]. The incidence of autoimmune thyroid diseases like GD and Hashimoto's thyroiditis is on the rise in tropical countries probably due to environmental immunological factors [3]. GD has systemic manifestations. Eyes's are involved to variable extent in more than half the patients. Treatment aims to restore to the thyroid hormones to normal levels along with achieving remission and care of ophthalmological manifestations. Anti-thyroid drugs (ATD), Radioactive Iodine (RAI) and surgery are the current modalities of treatment [1]. They have their unique indications, advantages, disadvantages and complications. ATD are the usual first line of treatment. Relapsing patients or GD with certain co existing conditions may require a definitive treatment. RAI or surgery are indicated in such patients. The choice of definitive therapy depends on the patient and treating physician. Patients involvement in decision making has been associated with increased patients satisfaction [4, 5].

2. Epidemiology and pathogenesis

The peak incidence of GD is observed between 30 to 50 years of age. Annual reported incidence of GD is 50 and of ophthalmopathy is 16 per 100000 population.

Orbital imaging if performed in all patients of GD will reveal changes of ophthalmopathy in upto 70% of patients. Approximately 3% of women and 0.5% of men during their life time can develop GD [6].

GD is an organ specific auto immune disease caused by thyroid stimulating hormone receptor (TSHR) circulating stimulating auto antibodies. The TSHR stimulating antibody binds to leucine rich extracellular domain of TSHR on surface of thyrocytes and orbital fibroblasts and IGF1 receptors. After binding it increases production of intracellular cyclic AMP causing thyrocyte growth and increased thyroid hormone production.

3. Diagnosis

Measurement of Free T4/Free T3 and TSH is the initial diagnostic test. In overt hyperthyroidism FT4 and FT3 are elevated but in milder hyperthyroidism FT4 may be normal with only FT3 elevation. TSH R antibody is sensitive (97%) and specific (98%) tool for accurate diagnosis of GD [7]. High resolution ultrasound reveals diffuse goiter and hypoechogenicity. Diagnosis is confirmed by thyroid scintigraphy by Tc^{99} pertechnatate or I^{123} scintigraphy. Scintigraphy is definitely needed for diagnosis.

4. Treatment options

Anti-thyroid drugs (ATD) are used in the initial management of GD with aim to achieve euthyroidism. Once patient is euthyroid it should be maintained to achieve remission. About half of the patients go into remission after 18 to 24 months of treatment with ATD. Patients without remission and recurrent disease (30–40% in the first 12 months and approximately 50–60% in long term) require definitive therapy. Definitive therapy is either surgical or medical ablation of all thyrocytes. The options are radioactive iodine (RIA) or thyroidectomy. After ablative therapy thyroid hormone replacement is provided to control hypothyroidism. There are reports of use of long term ATD to achieve remission. Choice between RIA and thyroidectomy are influenced by physician, patient, institutional and geographical beliefs and practice patterns. The most "effective" therapy for both physician's and patient perspective will be which will provide rapid euthyroidism and prevent recurrences.

Early and rapid euthyroidism is desirable in all GD patients as it decreases mortality and halts eye disease progression. In a retrospective cohort study of 4189 GD patients regardless of the method of treatment, low TSH at 1 year following GD diagnosis was associated with a 55% increase in cardiovascular mortality (atrial fibrillation, heart failure, pulmonary hypertension, angina pectoris, and stroke) [8]. Lillevang et al. in a cohort study of 235,547 individual investigated association between hyperthyroidism and mortality in both treated and untreated groups and concluded that decreased TSH increases mortality in both groups and with every duration of 6 months of suppressed TSH was associated with 11–13% increase in total mortality [9]. Dale et al. found that even transient hypothyroidism during treatment was associated with greater weight-gain during medical treatment in 162 consecutive hyperthyroid patients [10]. Even consensus statement of the European Group on Graves' orbitopathy (EUGOGO) recommends avoidance of hypothyroidism as it can cause exacerbation of thyroid eye disease [11].

Thyroidectomy is the only modality of treatment which can provide both rapid euthyroidism and prevent recurrence. There are reports of RAI worsening GD ophthalmopathy [12, 13]. In a systematic review of literature between 2001 and 2011which included retrospective and prospective studies (14,245 patients) on the comparison of RAI and surgery as best definitive treatment for GD, reported surgery to be 3.44 times more likely to be successful than RAI ($P < .001$). And total thyroidectomy (TT) was 95.45 times more successful than RAI ($P < .001$) and concluded thyroidectomy as the most successful modality for the management of GD [14].

5. Thyroidectomy

Thyroidectomy has been performed for GD since 19th century. However, the earlier years were fraught with significant morbidity and mortality. Introduction of RAI resulted in a rapid decline in popularity of thyroidectomy for GD. Improvements in medical management and refinements in surgical techniques along with knowledge of long term effects of RAI has renewed interests in surgery and it is re gaining the lost grounds [15–17].

6. Indications for surgery

Surgery is the treatment of choice in those with compressive symptoms attributable to goiter, large goiters, presence/suspicion of co-existing malignancy, GD with non-malignant nodule with no/reduced uptake of RAI which is large in size, co-existing parathyroid pathology. Those lactating, pregnant or desirous of pregnancy within next 6 months and presence of significant active ophthalmopathy are advised surgery [5, 18–20]. Pediatric patients failing ATD are more likely to undergo thyroidectomy compared to RAI [21]. Intolerance/non-compliance to ATD, patient preference is an indication in themselves for surgery as treatment of choice.

Indications of thyroidectomy in GD patients include following (6C's):

1. ATD **C**ontraindicated: Difficulty with adequate hormonal control on medications, or Intolerance, or recurrence after ATD treatment

2. RAI **C**ontraindicated: pregnant and nursing women, Large goiter with or without compressive symptoms (dysphagia, dysphonia, dyspnoea), Relatively low uptake of RAI, associated thyroid nodule with confirmed or suspected thyroid malignancy,

3. **C**oexisting moderate-to-severe active Graves' orbitopathy

4. Associated **C**oexiting disease: periodic paralysis

5. Other **C**onditions: Young or pediatric patients, women planning a pregnancy within 6 months, refusal or lack of facilities for RAI, individual preference for surgery

6. **C**igrette Smokers (increased risk of exacerbation of eye disease after definitive treatment with radioactive iodine).

7. Advantages of surgery

Surgery is considered the most effective treatment for GD. It results in prompt control of hyperthyroidism. Co-existing thyroid nodules a subset of which may be harboring malignancy are treated concurrently by surgery [22]. Surgery is said to have the best ophthalmological outcome in ophthalmopathy compared to ATD and RAI although these observations are based on expert opinion or non-randomized clinical trials [23–27]. Recurrence has been seen both after ATD and RAI with the former having a significantly higher recurrence rate. Though the recurrence rates after RAI and surgery are not significantly different, multiple doses of RAI may be required for cure in a given patient [23]. In a meta-analysis involving 1402 patients across 5 continents, surgery had the lowest recurrence rates even though a sub total thyroidectomy was the procedure performed in those with available surgical records [27]. More over surgery avoids the long-term systemic side effects of ATD and radiation exposure of RAI. Though a matter of debate, patients having chosen surgery as a definitive treatment are likely to be more satisfied compared to RAI [5, 28]. Patients preference should always be taken into consideration. Patients are likely to browse the internet for more information. However, the both reliability and comprehension of available information is occasionally questionable [29]. Hence, the treating physician should make available to the patient pertinent information so that patient can make an un biased decision which will further improve compliance and satisfaction to treatment.

8. Geographic variability in preferred treatment options

There are wide variations in the preferred first line treatment for GD. The choice is culmination of patient and physician preference along with disease status. In the US, RAI is likely to be the primary therapy though its popularity is decreasing. ATD are preferred in Latin America, Europe and Japan [30, 31]. Popularity of ATD has also surpassed RAI in New Zealand [32]. Once again ATD are the favored first line treatment in middle east and north African regions. Also, the physician practices were found to be that between European and American preferences, probably attributed to their training and affiliations [33].

9. Peri operative management

Imaging of thyroid is essential, and ultrasonography is useful. It aids in surgical planning and presence of nodule(s) mandates a fine needle aspiration cytology before surgery. Contrast enhanced CT scan (CECT) may be required for large goiters. Euthyroid state should be achieved in all patients before surgery [30]. This is achieved by ATD which is continued till the morning of surgery. Tachycardia if present is controlled by institution on beta blockers. The role of pre-operative Iodine solution remains controversial but the authors favor same [34]. Lugols Iodine/collosal Iodine/SSKI is given thrice a day for 7–12 days prior to surgery. Iodine has been shown to decrease the vascularity the thyroid and makes the gland firmer. These changes aid the surgeon [35]. Guidelines suggested by various professional bodies aid in management and peri operative preparation of hyperthyroid patients of which American Thyroid Association (ATA) seems to be most commonly followed. However, a study by Siddique Akram et al. found that adherence to ATA guidelines did not impact the outcome significantly but for increased intra operative tachycardia in patient not following ATA guidelines [36]. In fact, almost 28% of the cohort remained hyperthyroid at the time of surgery but no adverse impact was noted. Pre-operative vit D deficiency may result in higher incidence of post thyroidectomy hypocalcemia [37]. Vit D and calcium may be supplemented in pre-operative period to reduce the incidence of post-surgery hypocalcemia [38, 39]. However unpublished data from authors have not shown any advantage of supplementation in reducing post TT hypocalcemia.

DOI: http://dx.doi.org/10.5772/intechopen.96958

Surgery is best performed by a high-volume surgeon in a specialized unit for best outcome [40]. Surgical adjuncts may be utilized as per need, availability, cost constraints and surgeon preference. Meticulous surgery parathyroid vascularity is of prime importance in bettering outcomes. Parathyroid auto transplantation after inadvertent injury or excision results in increased occurrence of temporary hypocalcemia but not permanent hypocalcemia [41].

Post thyroidectomy, patients are kept under observation for development of hypocalcemia or risk of bleed. These were traditionally said to occur at a higher incidence after surgery performed for GD [41]. Hungry bone syndrome, Vitamin D deficiency, female sex are factors that have been associated with apparent higher incidence of post TT hypocalcemia in GD. However, recent studies have concluded that hypocalcemia and post thyroidectomy bleed do not occur at a significantly higher rate in GD [42]. Post TT PTH may be evaluated as per institutional protocols to predict hypocalcemia and plan early discharge. PTH gradient is said to better predict hypocalcemia than any single value. Same day safe discharge of patients is feasible for GD after surgery with no adverse outcomes [43]. ATD are discontinued and Beta blockers if prescribed are tapered gradually in the post-operative period. Thyroxine supplement is started between POD1–7 at a dose if 1.6–2.1 microgram/Kg.

10. Rapid preparation for Graves surgery

Patients are usually rendered euthyroid by ATD to reduce peri operative complications with thyroid storm being the most dreaded one. However, a subset of patients may require urgent/emergent surgery in view of significant compression, intolerance of drugs or failure of drugs. Such patients may be subjected to a rapid preparation protocol where in two or more of dexamethasone, beta blocker, sodium iopodate, iopanoic acid, collosal/lugols Iodine, cholestyramine, iodinated radiographic contrast agent, lithium and ATD if tolerated are used for 10–12 days prior to anticipated surgery. No significantly increased morbidity has been reported after surgery in the rapidly prepared patients and this strategy is required and is feasible in a subset of patients [44–46]. The occurrence of thyroid storm is rare and biochemically hyperthyroid patients may undergo thyroidectomy safely if the surgeon and anesthetist are comfortable [47]. However, the consensus remains that the outcome is best when surgery is performed on a euthyroid patient.

11. Choice of surgical procedure

Bilateral subtotal thyroidectomy (STT), Dunhill procedure (DP), near total thyroidectomy (NTT) and total thyroidectomy (TT) are the four procedures that have been or are being performed for GD. STT, DP, NTT were the procedure of choice till 21st century due to said higher incidence of hypoparathyroidism, nerve damage or hematoma [15]. However, these have not been verified in recent large studies or meta-analysis [48]. A retrospective cohort study 8032 patients of benign thyroid disease having undergone STT or TT found no difference in temporary of permanent nerve damage and permanent hypoparathyroidism though temporary hypocalcemia was significantly higher in TT compared to TT (13.12% Vs. 2.7%) [49]. A similar trend has been seen in most other studies. TT for GD has been found to have lower rates of recurrent hyperthyroidism compared to other procedures (STT more than DP) [17, 50]. The nerve damage rates have been higher however hypocalcemia rates have been slightly higher though they do not reach statistical significance [50]. The choice of surgical procedure did not have a difference in their effect on Graves' ophthalmopathy [17, 50]. RAI with steroid cover was found to be not inferior to surgery. The TT performed by trained surgeons at high volume center have no higher rates of these morbid complications. More and more TT are now being performed for benign diseases throughout world. Thomas WT et al. in an analysis of nationwide in patient analysis in US noted an increase in TT for benign diseases from 17.6% in 1993–1997 to 39.6 in 2003–2007 [51]. This trend is seen across the globe even in less developed regions [40, 52]. However TT may be avoided in in situations where lifelong thyroxine supplements may be un reliable, more common in the lesser developed countries [3]. Never the less, 2016 ATA guidelines for Hyperthyroidism suggest that a NTT of TT should be performed for GD if surgery is being contemplated [30].

12. Disadvantages of surgery

Patients would require lifelong thyroxine replacement after thyroidectomy and compliance may be an issue in some. Also, potential risk of permanent hypoparathyroidism and recurrent laryngeal nerve damage or neck hematoma are present. However, in trained hands, their incidence is no higher than after surgery for euthyroid goiters. Vis a vis ATD and RAI, surgery is the least cost effective first line treatment of Graves' Disease [53, 54]. In recurrent GD after ATT, surgery was more cost effective than RAI or lifelong ATD to a large extent [55]. The cost implications are likely to vary across the globe depending on various factors.

13. Surgical approach to thyroid

Though conventionally, open thyroidectomy through a transverse collar incision is the standard of care, heightened cosmetic demands of patients along with refinements in surgical instruments and surgical training has resulted in significant shift favoring minimally invasive procedures. Meta-analysis of 846 cases between 1999–2011 by Zhang et al. concluded that endoscopic thyroidectomy provides better cosmetic satisfaction along with lesser blood loss at the expense of higher costs and operative time with acceptable rates of hypocalcemia and nerve compromise [56].

Robotic surgery is now a feasible option for Graves' Disease with comparable complication rates [57]. Also, larger glands can be excised via robotic technique. Retrospective analysis of 44 robotic TT via bilateral axillo- breast approach was no inferior when compared to 144 cases of open thyroidectomy in terms of recurrence, hypocalcemia and nerve damage on prolonged follow up of 35 months [58]. This is now a valid option for those concerned about cosmesis.

14. Conclusion

Etiology of hyperthyroidism has to be determined thoroughly to determine the line of management. Radioactive iodine ablation (RAI) or surgery is the main modality of treatment in GD. Anti-thyroid drug is essential to make the patient euthyroid prior to definitive therapy. Prompt discussion with patients regarding delayed outcome and retreatment in those who opt for RAI is mandatory. Surgical treatment of choice in the form of NTT or TT ought to be performed in a high-volume centre to reduce complication and recurrence. Toxic adenoma and TMNG are managed similarly to GD i.e., rendering euthyroid with ATDs, followed by definitive therapy. Extent of surgery in toxic solitary adenoma depends on radiology, nuclear imaging after malignancy is ruled out. Newer ablative therapies like RFA, EA, LTA are considered as a substitute for definitive therapy in selective patients. Nonetheless malignancy should always be treated by surgery.

Conflict of interest

"The authors declare no conflict of interest."

Author details

Kul Ranjan Singh and Anand Kumar Mishra*
Department of Endocrine Surgery, King George's Medical University, Lucknow, U.P., India

*Address all correspondence to: mishra101@gmail com

References

[1] Terry J. Smith LH. Graves' Disease. N Engl Med. 2016;375(16):1552-1565.

[2] Nayak B, Hodak SP. Hyperthyroidism. Endocrinol Metab Clin North Am. 2007;36(3):617-656.

[3] Watters DA WJ. Thyroid surgery in the tropics. ANZ J Surg. 77(11):933-40.

[4] Hookham J, Truran P, Allahabadia A BS. Patients' perceptions and views of surgery and radioiodine ablation in the definitive management of Graves' disease. Postgr Med J. 2017;93(1099):266-270.

[5] Hookham J, Truran P, Allahabadia A, Balasubramanian SP. Patients ' perceptions and views of surgery and radioiodine ablation in the de fi nitive management of Graves ' disease. 2017;266-270.

[6] Bartalena L, Tanda ML. Graves'ophthalmopathy. N Eng J Med 2009;360:994-1001

[7] Kahaly GJ, Olivo PD. Graves' disease. N Eng J Med 2017;376:184

[8] Okosieme OE, Taylor PN, Evans C, Thayer D, Chai A, Khan I, Draman MS, Tennant B, Geen J, Sayers A, French R, Lazarus JH, Premawardhana LD, Dayan CM Primary therapy of Graves' disease and cardiovascular morbidity and mortality: a linked-record cohort study. Lancet Diabetes Endocrinol. 2019 Apr; 7(4):278-287.

[9] Lillevang-Johansen M, Abrahamsen B, Jørgensen HL, Brix TH, Hegedüs L Excess Mortality in Treated and Untreated Hyperthyroidism Is Related to Cumulative Periods of Low Serum TSH. J Clin Endocrinol Metab. 2017 Jul 1; 102(7):2301-2309.

[10] Dale J, Daykin J, Holder R, Sheppard MC, Franklyn JA. Weight gain following treatment of hyperthyroidism. Clin Endocrinol (Oxf). 2001 Aug; 55(2):233-239

[11] Bartalena L, Baldeschi L, Dickinson A, Eckstein A, Kendall-Taylor P, Marcocci C, et al, Consensus statement of the European Group on Graves' orbitopathy (EUGOGO) on management of GO.. Eur J Endocrinol. 2008 Mar; 158(3):273-285

[12] Bartalena L, Marcocci C, Bogazzi F, et al. Relation between therapy for hyperthyroidism and the course of Graves' ophthalmopathy. N Engl J Med. 1998;338:73-78 [PubMed] [Google Scholar]

[13] Tallstedt L, Lundell G, Torring O, et al. Occurrence of ophthalmopathy after treatment for Graves' hyperthyroidism. The Thyroid Study Group. N Engl J Med. 1992;326:1733-1738 [PubMed] [Google Scholar]

[14] Genovese BM, Noureldine SI, Gleeson EM, Tufano RP, Kandil E. What is the best definitive treatment for Graves' disease? A systematic review of the existing literature. Ann Surg Oncol. 2013;20:660-667.

[15] Bobanga ID, McHenry CR. Treatment of patients with Graves' disease and the appropriate extent of thyroidectomy. Best Pract Res Clin Endocrinol Metab [Internet]. 2019;33(4):101319. Available from: https://doi.org/10.1016/j.beem.2019.101319

[16] Kitahara CM, Berrington De Gonzalez A, Bouville A, Brill AB, Doody MM, Melo DR, et al. Association of Radioactive Iodine Treatment with Cancer Mortality in Patients with Hyperthyroidism. JAMA Intern Med. 2019;179(8):1034-1042.

[17] Stålberg, P., Svensson, A., Hessman O et al. Surgical Treatment of Graves'

Disease: Evidence-Based Approach. World J Surg. 2008;32:1269-1277.

[18] Stathopoulos P, Gangidi S, Kotrotsos G, Cunliffe D. Graves' disease: A review of surgical indications, management, and complications in a cohort of 59 patients. Int J Oral Maxillofac Surg [Internet]. 2015;44(6):713-717. Available from: http://dx.doi.org/10.1016/j.ijom.2015.02.007

[19] Zhang L, Li J, Tian Q, Liu S, Zhang H, Liu S, et al. Follow-up and evaluation of the pregnancy outcome in women of reproductive age with Graves ' disease after 131 Iodine treatment. 2016;57(6):702-8.

[20] Léger J, Oliver I, Rodrigue D, Lambert AS, Coutant R. Graves' disease in children. Ann Endocrinol (Paris) [Internet]. 2018;79(6):647-55. Available from: https://doi.org/10.1016/j.ando.2018.08.001

[21] Staniforth JUL, Erdirimanne S, Eslick GD. Thyroid carcinoma in Graves' disease: A meta-analysis. Int J Surg [Internet]. 2016;27(2016):118-125. Available from: http://dx.doi.org/10.1016/j.ijsu.2015.11.027

[22] Shi HH MC. Coexistent thyroid nodules in patients with graves' disease: What is the frequency and the risk of malignancy. Am J Surg. 216(5):980-4.

[23] De Bellis A, Conzo G, Cennamo G, Pane E, Bellastella G, Colella C, Iacovo AD, Paglionico VA, Sinisi AA, Wall JR, Bizzarro A BA. Time course of Graves' ophthalmopathy after total thyroidectomy alone or followed by radioiodine therapy: a 2-year longitudinal study. Endocrine. 2012;41(2):320-326.

[24] Bartalena L. The dilemma of how to manage Graves' hyperthyroidism in patients with associated orbitopathy. J Clin Endocrinol Metab. 2011;96(3):592-599.

[25] Burch HB, Cooper DS. Management of graves disease a review. JAMA - J Am Med Assoc. 2015;314(23):2544-2554.

[26] Genovese BM, Noureldine SI, Gleeson EM, Tufano RP KE. What is the best definitive treatment for Graves' disease? A systematic review of the existing literature. Ann Surg Oncol. 20(2):660-7.

[27] Sundaresh V, Brito JP, Wang Z, Prokop LJ, Stan MN, Murad MH, et al. Comparative effectiveness of therapies for graves' hyperthyroidism: A systematic review and network meta-A nalysis. J Clin Endocrinol Metab. 2013;98(9):3671-3677.

[28] Törring O, Watt T, Sjölin G, Byström K, Abraham-Nordling M, Calissendorff J, Cramon PK, Filipsson Nyström H, Hallengren B, Holmberg M, Khamisi S, Lantz M WG. No Title. Impair Qual Life After Radioiodine Ther Comp to Antithyroid Drugs or Surg Treat Graves' Hyperthyroidism A Long-Term Follow with Thyroid Patient-Reported Outcome Quest 36-Item Short Form Heal Status . 29(3):322-31.

[29] Purdy AC, Idriss A, Ahern S, Lin E ED. Dr Google: The readability and accuracy of patient education websites for Graves' disease treatment. Surgery. 162(5):1148-54.

[30] Ross DS, Burch HB, Cooper DS, Greenlee MC, Laurberg P, Maia AL, et al. 2016 American Thyroid Association Guidelines for Diagnosis and Management of Hyperthyroidism and Other Causes of Thyrotoxicosis. Thyroid. 2016;26(10):1343-1421.

[31] Unless R, Act P, Rose W, If T, Rose W. This is a repository copy of Variation in the use of definitive treatment options in the management of Graves ' disease : a UK clinician survey. White Rose Research Online URL for this paper : Version : Accepted Version Article : Hookham , J ., Collins ,. 2016;

[32] Cox SC, Tamatea JA, Conaglen JV EM. The management of Graves' disease in New Zealand 2014. N Z Med J.

[33] Beshyah SA, Khalil AB, Sherif IH, Benbarka MM, Raza SA, Hussein W, Alzahrani AS C. A SURVEY OF CLINICAL PRACTICE PATTERNS IN MANAGEMENT OF GRAVES DISEASE IN THE MIDDLE EAST AND NORTH AFRICA. Endocr Pr. 23(3):299-308.

[34] Mercier F, Bonal M, Fanget F, Maillard L, Laplace N, Peix JL, et al. Does Surgery Without Lugol's Solution Pretreatment for Graves' Disease Increase Surgical Morbidity? World J Surg [Internet]. 2018;42(7):2123-6. Available from: https://doi.org/10.1007/s00268-017-4443-3

[35] Calissendorff J, Falhammar H. Lugol's solution and other iodide preparations: perspectives and research directions in Graves' disease. Endocrine. 2017;58(3):467-473.

[36] Akram S, Elfenbein DM, Chen H, Schneider DF, Sippel RS. Assessing American Thyroid Association Guidelines for Total Thyroidectomy in Graves' Disease. J Surg Res [Internet]. 2020;245:64-71. Available from: https://doi.org/10.1016/j.jss.2019.07.029

[37] Tripathi M, Karwasra RK, Parshad S. Effect of preoperative vitamin D deficiency on postoperative hypocalcemia after thyroid surgery. Thyroid Res. 2014;7(1):4-9.

[38] Maxwell AK, Shonka DC, Robinson DJ, Levine PA. Association of preoperative calcium and calcitriol therapy with postoperative hypocalcemia after total thyroidectomy. JAMA Otolaryngol - Head Neck Surg. 2017;143(7):679-684.

[39] Jaan S, Sehgal A, Wani R, Wani M, Wani K, Laway B. Usefulness of pre-and post-operative calcium and Vitamin D supplementation in prevention of hypocalcemia after total thyroidectomy: A randomized controlled trial. Indian J Endocrinol Metab. 2017;21(1):51-55.

[40] Corvilain B, Hamy A, Brunaud L, Borson-Chazot F, Orgiazzi J, Bensalem Hachmi L, et al. Treatment of adult Graves' disease. Ann Endocrinol (Paris). 2018;79(6):618-635.

[41] Al Qubaisi M, Haigh PI. Hypocalcemia after Total Thyroidectomy in Graves Disease. Perm J. 2019;23:1-4.

[42] Kwon H. Increased risk of postoperative complications after total thyroidectomy with Graves ' disease. 2018;(December 2017):281-5.

[43] Mallick R, Asban A, Chung S, Hur J, Lindeman B CH. To admit or not to admit? Experience with outpatient thyroidectomy for Graves' disease in a high-volume tertiary care center. Am J Surg. 216(5):985-9.

[44] Ali A, Debono M, Balasubramanian SP. Outcomes After Urgent Thyroidectomy Following Rapid Control of Thyrotoxicosis in Graves' Disease are Similar to Those After Elective Surgery in Well-Controlled Disease. World J Surg [Internet]. 2019;43(12):3051-8. Available from: https://doi.org/10.1007/s00268-019-05125-5

[45] Nair GC, Babu MJC, Menon R, Jacob P. Preoperative preparation of hyperthyroidism for thyroidectomy - Role of supersaturated iodine and lithium carbonate. Indian J Endocrinol Metab. 2018;22(3):392-396.

[46] Panzer C, Beazley R, Braverman L. Rapid Preoperative Preparation for Severe Hyperthyroid Graves' Disease. J Clin Endocrinol Metab. 2004;89(5):2142-2144.

[47] Al Jassim A, Wallace T, Bouhabel S, Majdan A, Hier M, Forest VI, et al.

A retrospective cohort study: Do patients with graves' disease need to be euthyroid prior to surgery? J Otolaryngol - Head Neck Surg. 2018;47(1):3-7.

[48] Maurer E, Maschuw K, Reuss A, Zieren HU, Zielke A, Goretzki P, et al. Total Versus Near-Total Thyroidectomy in Graves Disease: Results of the Randomized Controlled Multicenter TONIG-trial. Ann Surg. 2019;270(5):755-761.

[49] Barczyński M, Konturek A, Stopa M, Cichoń S, Richter P NW. Total thyroidectomy for benign thyroid disease: is it really worthwhile? Ann Surg. 254(5):724-9.

[50] Liu ZW, Masterson L, Fish B, Jani P, Chatterjee K. Thyroid surgery for Graves' disease and Graves' ophthalmopathy. Cochrane Database Syst Rev. 2015;2015(11).

[51] Ho TW, Shaheen AA, Dixon E HA. Utilization of thyroidectomy for benign disease in the United States: a 15-year population-based study. Am J Surg. 201(5):570-4.

[52] Hu J, Zhao N, Kong R, Wang D, Sun B, Wu L. Total thyroidectomy as primary surgical management for thyroid disease: Surgical therapy experience from 5559 thyroidectomies in a less-developed region. World J Surg Oncol [Internet]. 2016;14(1):1-7. Available from: http://dx.doi.org/10.1186/s12957-016-0772-1

[53] Cooper DS. Hyperthyroidism. 2003;

[54] Donovan PJ, McLeod DSA, Little R, Gordon L. Cost-utility analysis comparing radioactive iodine, anti-Thyroid drugs and total thyroidectomy for primary treatment of Graves' disease. Eur J Endocrinol. 2016;175(6):595-603.

[55] In H, Pearce EN, Wong AK, Burgess JF, McAneny DB, Rosen JE. Treatment Options for Graves Disease: A Cost-Effectiveness Analysis. J Am Coll Surg [Internet]. 2009;209(2):170-179.e2. Available from: http://dx.doi.org/10.1016/j.jamcollsurg.2009.03.025

[56] Zhang Y, Dong Z, Li J, Yang J, Yang W, Wang C. Comparison of endoscopic and conventional open thyroidectomy for Graves' disease: A meta-analysis. Int J Surg [Internet]. 2017;40(2017):52-59. Available from: http://dx.doi.org/10.1016/j.ijsu.2017.02.054

[57] Garstka M, Kandil E, Saparova L, Bechara M, Green R, Haddad AB, Kang SW AP. Surgery for Graves' disease in the era of robotic-assisted surgery: a study of safety and feasibility in the Western population. Langenbecks Arch Surg. 2018;403(7):891-896.

[58] Kwon H, Yi JW, Song RY, Chai YJ, Kim SJ, Choi JY, et al. Comparison of Bilateral Axillo-Breast Approach Robotic Thyroidectomy with Open Thyroidectomy for Graves' Disease. World J Surg. 2016;40(3):498-504.

Chapter 12

Graves' Disease and Cardiac Complications

Abdulla Arslan and Hakan Altay

Abstract

Graves' Disease is an autoimmune thyroid disease and a common cause of hyperthyroidism. Thyroid hormones have multiple adverse effect on cardiovascular system through many direct and indirect mechanisms. They increases heart rate, cardiac contractility, systolic and mean pulmonary artery pressure, cardiac output, diastolic relaxation, and myocardial oxygen consumption, whereas decrease systemic vascular resistance and diastolic pressure. All these hemodynamic changes in cardiovascular system can eventually lead to heart failure, tachyarrhythmias, systemic and pulmonary hypertension, if left untreated. Cardiovascular complications of Graves' Disease are frequent and important cause of increased morbidity and mortality. This chapter reviews the cardiovascular complications of Graves' hyperthyroidism with underlying mechanisms and treatment.

Keywords: Graves' Disease, cardiac complications, heart failure, thyrotoxicosis, pulmonary hypertension

1. Introduction

Robert Graves identified the association of goiter, palpitations, and exophthalmos in 1835 [1]. Although the cause of Graves' hyperthyroidism was initially thought to be thyrotropin, it was later understood that Graves' hyperthyroidism was clearly caused by thyroid stimulating antibodies-IgG- which bind to and activate to thyrotropin receptors on thyroid cells [2]. Although the incidence is not known exactly, manifest hyperthyroidism is common and affects 2–5% of the population [3]. Approximately 60–80% of hyperthyroidism cases have Graves' Disease due to regional factors, particularly iodine intake. Over a period of 20 years, the incidence in women is around 0.5 per 1000 annually and the most frequent onset age gap is 40–60; hence, Graves' Disease is most common autoimmune disorder in the United States [4]. Graves' Disease rate in men is between 1/5 and 1/10 and equal to women; however, the disease is unusual in children. The prevalence is lower in African-Americans in reference to Asians and Whites [5]. Graves' Disease has similarities with autoimmune hypothyroidism, including high serum concentrations of antibodies against thyroglobulin, thyroid peroxidase, and possibly the sodium-iodide cotransporter in thyroid tissue. These antibodies' concentrations vary among patients, and the antibodies themselves may modify the stimulatory effects of thyroid-stimulating antibodies. In some patients, the simultaneous production of antibodies that block the thyrotropin receptor reduces the stimulatory action of thyroid-stimulating antibodies. For these reasons there is no direct correlation between serum concentrations of thyroid-stimulating antibodies and serum thyroid hormone concentrations in patients with Graves' hyperthyroidism [6].

Thyroid hormones have major effects on the heart and cardiovascular system through many mechanisms. They increase heart rate, cardiac contractility, systolic and mean pulmonary artery pressure, cardiac output, diastolic relaxation, and myocardial oxygen consumption, and reduce systemic vascular resistance and diastolic pressure [7]. Cardiovascular symptoms have been showing some signs of patients clinical presentation for the physicians: palpitations, exercise intolerance, dyspnoea, angina-like chest pain, peripheral edema and congestive heart failure are common symptoms of hyperthyroidism [8, 9]. In hyperthyroid patients mortality is increased by 20% and the major causes of death are cardiac problems [10].

2. Graves' hyperthyroidism

The clinical manifestation and the laboratory findings aid to establish the diagnosis of Graves' Disease in hyperthyroidism patients. Especially, serum thyrotropin levels is very beneficial marker in hyperthyroidism because secretion is thyrotropin is substantially reduced by small amount of elevation in thyroid secretion. Nevertheless, the diagnosis should be confirmed via the serum free thyroxine measurements [11]. However, in the early periods, only triiodothyronine increase may occur; considering this condition serum free triiodothyronine levels should be examined in the presence of normal serum free thyroxine and low serum thyrotropin concentrations. On the other hand, serum total thyroxine and triiodothyronine measurements are not as reliable as aforementioned markers because the certain drug use may cause elevated values in thyroid hormone–binding proteins. Establishing the diagnosis in a patient with hyperthyroidism is shown here:

3. Algorhythm for the diagnosis of suspected Hyperthyroidism

In the first step: Measure serum thyrotropin and free thyroxine

1. Low serum thyrotropin and normal free thyroxine- → Measure serum free triiodothyronine:

   A. Normal serum free triiodothyronine; Subclınıcal Hyperthyroidism

   B. High serum free triiodothyronine- → Triiodothyronine Hyperthyroidism

2. Low serum thyrotropin and high free thyroxine- → Hyperthyroidism

Diagnosis of Graves' hyperthyroidism was established for patients with biochemical evidence of overt hyperthyroidism, i.e. **high levels** of serum free T4, free T3, TSH < 0.1 mIU/l accompanied by at least two of following parameters: diffuse goiter, Graves' ophthalmopathy, **increased level** of anti-TSH receptor antibodies (TRAb), antithyroid peroxidase antibodies (TPOAb).

4. Pathogenesis

4.1 Cardiac effects, molecular and cellular mechanisms

Cellular and molecular mechanisms by which thyroid exerts its action on almost every cell and organ in the body have been well studied [12]. Thyroid gland maintains T4 and T3 excretion according to TSH levels. The thyroid gland primarily secretes T4 (≈85%), which is converted to T3 by 5′-monodeiodination in the liver, kidney, and skeletal muscle. The heart function is mainly based on T3, because of the absence of myocyte intracellular deiodinase activity and T3 migrates into the myocyte instead T4 [13]. Then, the activity of T3 is administered after binding to thyroid hormone nuclear receptors (THRs). Then, these receptor proteins binds to thyroid hormone response elements (TREs) in the promoter regions of positively regulated genes thus regulates the transcription [12, 14]. T3 acts on THRs in the nucleus, and creating dimers of 9-cis-retinoic acid receptor (RXR) [15]: the formed complexes recognize some specific DNA consensus sequences, TREs, located in the enhanced region of the genes to initiate the transcription [16]. Although, TRs considered as a steroid hormone receptors, unlikely, bind to TREs regardless of whether ligand is present or not. TRs connect to TREs with 1 of 3 isoforms of retinoid X receptor (RXRα, RXRβ, or RXR$^{\gamma}$) as homodimers or heterodimers [17]. While bound to T3, TRs induce transcription, and in the absence of T3 they repress transcription. Thyroid hormone upregulates α, but downregulates β-chain in myocytes [18]. Negatively regulated cardiac genes such as β-myosin heavy chain and phospholamban are induced in the absence of T3 and repressed in the presence of T3 [19, 20].

Thyroid hormone has a direct impact on cardiac activity through myocytes by achieving structural and regulatory gene expressions. The 2 isoforms of a contractile protein pertain to thick filament of cardiac myocyte is codified by myosin heavy chain gene.

The sarcoplasmic reticulum Ca^{2+}-ATPase and its inhibitor, phospholamban, regulate intracellular calcium cycling. Together they are largely responsible for enhanced contractile function and diastolic relaxation in the heart [21]. T3 levels are also intimately associated with the β –adrenergic receptors and sodium potassium ATPase.

Thyroid hormone cause extranuclear genome-free effects on both the cardiac myocyte and systemic vasculature. These effects of T3 can occur rapidly and do not involve

TRE-mediated transcriptional events [22]. These T3-mediated effects include changes in various membrane ion channels for sodium, potassium, and calcium, effects on actin polymerization, adenine nucleotide translocator-1 in the mitochondrial membrane, and a variety of intracellular signaling pathways in the heart and vascular smooth muscle cells (VSM) **A27**. The collaboration of the both genomic and nongenomic features of the T3 activity regulate the cardiovascular system.

Thyroid hormone express its activity in myocytes via various TREs, such as alpha myosin heavy chain fusion (MHC-α), sarcoplasmic reticulum calcium-activated ATPase (SERCA): which maintains calcium uptake during diastole, by calcium activated ATPase and phospholamban -the inhibitory cofactor- [23, 24] the cellular membrane Na-K pump (Na-K ATPase), β1 adrenergic receptor, cardiac troponin I, and atrial natriuretic peptide (ANP), and some genes are also suppressed, such as β-myosin heavy chain fusion (MHC-β), adenylyl cyclase (IV and V) and the Na-Ca antiporter [25–27]. The final effect of thyroid hormones in animal studies-and also similar effects have also been observed in preliminary human studies-is increased rate of V1 isoform of MHC (MHCα/α) synthesis that is characteristically faster in myocardial fiber shortening [28–30]. Thyroid hormones enhance myocardial relaxation by upregulating expression of SERCA, and downregulating expression of phospholamban. Cytoplasmic calcium concentration substantially decrease at the end of the diastole. This cause a higher magnitude of systolic transient of calcium; therefore heightens capacity for actin-myosin subunits activation. As a supportive evidence, a phospholamban deficient mice demonstrated no tachycardia in response to thyroid hormone treatment [31] on the plasma membranes, T3 has extragenic actions on various ion channels such as Na/K ATPase, Na/Ca++ exchanger, and voltage gated K channels (Kv 1.5, Kv 4.2, Kv 4.3) affecting cardiovascular hemodynamics [32].

For instance, Na channel activation period augments in myocardium; this cause prolonged intracellular Na uptake and increased secondary Na-Ca antiporter functions. Thus underlying mechanism under the inotropic effect may be comparatively revealed [33]. T3 effects on L-type calcium channels directly by abbreviating the action potential period [34, 35]. The augmentation of β-adrenergic receptors the may be the main reason for the intense inotropic response to the thyroid hormones [36]. Although, G protein and β-receptors increased; circulating cathecolamine measurements remained similar [37]. The sensitivity of the cardiovascular system to adrenergic stimulation is not changed by thyroid hormones. The changes in the heart rate result from both an increase in sympathetic tone and decrease in parasympathetic tone [38, 39]. Rapid response for the Cardiac and vascular structures of the thyroid hormone response was not sufficiently clarified by genomic effects [40–42].

Hyperthyroidism elicits rapid hemodynamic response as well as non-genomic changes in plasma membranes. Authors, indicate that thyroid hormone stimulates acute phosphorylation of phospholamban. This pathway may be slightly responsible the collaboration between thyroid hormone and the adrenergic effects on the heart [43].

The use of β-adrenergic receptor antagonists in hyperthyroidism reduced heart rate, but systolic or diastolic contractile performance remained similar, supporting the direct cardiac muscle effect of thyroid hormone [44]. Meanwhile, thyroid hormone impacted on the sinoatrial node and caused oxidative stress in experimental studies. The heart rate is parallel to the sinoatrial activity, lower threshold for atrial activity, and shortened atrial repolarization [45]. Hemodynamic changes such as volume preload increase following the renin-angiotensin system activation or augmented contractility due to improved metabolic demand or the reduction in the direct effect of the thyroid hormone on heart muscle, decreased systemic vascular resistance caused by triiodothyronine-induced peripheral vasodilatation, lead to a dramatic impairment in cardiac output [7, 46, 47].

Preload is increased in a state of hyperthyroidism, and the reduced peripheral vascular resistance and elevated heart rate lead to increased cardiac output. The reduction in systemic vascular resistance lead to impaired renal perfusion pressure thus activates renin-angiotensin-aldosterone system (RAAS), hence sodium reabsorption and blood volume increase. In turn, this leads to increased preload, decreased afterload, and **ultimately** a significant increase in stroke volume [48]. Furthermore, it is suggested that T3 enhances renin substrate synthesis in liver and stimulates the cardiac expression of renin mRNA, leading to elevated cardiac renin levels and angiotensin II independent from the circulating renin and angiotensin. The expression of angiotensin II receptors in the myocardium increases in the hyperthyroid state [49]. These hemodynamic responses trigger atrial stretch trigger and stimulate atrial natriuretic peptide (ANP) secretion, resulting in more vasodilation. Such changes figure out a critical role of the myocardial RAAS in thyroxine-induced cardiac hypertrophy as well as potential therapeutic implications of agents that block this system.

Adrenomedullin, a polypeptide of 52 amino acids, is a potent vasodilator and thyroid gland is responsible for regulation transcription of adrenomedullin. Serum levels therefore proportionally increase in thyrotoxicosis [50]. Interestingly, however, Diekman and colleagues demonstrated that although systemic vascular resistance (SVR) is decreased and adrenomedullin is increased in thyrotoxicosis, restoration of euthyroidism normalized SVR but was not correlated with plasma adrenomedullin levels [51]. In the present study, only T3 was an independent determinant of SVR.

5. Clinical manifestations and Hemodynamic Effects of Thyroid Hormones

The clinical manifestations and the severity of the disease are strongly correlated to the duration of Graves' Disease and the patient age. More than half of the patients are symptomatic in time of diagnosis. The most frequent findings may be counted as nervousness, fatigue, a rapid heartbeat or palpitations, heat intolerance, and weight loss respectively. By age, weight loss and decreased appetite are frequently observed, whereas irritability and heat intolerance are less frequent. Atrial fibrillation is occasional below age 50. A firm, diffuse goiter of variable size presents in the 90% and 75% patients, respectively; when 50 years of age was hold as threshold [52].

Thyroid hormone has cardiovascular effects that include decreased SVR and increased resting heart rate, left ventricular contractility, and blood volume. Thyroid hormone reduce the peripheral arteriolar resistance and decrease mean arterial pressure, through the renin-angiotensin-aldosterone system. Also, T3 increases erythropoietin synthesis, which leads to an increase in red cell mass. Harmony of these effects contribute to increase in blood volume and preload. In hyperthyroidism, these combined mechanisms maximize cardiac output up to 300% higher when compared to control group. In hypothyroidism, the cardiovascular effects are diametrically opposite and cardiac output may decrease by 30–50% [53].

Thyroid hormone shows its affects rapidly and non-genomic pathway through heart and blood vessels. Beyond what is reported above, In the peripheral vascular system, the elevated oxygen consumption, metabolic remnants and relaxation of arterial smooth muscle fibers by thyroid hormone eventuate in peripheral vasodilatation [32]. This dramatical decrease in peripheral vascular resistance (PVR) has a great role in hemodynamic changes caused by thyroid hormones [54]. Decreased PVR results in bradycardia, a selective increased blood flow towards visceral organs eventually, cause a decrease in diastolic pressure thus widen pulse pressure. Vasodilatation without elevated renal blood flow results in a reduction in renal perfusion thus activates the renin-angiotensin cascade. Hence, sodium retention and increased blood volume occurs [46]. Moreover, thyroid hormones effects on erythropoietin secretion; hence cause to increase in red cell mass and the blood volume [55]. Increased diastolic relaxation and blood volume improves left ventricular end-diastolic volume (LVEDV). Reduced PVR and increased LVEDV in together, augment preload and impair afterload; thus the stroke volume increases. Improved stroke volume and heart rate increase cardiac output, which cannot be only a consequence of an increased metabolic rate [56]. The correlation between systemic vascular resistance and systemic blood flow in hyperthyroidism is investigated previously, focusing on arterial vasoconstrictors in particular. On the contrary to the normal subjects, atropine and phenylephrine succeeded to decrease peripheral blood flow and cardiac output by 34% in hyperthyroidism group [57].

Studies including large cohorts determined that blood pressure levels widened throughout the entire spectrum of thyroid function [58]. In this study, Asvold et al. reported a linear correlation between TSH and both systolic and diastolic blood pressure, however other studies did not find a correlation [59]. Basal metabolism is triggered by thyroid hormones and a complete response develops in almost every tissue and organ system in the body, as a consequence of increased metabolic demands, hemodynamic changes in cardiac output, SVR, and blood pressure occur. On several counts, such changes are similar to the physiological response to exercise [60]. Pulse pressure tends to be widened in case of hyperthyroidism. Some current reports have determined that despite the low SVR in hyperthyroidism, arterial stiffness is increased [61]. Thus excess thyroid hormone typically enforce systolic blood pressure to rise, the increase can therefore be quite dramatic in older patients with atherosclerosis led to impaired arterial compliance. Hyperthyroidism has been identified as the second most common reason for isolated systolic hypertension [62]. Efficient hyperthyroidism treatment and the administration of β-blockade to achieve normocardia reverses these changes. In hypothyroidism, endothelial dysfunction and impaired VSM relaxation eventuate in lower SVR [63]. These effects lead to diastolic hypertension in ≈30% of patients, and thyroid hormone replacement therapy restores endothelial-derived vasorelaxation and blood pressure to normal in most [64].

Sinus tachycardia is the most frequent ECG disorder. Intraventricular conduction delay in the form a right bundle branch block is observed in approximate of 15% patients.

Alternative, unknown reasons may also be present for the occurrence of atrioventricular block Increased dispersion of QT interval corrected by the heart rate (QTcD) and pulmonary hypertension may also be present, however underlying mechanisms are yet unclear; the similar cardiac and hemodynamic changes accompanying with the autoimmune disorders in Graves' patients probably contribute to conduction problems [65]. Hyperthyroidism leads to shortened action potential and altered expression of L-type calcium channel 1D, enhances Na and K permeability, and affects Na pump density [66]. The forced preload increase and altered total blood volume impose burden on cardiac workload, hence frequently myocardial hypertrophy develops.

6. Graves' Disease and atrial fibrillation

Patients with hyperthyroidism manifest more premature supraventricular depolarization and premature atrial complex (PAC; also referred to a premature atrial beat, premature supraventricular complex, or premature supraventricular beat), more nonsustained supraventricular tachycardias, and reduced heart rate variability [67]. The reduced variability is probably occurs as a consequence of decreased parasympathetic tone. These electrical stimulates may lead to paroxysmal atrial tachycardia, atrial fibrillation, and atrial flutter. The most frequent rhythm disorder is sinus tachycardia in hyperthyroidism [43]. Its clinical impact is overshadowed by atrial fibrillation. The rate of atrial fibrillation (AF) and other rare forms of supraventricular tachycardia in this disease varies between 2% and 20% The prevalence of atrial fibrillation in hyperthyroidism was determined as 13.8%, however peaked at up to 15% in patients over the age of 70 years. These results is significantly higher when compared to the rate of 2.3% in control group [66–69]. Atrial fibrillation often coexists with a rapid ventricular response. The occurrence of AF is more frequent in men and significantly increases with age, over 40 years in particular [69]. A current study revealed that the AF rate was below 2% in a cohort includes more than 13 k cases with hyperthyroidism. Early stage of disease or recognition may contribute to these result [70]. A stepwise increase in the prevalence was observed in the analysis based on age, especially peaked at ≈15% in patients >70 years old. This findings support data from the cohort of 40.628 hyperthyroid patients in the Danish National Registry. This database revealed that although 8.3% of the patients demonstrated an atrial fibrillation; male gender, the presence of ischemic or valvular heart disease or congestive heart failure were associated with the highest risk rates. Apparently, subclinical (mild) hyperthyroidism involves similar relative risk for atrial fibrillation as does overt disease [68]. This dilemma may be interpreted in favor of other accompanying diseases that occur in the older population. In unselected patients with atrial fibrillation, less than 1% were the consequence of over-hyperthyroidism [71]. Consequently, although the abnormal thyroid function levels seems less reliable and indicative in the new-onset atrial fibrillation, establishing an euthyroid state and achieving sinus rhythm, justifies the value of TSH examining [7].

The left atrial size is enlarged in most of the patients with hyperthyroidism and AF rather than hyperthyroid people with sinus rhythm. Hyperthyroidism should not be accepted as the only reason for developing the new onset AF and possible underlying organic heart diseases should be investigated to avoid as serious cardiovascular events such as angina or heart failure. In an experimental study, connexin-40, a gap junction protein of myocardium which is essential for the transport of electrical activity upregulated by thyroid hormone in rats. This pathway may contribute to atrial fibrillation development in hyperthyroidism [72].

Atrial fibrillation generally reverts to sinus rhythm when an euthyroid state established. On the other hand, in young and early diagnosed patients β-Adrenergic blockade may be sufficient to regulate the ventricular rate. Higher dose may be required in case of elevated plasma clearance of β-blockers. Propranolol has an additional advantage by blocking T4 - T3 conversion in peripheral tissues. Nevertheless, cardio-selective β-blockers have a longer half-life and have similar cardiac effects. Intravascular administration of calcium blockers should be avoided considering the possible risk of a further fall in PVR: channel blockers, may cause potential adverse cardiovascular events such as blood pressure reduction via developing relaxation through smooth muscle cells of the resistance arterioles. Such treatment has been linked to acute hypotension and cardiovascular collapse [73]. Treatment of atrial fibrillation in the setting of hyperthyroidism includes β -adrenergic blockade. This can be accomplished with β 1-selective or nonselective agents, even in peroral usage, whereas treatments such as antithyroid therapy or radioiodine, which lead to a restoration of a chemical euthyroid state [7]. Although digitalis was an option in the treatment of hyperthyroidism and coexisting atrial fibrillation, due to the increased digitalis clearance and decreased sensitivity of the hyperthyroid heart to digitalis necessitated higher doses for optimal treatment beside leading to less predictable responses [74, 75]. How much risk does the systemic embolization include in the setting of thyrotoxicosis is yet unclear. It is still controversial whether to administer an anticoagulant therapy in patients with AF is efficient to prevent systemic embolization. Accordingly, each patient should be evaluated individually considering the risk of bleeding over embolization [76]. Hyperthyroidism in younger patients without any cardiac disease except for AF, the risk of anticoagulant therapy **may exceed its benefits**. However, it would be wise to administer anticoagulant drugs to older patients with previously diagnosed or suspected heart diseases or AF with longer duration. Oral anticoagulants doses should be trimmed considering that hyperthyroid patients will require less medication than euthyroid ones, **due to faster elimination of vitamin-K** dependent clotting factors [77]. Early diagnosis and full treatment radioiodine or thioureas demonstrated a reversion to sinus rhythm most patients within 2 to 3 months [70]. Older patients (>60 years old) with atrial fibrillation with longer duration are more resistant to spontaneous reversion to sinus rhythm. For this reason, electrical or pharmacological cardioversion are advised to attempt if the AF continues after an euthyroid state achieved chemically. Following an adequate treatment most of the patients turn into sinus rhythm permanently. Disopyramide (300 mg/d) administration after successful cardioversion, contribute to remain in sinus rhythm when compared to those not treated [76].

Reversion and maintenance from AF to sinus rhythm is unusual before the euthyroid state is achieved; therefore electrical cardioversion should be avoided before euthyroid condition. In another experimental study, the authors remarked the downregulator effects T3 via connexin-43 phosphorylation in diabetic rats. Thus, cardiac adaption to hyperglycemia reduced and the heart become **prones** to ventricular arrhythmias [78].

7. Graves' Disease and heart failure

Early manifestations regarding heart failure may be present in patients with hyperthyroidism [7, 14, 79]. Majority of the patients with hyperthyroidism suffer from exercise intolerance and exertional dyspnea, due to the loss of skeletal and respiratory muscle strength. Hyperthyroid patients can demonstrate congestive heart failure symptoms regardless of prior cardiac injury. This phenomenon has inaccurately identified "high-output heart failure," in the presence of paradoxical features involving enhanced cardiac contractility and output characterized by thyroid hormone excess [7]. Decreased cardiac contractility, reduced diastolic compliance, and pulmonary congestion are true manifestations of the heart failure however these can be consequences of severe and chronic hyperthyroidism, tachycardia, and **atrial fibrillation also** [80–82]. The use of "high output heart failure" has not abandoned in late decades, considering the potential of the heart to enhance the output at both rest and exercise. However, In the setting of low vascular resistance and decreased preload, cardiac functional reserve is compromised thus lose the capacity of accommodating the demands of maximal or even submaximal exercise [83]. High-output heart failure may demonstrate dyspnea on exertion, fatigue, and fluid retention with peripheral edema, pleural effusion, hepatic congestion, and PAH [82]. Heart failure develops approximately in the 6% of thyrotoxic patients. Beyond that, dilated cardiomyopathy with reduced left ventricular systolic dysfunction occurs less than 1%, due to a tachycardia-mediated mechanism causing an elevated cytosolic calcium levels during diastole with impaired contractility of the ventricle and diastolic dysfunction, often with tricuspid regurgitation [84]. A research conducted by Yue *et al.*, diastolic dysfunction was found to be more prominent in thyrotoxic patients older than 40 years of age, whereas in younger ones a demonstrated a reduction in peripheral vascular resistance and improved cardiac output were outstanding [85]. However, severe and chronic hyperthyroidism may exaggerate sinus tachycardia or atrial fibrillation; hence, produce rate-related left ventricular dysfunction and heart failure [86]. This clarifies the reason why several patients manifesting the combination of hyperthyroidism, low cardiac output, and impaired left ventricular function had AF at the time of diagnosis [7]. However, pre-existent ischemic or hypertensive heart disease may also contribute the to the development of heart failure in hyperthyroid patients [14, 86].

Mitral valve prolapse is more frequently reported in patients with Graves' Diseases. The latter may be a predisposing factor for the elonged the left atrial diameter and atrial fibrillation [87]. The risk for AF which may lead to congestive heart increases in the presence of low TSH levels, especially among patients over 60 years old [88, 89]. The high prevalence of pulmonary artery hypertension that comprises several signs of heart failure, such as neck vein distension and peripheral edema, may be caused by right heart strain [90, 91]. Similarly, reduced pulmonary compliance and skeletal muscle dysfunction may lead to the exercise intolerance and exertional dyspnea in such patients [14]. Distinctively, thyrotoxic cardiomyopathy represents a myocardial damage that caused by toxic effects as a result of excessive thyroid hormone activation. This condition leads to dynamic and structural changes such as myocyte energy production, intracellular metabolism, and myofibril contractile function. Left ventricular hypertrophy, heart rhythm disturbances, primary atrial fibrillation, dilation of the heart chambers, heart failure, PAH, and diastolic dysfunction constitutes the main manifestations [48].

Although, β-adrenergic blockage was contraindicated in previous decades in the treatment of thyrotoxic cardiac events, nowadays the use of such drugs considered as first-line therapy [92]. Digitalis and diuretics are not recommended in the heart failure accompanying pulmonary congestion [60].

The definitive treatment option for the hyperthyroidism is 131I-radioiodine [93]. Optimal hyperthyroidism treatment goals to establish an euthyroid state commonly represents a recovery from atrial fibrillation to sinus rhythm and a dissolution of the cardiac manifestations [76, 79]. Studies pointing out how crucial is an adequate and sufficient treatment concluded that the cardiovascular complications arising from thyrotoxicosis are the primary cause of death [94].

8. Graves' Disease and arterial hypertension

Thyroid hormone causes decreased resistance in peripheral arterioles through a direct effect on VSM cells and decreased mean arterial pressure, which, when sensed in the kidneys, activates the renin-angiotensin-aldosterone system and increases renal sodium absorption. T3 also induces erythropoietin synthesis, which leads to an increase in red cell mass. These changes combine to promote an increase in blood volume and preload. Hyperthyroidism has been identified as the second most common reason for isolated systolic hypertension [62]. Because of the reversible effects of hyperthyroidism hypertension, efficient hyperthyroidism treatment and the administration of β-blockade to achieve normocardia reverses hypertension, heart rate variability and arrhythmias. Iryna Tsymbaliuk et al. [95] reported that there are 95% arterial hypertension between Graves' hyperthyroidism patients, especially demonstrating high systolic blood pressure, as result of low vascular resistance, elevated resting heart rate and blood volume due to excess of thyroid hormones [95, 96]. Moreover, they showed that arterial hypertension was developed secondary to Graves' hyperthyroidism and associated with diminished quality of life. Restoring of euthyroid state resulted in elimination of arterial hypertension or stabilization of blood pressure levels in patients with a history of arterial hypertension, which is consistent with other studies.

The role of euthyroidism restoration is supported by findings from other studies showing the direct effect of hyperthyroid state on the cardiovascular system; in animal studies, the excess of thyroid hormones had a major impact on the cardiomyocytes, whereas beta-adrenergic or angiotensin receptor stimulations played a minor role [79, 97]. And in the study, as a result, improvement of cardiovascular parameters in relatively short follow up time was achieved after restoring of euthyroid state by antithyroid therapy accompanied by administration of beta-blockers and ACE inhibitors.

9. Graves' Disease and pulmonary hypertension

About 1/5 of pulmonary hypertension cases are shown to be concomitantly occurring with thyroid disease [98]. Pulmonary artery hypertension (PAH) is identified as mean pulmonary arterial pressure levels higher than 25 mm Hg at rest [81]. Increased pressure in the left atrium is transmitted backwardly to pulmonary veins. This activates baroreceptors ending up with a reflex contraction in the arterioles. Elevated pulmonary artery pressure aggravates the right ventricular workload. This overload forces the right ventricle to contract laboriously to maintain blood flow towards pulmonary vasculature. However, this process eventually leads to increased pulmonary resistance and PAH [48]. Although, current knowledge regarding hemodynamics of

PAH in hyperthyroidism has not well explained yet, decrease in PAH after establishing an euthyroid state may be considered as a supportive evidence for a causal relationship [99]. A current study asserts a direct relation between TSH receptor antibodies and PAH, thus a possible autoimmune-mediated pulmonary vascular remodeling may be conducted [101]. Hyperthyroidism should be excluded in patients with PAH; moreover, in case of coexisting hyperthyroidism and dyspnea, every patient should be examined for PAH either [98, 100].

PAH has been associated with thyroid dysfunction, mainly hyperthyroidism. It has been suggested that SVR lowering effect of thyroid hormone may not occur in the pulmonary vasculature [60]. PAH and atrioventricular valve regurgitation have been both documented with a high prevalence [90]. Various articles have revealed that hyperthyroidism may manifest as right heart failure and tricuspid regurgitation [91]. A research including of 23 cases with hyperthyroidism originating from Graves' Disease documented that 65% of those patients had PAH. Following an adequate treatment for the Graves' Disease, pulmonary artery pressure levels returned to normal values in almost all patients [100, 101].

Right heart failure and peripheral edema accompanying hyperthyroidism may be reasoned by this reversible increase in pulmonary artery pressure [60, 91]. Primary pulmonary hypertension is defined as the levels of pulmonary artery pressure above 25 mm Hg at rest and 30 mm Hg during exercise and frequently seen in young women. It has a progressive nature and mostly leads to right heart failure. A link between pulmonary hypertension and thyroid disease (i.e., hypothyroidism and hyperthyroidism) has been elucidated in recent [102]. Hypothyroidism rate was determined as 22% in a study including 40 patients with primary pulmonary hypertension [103]. There are several evidences indicating the importance of the autoimmune disease's role in both hypothyroid and hyperthyroid linked cases of primary pulmonary hypertension [91, 101, 103]. Thyroid dysfunction therefore should always be examined in the presence of primary pulmonary hypertension.

10. Thyroid hormone effects on lipid metabolism

Increased serum lipid levels in hypothyroidism is well-known. Hypothyroidism causes hypercholesterolemia especially augments low-density lipoproteins (LDL) and apolipoprotein B. Although, estimated prevalence of overt hypothyroidism in patients with hypercholesterolemia is between 1.3% to 2.8%, hypercholesterolemia is observed in 90% of the patients with hypothyroidism [104]. Altered lipid profile levels manifest even in subclinical hypothyroidism. Some authors revealed reversible increased LDL levels in subclinical hypothyroidism after thyroid hormone replacement. On the contrary, some other studies have determined no changes in LDL levels despite increased total cholesterol levels in subclinical hypothyroidism [105]. The underlying mechanisms of the hypercholesterolemia in hypothyroidism involves impaired fractional clearance of LDL by decreased LDL receptors and receptor activity in the liver [106]. Cholesterol catabolism is regulated by cholesterol 7α-hydroxylase [107]. This liver-origin enzyme has a negative correlation with T3 and may reduce catabolism and cause elevated serum cholesterol levels associated with hypothyroidism [103]. The increased serum lipid levels in subclinical hypothyroidism are strongly associated with increased cardiovascular risk [108]. This high risk may be reversed by thyroid hormone replacement therapy to establish euthyroid condition [106]. If left untreated, the dyslipidemia accompanying with the diastolic hypertension associated with hypothyroidism lead the patient prone to atherosclerosis [53, 86].

11. Subclinical hyperthyroidism and heart

The impact of thyroid hormones especially the subclinical hyperthyroidism on cardiovascular system faces an ever-increasing interest in last decades. Subclinical hyperthyroidism represents low serum TSH levels accompanying with normal serum free T4 and T3 concentration and its prevalence varies from 0.6–16% [109]. Persistent abnormal TSH measurements have to be re-examined within 2–3 months from initial values [109, 110]. There are two main categories regarding subclinical hyperthyroidism: Grade 1 defines a mildly low serum TSH (0.1–0.45 mIU/L) levels whereas Grade 2 represent lower levels of serum TSH (< 0.1 mIU/L). Subclinical hyperthyroidism may have exogenous or endogenous etiology. Exogenous origin mainly occurs as a result of a TSH suppressive therapy (or excessive use of levothyroxine) for thyroid carcinoma. Endogenous reasons resembles overt hyperthyroid state causes including mild Graves' Disease, multinodular goiter, and autonomous functioning thyroid nodule. Various authors have evaluated the effects of subclinical hyperthyroidism on cardiovascular and skeletal systems, particularly in older populations. Nanchen et al. analyzed conducted a study with a large cohort composed of patients with subclinical hyperthyroidism and observed a significantly higher hospitalizations rate due to heart failure in older patients, especially in those with grade 2 subclinical hyperthyroidism [111]. A distinct inverse proportion between TSH level and the risk of AF have been concluded in previous studies [112]. Furthermore, current retrospective studies with large cohorts have obviously determined a link between subclinical hyperthyroidism and cardiovascular events especially heart failure. More importantly, all-cause mortality observed higher in this group [113]. The European Thyroid Association recommends full treatment in patients older than 65 years with grade 2 subclinical hyperthyroidism. Beyond that, same guideline suggests to treat milder grade if any additional heart disease or other significant comorbidities or risk factors present [110].

12. Treatment

Recent treatment options for Graves' hyperthyroidism include antithyroid drugs, radioactive iodine, and surgery. In addition β-adrenergic blockade is targeted to blockade cathecolamine discharge. The cardiovascular symptoms stimulated by hyperthyroidism resolve after an adequate treatment regardless of utilizing radioactive iodine or antithyroid drug. Hyperthyroidism may exaggerate preexisting cardiovascular diseases by increasing demand for myocardial oxygen, contractility and heart rate. In such circumstances, silent coronary artery disease, angina or compensated heart failure and even endothelial dysfunction develop [114]. Tachycardia control by using β-blockers should be added into treatment in the management of heart failure. Nevertheless, possible contraindications have to be considered in each individuals. Furosemide may aid to reduce volume overload. However, requirement of more Na-K-ATPase in the myocardium due to İncreased blood volume (distribution) in euthyroid heart failure patients result in relative resistance to digoxin [77]. Beta blockers, especially propranolol and atenolol aid to control palpitations by decelerating the heart rate in case of sinus tachycardia [115]. Although, all types of calcium channel blockers are utilized in the management of newly emerged atrial fibrillation, in the presence of thyrotoxicosis, intravenous administration increase adverse effects. The vasodilator and negative inotrope effects of these drugs may cause hypotension and even cardiovascular collapse [116]. Further precautions are required in case of atrial fibrillation, marked palpitations, or severe tachycardia [7, 92].

In case of heart failure resisting despite the heart rate decelerated, or if the patient is in advanced age, or has diagnosed or suspected preexisting heart disease, or has hypertension standard treatment protocols should be applied. In occasional conditions such as hyperthyroidism or thyroid storm requires close cardiovascular monitoring and management of other comorbidities (infection, trauma, acute psychiatric illness) [92, 117]. The efficacy of anticoagulant drugs has been less investigated into correctable causes of AF such as hyperthyroidism. Our clinical routine tends to initiate antithrombotic agents as in general population. After euthyroid state established, and in the documented absence of AF during at least three months, terminating the anticoagulant therapy should be concluded. However, the patients should be kept in close follow-up with routine intervals in terms of heart rate. Although, some clinics demand further documentation, 24 hours of continuous monitoring without AF and the absence of any sign and symptoms regarding AF is sufficient to terminate anticoagulant therapy in our protocol. However, two clinicians decide whether to discontinue anticoagulant treatment according to CHA_2DS_2-VASc score, regardless of rhythm.

13. Conclusion

It's important to bear in mind that significant cardiac complications of Graves' Disease (dilated cardiomyopathy, atrial fibrillation, systemic hypertension and pulmonary hypertension) may occur in previously fit young patients without cardiac disease. All these cardiac complications increase mortality and morbidity in patients with Graves' Disease. Most of the time cardiac function recovers if Graves' Disease is specifically treated and cardiac interventions are done in a timely fashion. Therefore early diagnosis and definitive treatment of hyperthyroidism is crucial for prevention of the development of thyrotoxic cardiomyopathy.

Author details

Abdulla Arslan* and Hakan Altay
Department of Cardiology, Faculty of Medicine, Baskent University, Istanbul, Turkey

*Address all correspondence to: apaslan@msn.com

References

[1] Anthony P. Weetman , MD, D.SC GRAVES' DISEASE Review Article, The New England Journal of Medicine

[2] Rapoport B, Chazenbalk GD, Jaume JC, McLachlan SM. The thyrotropin (TSH) receptor: interaction with TSH and autoantibodies. Endocr Rev 1998;19:673-716. [Erratum, Endocr Rev 1999;20:100.]

[3] Bulow PI, Laurberg P, Knudsen N, et al. Increase in incidence of hyprthyroidism predominantly occurs in young people after iodine fortification of salt in Denmark. J Clin Endocrinol Metab 2006; 91: 3830-3834

[4] Jacobson DL, Gange SJ, Rose NR, Graham NM. Epidemiology and estimated population burden of selected autoimmune diseases in the United States. Clin Immunol Immunopathol 1997;84:223-243.

[5] Vanderpump MPJ, Tunbridge WMG. The epidemiology of autoimmune thyroid disease. In: Volpe R, ed. Autoimmune endocrinopathies. Vol. 15 of Contemporary endocrinology. Totowa, N.J.: Humana Press,1999:141-62.

[6] Takata I, Suzuki Y, Saida K, Sato T. Human thyroid stimulating activity and clinical state in antithyroid treatment of juvenile Graves' disease. Acta Endocrinol (Copenh) 1980;94:46-52.

[7] Klein I, Ojamaa K. Thyroid hormone and the cardiovascular system. N Engl J Med 2001; 344:501.

[8] Ghandour A, Reust C. Hyperthyroidism: a stepwise approach to treatment. J Fam Pract 2011; 60: 388-395

[9] Palitzsch KD. Prevention and multimodal therapy of hyperthyroidism. Internist (Berl) 2008; 49: 1428-1436

[10] Brandt F, Green A, Hegedüs L, Brix TH. A critical review and meta-analysis of the association between overt hyperthyroidism and mortality. Eur J Endocrinol 2011; 165:491-497.

[11] Singer PA, Cooper DS, Levy EG, et al. Treatment guidelines for patients with hyperthyroidism and hypothyroidism. JAMA 1995;273:808-812.

[12] Brent G. The molecular basis of thyroid hormone action. N Engl J Med. 1994;331:847-853

[13] Everts ME, Verhoeven FA, Bezstarosti K, Moerings EP, Hennemann G, Visser TJ, Lamers JM. Uptake of thyroid hormones in neonatal ratcardiac myocytes. Endocrinology. 1996;137:4235-4242

[14] Kahaly GJ, Dillmann WH. Thyroid hormone action in the heart. Endocrine Rev. 2005;26:704-728.

[15] Leng X, Bianco J, Tsai SY, Ozato K, O'Malley BW, Tsai MJ. Mechanisms for synergic activation of thyroid hormone receptor and retinoid X receptor on different response elements. J Biol Chem 1994; 269: 31436-31442

[16] Ribeiro RC, Apriletti JW, West BL, et al. The molecular biology of thyroid hormone action. Annual N Y Acad Sci 1995; 758: 266-289

[17] Lazar MA, Chin WW. Nuclear thyroid hormone receptors. J Clin Invest.1990;86:1777-1782

[18] Ojamaa K, Klemperer JD, MacGlivray SS. Thyroid hormone and hemodynamic regulation of beta-myosin heavy chain promoter in the heart. Endocrinology 1996; 137: 802-808

[19] Wu Y, Koenig RJ. Gene regulation by thyroid hormone. Trends EndocrinolMetab. 2000;11:207-211.

[20] Hu X, Lazar MA. Transcriptional repression by nuclear hormone receptors. Trends Endocrinol Metab. 2000;11:6-10

[21] Mintz G, Pizzarello R, Klein I. Enhanced left ventricular diastolic function in hyperthyroidism: noninvasive assessment and response to treatment. J Clin Endocrinol Metab. 1991;73:146-150

[22] Hiroi Y, Kim H-H, Ying H, Furuya F, Huang Z, Simoncini T, Noma K, Ueki K, Nguyen N-H, Scanlan TS, Moskowitz MA, Cheng S-Y, Liao JK. Rapid nongenomic actions of thyroid hormone. Proc Natl Acad Sci U S A. 2006;103:14104-14109

[23] Dillman WH. Biochemical basis of thyroid hormone action in the heart. Am J Med 1990; 88: 626-630

[24] Kiss E, Jakab G, Kranias EG, et al. Thyroid hormoneinduced alteration in phospholamban protein expression: regulatory effects on sarcoplasmic reticulum Ca2+ transport and myocardial relaxation. Circ Res 1994; 75:245-251

[25] Tsika RW, Bahl JJ, Leinwand LA, Morkin E. Thyroid hormone regulates expression of a transfected human alphamyosin heavy chain fusion gene in fetal rat heart cells. Proc Natl Acad Sci USA 1990; 87: 379-383.

[26] Averyheart-Fullard V, Fraker LD, Murphy AM, Solaro RJ. Differential regulation of slow skeletal and cardiac troponon I mRNA during development and by thyroid hormone in rat heart. J Mol Cell Cardiol 1994; 26: 609-616

[27] Morkin E. Regulation of myosin heavy chain genes in the heart. Circulation 1993; 87: 1451-1460.

[28] Izumo S, Nadal-Ginard B, Mahdavi V. All members of the MHC multigene family respond to thyroid hormone in a highly tissue-specific manner. Science 1986; 231:597-600

[29] Ladenson PW, Sherman SI, Boughman RL. Reversible alterations in myocardial gene expression in a young man with dilated cardiomyopathy and hypothyroidism. Proc Natl Acad Sci USA 1992; 89: 5251-5255

[30] Magner J, Clarck W, Allenby P. Congestive heart failure and sudden death in a young woman with thyrotoxicosis. West J Med 1988; 110: 759-760

[31] Kiss E, Brittsan AG, Elds I, et al. Thyroid hormone-induced alterations in phospholamban deficient mouse hearts. Circ Res 1998; 83: 608-13

[32] Panagoulis C, Halapas A, Chariatis E, Driva P, Matsakas E. Hyperthyroidism and heart. Hellenic J Cardiol 2008; 49:169-175

[33] Kasturi S, Ismail-Beigi F. Effect of thyroid hormone on the distribution and activity of Na, K ATPase in ventricular myocardium. Arch Biochem Biophys 2008; 475: 121-127

[34] Ojamaa K, Sabet A, Kenessey A, et al. Regulation of rat cardiac Kv 1.5 gene expression by thyroid hormone is rapid and chamber specific. Endocrinology 1999; 140: 3170-3176.

[35] Chen WJ, Yeh YH, Lin KH, Chang GJ, Kuo CT. Molecular characterisation of thyroid hormone-inhibited atrial Ltype calcium channel expression: implication for atrial fibrillation in hyperthyroidism. Basic res Cardiol 2011; 106:163-174

[36] Hammond HK, White FC, Buxton IL, Salzstein P, Brunton LL, Longhurst JC. Increased myocardial beta-recepors and adrenergic responses in hyperthyroid pigs. Am J Physiol 1987; 252: H283–H290

[37] Levey GS, Klein I. Cathecholamine thyroid hormone interactions and the cardiovascular manifestations of hyperthyroidism. Am J Med 1990; 88: 642-646

[38] Ojamaa K, Klein I, Sabet A, Steinberg SF. Chnages in adenylyl cyclase isoforms as a mechanism for thyroid hormone modulation of cardiac beta adrenergic receptor responsiveness. Metabolism 2000; 49: 275-279

[39] Klein I, Ojamaa K. Thyrotoxicosis and the heart. Endocrinol Metab Clin North Am 1998; 27: 51-62

[40] Davis PJ, Davis FB. Acute cellular actions of thyroid hormone and myocardial function. Ann Thorac Surg 1993; 56 (Suppl.): S16-23

[41] Klemperer JD, Klein I, Gomez M, et al. Thyroid hormone treatment after coronary artery by-pass surgery. N Eng J Med 1995; 333: 1522-1527

[42] Walker JD, Crawford FA, Kato S, et al. The novel effects of 3,5,3′-triiodo-L-thyronine on myocyte contractile function and beta adrenergic responsiveness in dilated cardiomyopathy. J Thorac Cardiovasc Surg 1994; 108: 672

[43] Cacciatori V, Bellavere F, Pessarosa A, et al. Power spectral analysis of heart rate in hyperthyroidism. J Clin End Metab 1996; 81: 2828

[44] Ojamaa K, Kenessey A, Klein I. Thyroid hormone regulation of phospholamban phosphorylation in the rat heart. Endocrinology 2000; 141: 2139-2144

[45] Messarah M, Saoudi M, Boulakaud MS, Feki AE. Oxidative stress induced by thyroid dysfunction in rat erythrocytes and heart. Environ Toxicol Pharmacol 2011; 31: 33-41

[46] Resnick LM, Laragh JH. Plasma rennin activity in syndromes of hyroid hormone excess and deficiency. Life Sci 1982; 30: 585-586

[47] Ojamaa K, Klemperer JD, Klein I. Acute effects of thyroid hormone on vascular smooth muscle. Thyroid 1996; 6:505

[48] Vargas-Uricoechea H, Bonelo-Perdomo A, Sierra-Torres CH. Effects of thyroid hormones on the heart. Clin Investig Arterioscler. 2014 Nov-Dec;26(6):296-309

[49] Nabbout LA, Robbins RJ. The cardiovascular effects of hyperthyroidism.Methodist DeBakey Cardiovasc J. 2010 Apr-Jun;6(2):3-8

[50] Imai T, Hirata Y, Iwashina M, Marumo F. Hormonal regulation of rat adrenomedullin gene in vasculature. Endocrinology. 1995;136:1544-1548

[51] Diekman MJ, Harms MP, Endert E, Wieling W, Wiersinga WM. Endocrine factors related to changes in total peripheral vascular resistance after treatment of thyrotoxic and hypothyroid patients. Eur J Endocrinol. 2001;144:339-346

[52] Nordyke RA, Gilbert FI Jr, Harada ASM. Graves' disease: influence of age on clinical findings. Arch Intern Med 1988;148:626-631

[53] Danzi S, Klein I. Thyroid hormone and the cardiovascular system. Minerva Endocrinologica. 2004;29:139-150

[54] Park KW, Dai HB, Ojamaa K, Lowenstein E, Klein I, Sellke FW. The direct vasomotor effect of thyroid hormones on rat skeleteal muscle resistance arteries. Anesth Analog 1997; 85: 734-738

[55] Klein I, Levey GS. Unusual manifestations of hypo thy roidism. Arch Intern Med 1984; 144: 123-128

[56] Fadel BM, Ellahham S, Ringel MD, Lindsay J, Wartofsky L, Burman KD. Hyperthyroid heart disease. Clin Cardiol 2000; 23: 402-408

[57] Theilen EO, Wilson WR. Hemodynamic effects of peri pheral vasoconstriction in normal and thyrotoxic subjects.J Appl Physiol 1967; 22: 207-210

[58] Asvold BO, Bjoro T, Nilsen T, Vatten LJ. Association between blood pressure and serum TSH concentration within the reference range: a population-based study. J Clin Endocrinol Metab. 2007;9:841-845

[59] Volzke H, Alte D, Dorr M, Wallaschofski H, John U, Felix SB, Rettig R. The association between subclinical hyperthyroidism and blood pressure in a population-based study. J Hypertens. 2006;24:1947-1953

[60] Danzi S, Klein I. Thyroid hormone and blood pressure regulation. Cur Hypertens Rep. 2003;5:513-520

[61] Palmieri EA, Fazio S, Palmieri V, Lombardi G, Biondi B. Myocardial contractility and total arterial stiffness in patients with overt hyperthyroidism: acute effects of beta1-adrenergic blockade. Eur J Endocrinol.2004;150:757-762

[62] Prisant LM, Gujral JS, Mulloy AL. Hyperthyroidism: a secondary cause of isolated systolic hypertension. J Clin Hypertens. 2006;8:596-599

[63] Napoli R, Biondi B, Guardasole V, Matarazzo M, Pardo F, Angelini V, Fazio S, Sacca L. Impact of hyperthyroidism and its correction on vascular reactivity in humans. Circulation. 2001;104:3076-3080

[64] Taddei S, Caraccio N, Virdis A, Dardano A, Versari D, Chiadoni L, Salvetti A, Ferrannini E, Monzani F. Impaired endothelium-dependent vasodilatation in subclinical hypothyroidism: beneficial effect of levothyroxine therapy. J Clin Endocrinol Metab. 2003;88:3731-3737

[65] Guntekin U, Gunes Y, Tuncer M, et al. QTc dispersion in hyperthyroidism and its association with pulmonary hypertension. Pacing Clin Electrophysiol 2009; 32: 494-499

[66] Bielecka-Dabrowa A, Mikhailidis DP, Rysz J, Banach M. The mechanisms of atrial fibrillation in hyperthyroidism. Thyroid Res 2009; 2: 4

[67] Wustmann K, Kucera JP, Zanchi A, et al. Activation of electrical triggers of atrial fibrillation in hyperthyroidism. J Clin Endocrinol Metab 2008; 93:2104

[68] Auer J, Scheibner P, Mische T, et al. Subclinical hyperthyroidism as a risk factor for atrial fibrillation. Am Heart J 2001; 142: 838

[69] Vardas PE, Mavrakis HE. Atrial fibrillation: a symptom treated as a disease? Hellenic J Cardiol 2006; 47: 191-193

[70] Nakazawa H, Lythall DA, Noh J, Ishikawa N, Sugino K, Ito K, Hardman SM. Is there a place for the late cardioversion of atrial fibrillation? A long-term follow-up study of patients with post-thyrotoxic atrial fibrillation. Eur Heart J. 2000;21:327-333

[71] Krahn AD, Klein GJ, Kerr CR, Boone J, Sheldon R, Green M, Talajic M, Wang X, Connolly S. How useful is thyroid function testing in patients with recent-onset atrial fibrillation? The Canadian Registry of Atrial Fibrillation Investigators. Arch Intern Med. 1996;156:2221-2224

[72] Almeida NA, Corderio A, Machado DS, et al. Connexin 40 messenger ribonucleic activity is posotovely regulated by thyroid hormone (TH)acting in cardiac atria via

the THreceptor. Endocrinology 2009; 150: 546-554

[73] Nakazawa HK, Sakurai K, Hamada N, Momotani N, Ito K. Management of atrial fibrillation in the post-thyrotoxic state. Am J Med 1982; 72: 903-906

[74] Kim D, Smith TW. Effects of thyroid hormone on sodium pump sites, sodium content, and contractile responses to cardiac glycosides in cultured chick ventricular cells. *J Clin Invest*. 1984;74:1481-1488. 87

[75] Roti E, Montermini M, Roti S, Gardini E, Robuschi G, Minelli R, Salvi M, Bentivoglio M, Guiducci U, Braverman LE. The effect of diltiazem, a calcium channel-blocking drug, on cardiac rate and rhythm in hyperthyroid patients. Arch Intern Med. 1988;148:1919-1192

[76] Shimizu T, Koide S, Noh JY, Sugino K, Ito K, Nakazawa H. Hyperthyroidism and the management of atrial fibrillation. Thyroid. 2002;12:489-493.

[77] Chaudhury S, Ismail-Beigi F, Gick GG, Levenson E, Edel man IS. Effect of thyroid hormone on the abundance of Na,K,ATPase alpha subunit messenger ribonucleic acid.Mol Endocrinol 1987; 1: 83-89

[78] Lin H, Mitasikova M, Dlugosova K, et al. Thyroid hormones suppress epsilon PKC-signalling, downregulate connexin- 43 and increase lethal arrhythmia susceptibility in nondiabetic and diabetic rats. J Phsiol Pharm 2008; 59: 271-285

[79] Osman F, Franklyn JA, Holder RL, Sheppard MC, Gammage MD. Cardiovascular symptoms and cardiac rate and rhythm abnormalities improve with treatment in patients with hyperthyroidism. J Am Coll Cardiol. 2007;49:71-81

[80] Danzi S, Klein I. Thyroid disease and the cardiovascular system. Endocrinol Metab Clin North Am. 2014 Jun;43(2):517-528

[81] Klein I, Danzi S. Thyroid disease and the heart. Curr Probl Cardiol. 2016 Feb;41(2):65-92

[82] Biondi B. Mechanisms in endocrinology: Heart failure and thyroid dysfunction. Eur J Endocrinol. 2012 Nov;167(5):609-618

[83] Kahaly GJ, Kampmann C, Mohr-Kahaly S. Cardiovascular hemodynamics and exercise tolerance in thyroid disease.Thyroid 2002; 12: 473

[84] Dahl P, Danzi S, Klein I. Thyrotoxic cardiac disease. Curr Heart Fail Re 2008; 5: 170-176.

[85] Yue WS, Chong BH, Zhang XH, et al. Hyperthyroidisminduced left ventricular diastolic dysfunction: implication in hyperthyroidism-related heart failure. Clin Endocrinol (Oxf) 2011; 74: 636-643

[86] Klein I. Endocrine disorders and cardiovascular disease. In: Zipes DP,Libby P, Bonow R, Braunwald E, eds. *Braunwald's Heart Disease: ATextbook of Cardiovascular Medicine*. 7th ed. Philadelphia, Pa. W.B.Saunders; 2005:2051-2065.

[87] Evangelopoulou ME, Alevizaki M, Toumanidis S, Piperingos G, Mavrikakis M, Sotou D, Evangelopoulou K, Koutras DA. Mitral valve prolapse in autoimmune thyroid disease: an index of systemic autoimmunity? Thyroid. 1999;9:973-977

[88] Frost L, Vestergaard P, Mosekilde L. Hyperthyroidism and risk of atrial fibrillation or flutter: a population-based study. Arch Intern Med. 2004; 164:1675-1678

[89] Sawin CT, Geller A, Wolf PA, Belanger AJ, Baker E, Bacharach P, Wilson PW, Benjamin EJ, D'Agostino RB. Low serum thyrotropin concentrations as a risk factor for atrial fibrillation in older persons. N Engl J Med. 1994;331:1249-1252

[90] Merce J, Ferras S, Oltra C, Sanz E, Vendrell J, Simon I, Camprubi M, Bardaji A, Ridao C. Cardiovascular abnormalities in hyperthyroidism: a prospective Doppler echocardiographic study. Am J Med. 2005;118:126-133

[91] Paran Y, Nimrod A, Goldin Y, Justo D. Pulmonary hypertension and predominant right heart failure in thyrotoxicosis. Resuscitation. 2006; 69:339-341.

[92] Ventrella S, Klein I. Beta-adrenergic receptor blocking drugs in the management of hyperthyroidism. The Endocrinologist. 1994;4:391-399

[93] Delit C, Silver S, Yohalem SB, Segal RL. Thyrocardiac disease and its management with radioactive iodine I-131. JAMA. 1961;29:262-267

[94] Franklyn JA, Sheppard MC, Maisonneuve P. Thyroid function and mortality in patients treated for hyperthyroidism. JAMA. 2005;294:71-80

[95] Tsymbaliuk I, Unukovych D, Shvets N, Dinets A (2015) Cardiovascular Complications Secondary to Graves' Disease: A Prospective Study from Ukraine. PLoS ONE 10(3): e0122388. doi:10.1371/journal.pone.0122388

[96] Scerrino G, Morfino G, Paladino NC, Di Paola V, Amodio E, Gulotta G, et al. Does thyroid surgery for Graves' disease improve health-related quality of life? Surgery today. 2013; 43(12):1398-405. Epub 2012/12/12. doi: 10.1007/s00595-012-0442-z PMID: 23229839

[97] Jiang SY, Xu M, Ma XW, Xiao H, Zhang YY. A distinct AMP-activated protein kinase phosphorylation site characterizes cardiac hypertrophy induced by L-thyroxine and angiotensin II. Clin Exp Pharmacol Physiol. 2010; 37(9):919-25. doi: 10.1111/j.1440-1681.2010.05404.x PMID: 20497424

[98] Vallabhajosula S, Radhi S, Cevik C, Alalawi R, Raj R, Nugent K. Hyperthyroidism and pulmonary hypertension: an important association. Am J Med Sci. 2011 Dec;342(6):507-512

[99] Siu CW, Zhang XH, Yung C, Kung AW, Lau CP, Tse HF. Hemodynamic changes in hyperthyroidism-related pulmonary hypertension: a prospective echocardiographic study. J Clin Endocrinol Metab. 2007 May;92(5):1736-1742

[100] Sugiura T, Yamanaka S, Takeuchi H, Morimoto N, Kamioka M, Matsumura Y. Autoimmunity and pulmonary hypertension in patients with Graves' disease. Heart Vessels. 2015 Sep;30(5):642-646

[101] Marvisi M, Zambrelli P, Brianti M, Civardi G, Lampugnani R, Delsignore R. Pulmonary hypertension is frequent in hyperthyroidism and normalizes after therapy. Eur J Intern Med. 2006;17:267-271

[102] Ma RC, Cheng AY, So WY, Hui DS. Thyrotoxicosis and pulmonary hypertension. Am J Med. 2005;118:927-928

[103] Curnock AL, Dweik RA, Higgins BH, Saadi HF, Arroliga AC. High prevalence of hypothyroidism in patients with primary pulmonary hypertension. Am J Med Sci. 1999;318:289-292

[104] Duntas LH. Thyroid disease and lipids. Thyroid. 2002;12:287-293

[105] Razvi S, Ingoe L, Keeka G, Oates C, McMillan C, Weaver JU. The beneficial effect of L-thyroxine on cardiovascular risk factors, endothelial function and quality of life in subclinical hypothyroidism: randomised, crossover trial. J Clin Endocrinol Metab. 2007;92:1715-1723

[106] Rush J, Danzi S, Klein I. Role of thyroid disease in the development of statin-induced myopathy. The Endocrinologist. 2006;16:279-285

[107] Drover VAB, Agellon LB. Regulation of the human cholesterol 7α-hydroxylase gene (*CYP7A1*) by thyroid hormone in transgenic mice. Endocrinology. 2004;145:574-581

[108] Hak AE, Pols HA, Visser TJ, Drexhage HA, Hofman A, Witteman JC. Subclinical hypothyroidism is an independent risk factor for atherosclerosis and myocardial infarction in elderly women: the Rotterdam Study. Ann Intern Med. 2000;132:270-278

[109] Biondi B, Palmieri EA, Lombardi G, Fazio S. Effects of subclinical thyroid dysfunction on the heart. Ann Intern Med. 2002 Dec 3;137(11):904-914.

[110] Biondi B, Bartalena L, Cooper DS, Hegedus L, Laurberg P, Kahaly GJ. The 2015 European Thyroid Association Guidelines on Diagnosis and Treatment of Endogenous Subclinical Hyperthyroidism. Eur Thyroid J. 2015 Sep;4(3):149-163

[111] Nanchen D, Gussekloo J, Westendorp RG, et al. Subclinical thyroid dysfunction and the risk of heart failure in older persons at high cardiovascular risk. J Clin Endocrinol Metab. 2012 Mar;97(3):852-861

[112] Selmer C, Olesen JB, Hansen ML, et al. The spectrum of thyroid disease and risk of new onset atrial fibrillation: a large population cohort study. BMJ. 2012 Nov 27;345: e7895

[113] Selmer C, Olesen JB, Hansen ML, et al. Subclinical and overt thyroid dysfunction and risk of all-cause mortality and cardiovascular events: a large population study. J Clin Endocrinol Metab. 2014 Jul;99(7):2372-2382

[114] Gu LQ, Zhao L, Zhu W, et al. Relationships between serum levels of thyroid hormones and serum concentrations of symmetric dimethylarginine (ADMA) and N-terminal-pro B-type natriuretic peptide (NT-proBNP) in patients with Graves' disease. Endocrine 2011; 39: 266-271

[115] Ross DS, Burch HB, Cooper DS, et al. 2016 American Thyroid Association Guidelines for Diagnosis and Management of Hyperthyroidism and Other Causes of Thyrotoxicosis. Thyroid 2016; 26:1343}}

[116] Subahi A, Ibrahim W, Abugroun A. Diltiazem-Associated Cardiogenic Shock in Thyrotoxic Crisis. Am J Ther 2018; 25:e666.

[117] Klein I, Biondi B. Endocrine disorders and cardiovascular disease. In: Braunwald's Heart Disease: A Textbook of Cardiovascular Medicine, Bonow RO, Mann DL, Tomaselli GF, Bhatt D (Eds), Saunders Elsevier, Philadelphia 2019. p.1807.

Section 4

Graves' Disease in Pregnancy

Chapter 13

Graves' Disease and Pregnancy

Nikolay Petrov Botushanov, Aleksandar Nikolaev Botushanov and Albena Dimitrova Botushanova

Abstract

Graves' Disease is an autoimmune organ specific disease characterized by excessive production of hormones from the thyroid gland and by its diffuse enlargement. The growth and function of the thyroid gland are stimulated by autoantibodies directed against the thyroid-stimulating hormone receptor. Pregnancies complicated by Graves' Disease are characterized with higher incidence of abortion, preterm delivery, low-birth- weight infants and neonatal mortality, as well as maternal complications such as heart failure, eclampsia and rarely thyroid storm. When fully controlled hyperthyroidism have excellent outcomes. Different therapeutic approaches are used in women with Graves' planning pregnancy and in those when the disease is diagnosed after they became pregnant. Thionamides are the first choice for treatment, with Propylthyouracil being preferred for the first trimester and Methimazole for the second and third trimester. Aplasia cutis and some other malformations were associated with methimazole use during pregnancy. Monitoring the effect of treatment should ensure keeping maternal FT4 in the high normal range. Block-and replace regimen is not recommended and rdioiodine therapy is absolutely contraindicated. Thyroidectomy may be considered before pregnancy or in rare cases in the second trimester. Iodine is avoided because of the risk of fetal hypothyroidism and goiter. The use of beta-blockers is controversial. Noenatal thyrotoxicosis may occur in association with maternal Graves' Disease due to maternal TSAbs cross through the placenta.

Keywords: Graves' Disease, pregnancy, thionamides, iodine, surgery

1. Introduction

Graves' Disease (GD) is an autoimmune organ specific disease characterized by excessive production of hormones from the thyroid gland (hyperthyroidism) and by its diffuse enlargement. The growth and function of the thyroid gland are stimulated by autoantibodies directed against the thyroid-stimulating hormone (TSH) receptor (TSHR). Nevertheless, other autoantibodies against thyroid peroxidase (TPO) and thyroglobulin (Tg) may also be present, TSHR is the major autoantigen of Graves' Disease, making antibodies against it (TRAb) the most characteristic for the disease. Graves' Disease (GD) is the most frequent cause of thyrotoxicosis in iodine sufficient countries [1], although the exact frequency of GD in general population is difficult to be established and differs from country to country. A meta-analysis of various studies has estimated the general prevalence of GD to be around 1% [2], which makes it one of the most frequent clinically relevant autoimmune disorders. Graves' Disease is a multifactorial disorder. Like all autoimmune diseases, GD is characterized with the loss of immune tolerance to thyroid antigens and the initiation of a sustained autoimmune reaction caused by a complex interplay of genetic, hormonal and environmental factors. While detailed discussion of these factors is beyond the scope of this chapter, it is worth to mention that GD is typically a disease of women, with the female-to- male ratio ranges in different studies from 5 to 10 at any age [2, 3]. Autoimmune disorders are in general more prevalent in women and genetic and nongenetic factors may play role for that [4, 5]. Male hormones are considered to down-regulate immunity and thus play a protective role from autoimmunity, whereas the effect of estrogen is not always unequivocal [4, 5]. Despite this, little evidences in the literature are backing the role for sex hormones in the high prevalence of GD in women. Moreover thyroid autoimmunity often accompanies patients with Turner's syndrome, who have low estrogen levels [6]. Besides sex hormones, some genetic factors linked with the X chromosome could explain the epidemiologic evidence of a female preponderance in GD. In families with GD, a putative Graves' Disease susceptibility locus on the long arm of X chromosome was located by an linkage analysis [7]. Inactivation of the X chromosome, an epigenetic phenomenon, has been suggested to determine the female predisposition to thyroid autoimmunity. One study showed that this phenomenon is more frequently observed in patients with GD or autoimmune thyroiditis than in healthy controls [8]. Never mind, what the predisposing factors for GD could be, pregnancy, itself, is a well-known risk factor for thyroid autoimmunity. Pregnancy can influence and change the course of a pregestational Graves' Disease or can become a reason for the development of GD during the pregnancy or after delivery. The risk of development of GD in postpartum year increases fourfold to eightfold [9]. The reasons for this could be explained by the observed abrupt fall in the level of pregnancy-associated immunosuppressive factors immediately after delivery (rebound immunity) [9]. The factors involved in the immune alterations of the postpartum period may include, but are not limited to estrogen and progestin [9, 10]. Approximately 2–3% of all pregnancies are complicated by thyroid disease [11], making thyroid disorders the second most common significant pathology affecting women during pregnancy after diabetes mellitus [12]. Detailed understanding of the physiology, pathophysiology, diagnosis and treatment is required to limit the effects on both maternal and fetal health.

2. Physiology of maternal and fetal thyroid in pregnancy

Pregnancy induces several major changes to thyroid morphology and physiology. Diagnosis of thyroid dysfunction during pregnancy is complicated by the hormonal changes that take place, posing specific challenges for both detection and management. During pregnancy, thyroid gland physiologically undergoes moderate enlargement, typically increasing in size between 10 and 40% of volume, and increasing of vascularization. This enlargement can be more pronounced if there is underling iodine deficiency [13]. At the same time there are transient, reversible after delivery, changes in thyroid hormone physiology and iodine metabolism. In early gestation, the thyroid gland is stimulated not only by TSH, but also by the alpha subunit of human chorionic gonadotropin (hCG), produced by the syncytiotrophoblasts of the developing placenta, which binds to and stimulates the TSH receptor, increasing thyroid hormone production and resulting in a subsequent reduction in serum TSH concentration [14]. Normally, hCG starts to rise from the very beginning of pregnancy and peaks at around 9–11 weeks of gestational age. Due to this, there is a parallel decrease in serum

TSH in the first trimester. Generally, TSH concentrations in pregnant women are lower than in non-pregnant women. Physiologically TSH concentrations fluctuate during different periods of gestation. During the first trimester, approximately 15% of healthy women have TSH level below the lower limit of the reference range of 0.4 mU/L [15, 16]. The percentage of women with suppressed TSH falls to about 10% in the second trimester, and 5% in the third trimester [17]. The upper limit of TSH reference range during pregnancy is also decreased by about 0.5–1.0 mU/L, in comparison to the typical nonpregnant TSH reference range and this downward shift usually occurs in the latter first trimester of pregnancy but typically not before week 7 [18]. Levels of hCG then decline until approximately 20 weeks of gestation and remain stable for the remainder of the pregnancy [19], which is followed by a slight increase of TSH levels. The level of decrease of TSH depends on number of the developing fetuses, because hCG concentrations are higher in multiple pregnancies than in singleton pregnancies, and downward shift in the TSH reference interval is greater in twin pregnancies [20]. The degree of the lowering of TSH concentrations during pregnancy varies significantly between different racial and ethnic groups, that is why the recommended by American Thyroid Association (ATA) trimester-specific reference ranges for TSH levels shown on **Table 1** [21], require determination of population-based trimester-specific reference ranges for serum TSH through assessment of local population data.

The reduction of the lower TSH reference range, observed during pregnancy should be regarded in the light of the data that even if this represents an undergoing subclinical hyperthyroidism, it has not been associated with adverse pregnancy outcomes. In a small percentage of women, TSH can be undetectable (<0.01 mU/L), but this is still represent a normal pregnancy. Therefore, a maternal TSH concentration that is low but detectable is likely not to be clinically significant [22].

Starting from the fourth week of gestation, the increase of estrogens causes the rise of circulating level of thyroid-binding globulin (TBG). Estrogens induce increase in the sialylation of the TBG, which is followed by a decrease of its hepatic clearance and by a prolongation of its serum half-life from 15 minutes to 3 days in comparison with the nonpregnancy time. TBG level reaches a plateau during mid-gestation and remain elevated until delivery. In the postpartum period TBG tend to normalize [23]. This rise of TGB level is followed by an increase of the total concentrations of thyroxine (TT4) and of triiodothyronine (TT3) in early pregnancy. There levels achieve a plateau early in the second trimester, at a concentrations value of 30–100% greater than prepregnancy [24]. To continue to maintain normal unbound thyroid hormone levels, thyroid gland needs to increase its thyroid hormone production. Some studies have reported a decrease, whereas others have stated even an increase of free T4 (FT4) and T3 (FT3) making the changes in free-hormone levels during pregnancy controversial. Despite this, pregnant women in general have lower free-hormone concentrations at term than nonpregnant women [17, 25, 26]. Because

	TSH range
First trimester	>0.1 mIU/L and < 2.5 mIU/L
Second trimester	>0.2 mIU/L and < 3.0 mIU/L
Third trimester	>0.3 mIU/L and < 3.0 mIU/L
TSH, thyroid-stimulating hormone.	

Table 1.
Generalized trimester-specific reference ranges for TSH levels [21].

FT4 reference intervals in pregnancy vary widely between methods, interpretation of FT4 values requires method-specific as well as trimester-specific ranges.

The placenta is also an active player in thyroid hormone metabolism. It is a site for the inner ring deiodination of T4 and T3, generating the inactive iodothyronines, reverse T3 and 3,3′-T2, respectively, and thus modulating the amount of active hormone that passes to the fetus [27]. Because of the increased thyroid hormone requirements and iodine glomerular filtration rate during pregnancy [28], adequate iodine availability is strongly necessary to meet these needs. In iodine-replete regions, women are able to meet the increased demands of pregnancy. If adequate iodine is not available, TSH rises and consequently goiter develops [29]. Thyroid hormones play a vital role in the early embryogenesis. They are essential for neurodevelopment, somatic growth, and tissue differentiation. Because, organogenesis of fetal thyroid gland occurs by around 12-th week of gestation and the gland becomes functionally active approximately eight weeks later by the 20-th week of gestation, till then, the fetus fully relay on maternal T4, which is the only thyroid hormone that can cross the placenta. Fetal deiodinase converts maternal T4 to the bioactive T3The [30].

After his thyroid gland becomes active and starts to produce hormones, fetal thyroidal turnover of iodine increases and becomes much higher than that in adults [30]. Fetal iodine store, which exclusively depends from maternal intake, must be continuously refilled. Iodine homeostasis, following fluctuating metabolic needs varies across the different trimesters. After parturition, maternal iodine continues to be the only source of iodine to the breast-fed neonate. Sodium Iodine symporter (NIS) is present in breast tissue and is responsible for concentrating iodine in colostrum and breast milk [31].

3. Thyroid autoimmunity in pregnancy

In around 10% of the women with childbearing potential thyroid antibodies could be found and they represents the most common autoimmune disease. Stagnaro-Green et al. in 1990 first demonstrated an association between pregnancy loss and thyroid antibodies. They showed, that there was a 2-fold increase in the risk of pregnancy loss (17% vs. 8.4%) in women with thyroid antibodies [32]. One meta-analysis discovered, that the presence of thyroid antibodies in pregnant women was connected with a 4-fold increased risk of miscarriage in cohort studies, and a 1.8-fold increased risk in case–control studies [33]. The association of thyroid autoimmunity and preterm birth is not unambiguously as the studies showed conflicting results. Some found significant association [33–36], while others [37] didn't show such correlation.

Following the changes of the activity of the immune system through pregnancy, the activity of Graves' Disease fluctuates. Concomitant changes of the TSH receptor antibody (TRAb) levels, generally reflecting the clinical course of the disease, are observed [38]. During the first trimester TRAb levels are usually elevated with a subsequently fall to even undetectable values during the second and third trimesters and may increase again postpartum [39, 40]. Due to this pattern of fluctuations of TRAb levels, exacerbation of the clinical symptoms of Graves' Disease may occur in the first trimester of gestation, followed by a remission in the second and third trimesters, because of the observed immune tolerance [41]. The decrease in TRAb levels, rather than increases in inhibitory anti-TSH receptor antibodies determines this clinical pattern [39]. From a clinician's point of view, the dosage of antithyroid drugs can be reduced or even discontinued late in gestation and restarted in the postpartum period [41].

4. Hyperthyroidism and pregnancy

Hyperthyroidism is defined as an excessive production of thyroid hormones caused by immune or nonimmune thyroid disease. Hyperthyroidism is less common than hypothyroidism, but nevertheless, it represents a great challenge for the physician, pregnant woman and developing fetus. Specific knowledge is required by healthcare providers and a team approach is necessary to provide the best possible cares for pregnant women with GD. Caring physicians (gynecologists, endocrinologists, cardiologists) must be aware of the symptoms of thyrotoxicosis, often overlapping with the pregnancy itself and of specific changes of the thyroid hormones during pregnancy. Knowing the fact, that any pregnancy complicated with hyperthyroidism carries a greater risk for complications for both mother and developing fetus, proper diagnosis and treatment are necessary. Adequate decisions about when to start treatment and with what to start are required, following the ancient principle of *primium non nocere*. Although our therapeutic approaches didn't change very substantially during the last fifty years, our understanding of the pathophysiology, hormonal changes, immunology and obstetric outcomes have changed dramatically. We still have at our disposal only two types of antithyroid drugs (ATD) (see later in the text), which are the same that had been in use since the 1950's and still remain the cornerstone of treatment of GD in pregnancy. Rarely, other approaches are necessary, like surgery during the second trimester. Radioiodine ablation is absolutely contraindicated. Close monitoring of thyroid hormone levels and frequent adjustment of the dose are necessary to avoid both overdosage or subdosage of antithyroid drugs.

The reasons for thyrotoxicosis during pregnancy can be divided in such typical for all patients and such specific for the pregnancy. The common causes for thyrotoxicosis include: Graves' Disease, chronic thyroiditis, painless thyroiditis, subacute thyroiditis, toxic adenoma, multinodular goiter; excessive levothyroxine (LT4) intake and drug induced thyrotoxicosis caused by iodine, amiodarone, lithium. The causes of thyrotoxicosis specific for the pregnancy are: gestational transient thyrotoxicosis, multiple gestations, trophoblastic disease, hyperplacentosis, hyperreactio luteinalis [22]. Graves' Disease and gestational transient thyrotoxicosis (GTT) account for the majority of hyperthyroidism in pregnancy. Graves' Disease affects 0.2% of pregnant women [42]. Thyrotoxicosis during pregnancy could affect both pregnant woman and developing fetus. Hyperthyroidism may cause both maternal complications such as heart failure, eclampsia and thyroid storm and also higher incidence of abortion, preterm delivery, low-birth-weight infants and neonatal mortality [43]. Distinguishing between different causes of hyperthyroidism is relevant, because some of them, like GTT, are transient, lead to mild thyrotoxicosis and do not require treatment with antithyroid drugs and are not associated with adverse pregnancy outcomes [44]. The Endocrine Society recommends that screening for thyroid conditions in pregnancy is performed in women >30 years, those with previous personal or family history of thyroid disease, women with issues with conception and existing autoimmune conditions [45].

5. Graves' Disease and pregnancy

As it has been already discussed, generally there are three scenarios in which Graves' Disease may affect a pregnancy. *First*, women with preexisting active Graves' Disease. *Second,* women in remission, who may experience a relapse during pregnancy. *Third*, Graves' Disease may occur for the first time during gestation

[46]. The women with prepregnancy active disease (either treated or untreated) may undergo exacerbation during the first trimester. Those, with previously diagnosed GD, who stayed in clinical remission and remained euthyroid throughout the whole pregnancy, hyperthyroidism may recur in the postpartum period. We must be very careful in this situation, because this may represent either the thyrotoxic phase of postpartum thyroiditis (PPT) or in up to 25% or relapse of Graves' Disease. Even in those with PPT, Graves' Disease may recur after resolution of PPT, triggered by the destruction of the thyrocytes [47].

5.1 Diagnosis

Diagnosis should begin with taking complete case history, medical history and family history. The clinical diagnosis of hyperthyroidism may be *difficult* because pregnancy is itself a hypermetabolic state with symptoms of palpitations and heat intolerance. In addition, patients will usually have increased irritability, decreased exercise tolerance, heat intolerance, fatigue and increasing shortness of breath during physical activity. The examination usually reveals the presence of a diffuse goiter, sometimes with a bruit or thrill and eye changes. The clinician must recognize this constellation of symptoms so that the patient can be appropriately screened for hyperthyroidism. Once, hormonally hyperthyroidism has been established, it is very important to go deeper into the specific reason which causes it, because all types of thyrotoxicosis are characterized with similar changes of thyroid hormones. Different reasons for hyperthyroidism during pregnancy require different therapeutic approaches. Some are self-limiting and do no require treatment with ATD but only follow up.

5.2 Differential diagnosis

The most common cause of nonautoimmune hyperthyroidism is gestational transient thyrotoxicosis (GTT), defined as transient hyperthyroidism, limited to the first trimester of pregnancy. It is associated with hyperemesis gravidarum (HG) and is characterized by elevated serum FT4 and suppressed or undetectable serum TSH. It is differentiated from Graves' Disease by the absence of anti-TSH-receptor antibody (TRAb) [48]. Hyperemesis gravidarum often presents in the first trimester of pregnancy with severe nausea and vomiting [49]. It may result in dehydration and ketonuria. Thyroid hormones return to their normal trimester specific reference ranges within 15 weeks, due to resolution of vomiting. Initially FT4 normalized spontaneously; however, serum TSH may remain suppressed for several other weeks and does not require ATD therapy, because this condition is self-limiting [50]. Rarely, for example in the case of dual or triple pregnancy, connected with very high level hCG, the use of ATD is required due to the severity of symptoms. For the clinical practice, it is very important to differentiate between GTT and Graves' Disease. The presence of goitre, thyroid eye disease (Graves' orbitopathy) and TRAbs in Graves' Disease and their absence in GTT can help for proper diagnosis. Because in both conditions there are similar changes of TSH (low) and FT4(high) levels, using a free T3/free T4 ratio could be discriminatory. Often the patients with gestational thyrotoxicosis have significantly lower or even normal T3 values [51].

Subclinical hyperthyroidism, defined as a serum TSH concentration below the lower limit of reference range, with FT4 and FT3 concentrations within normal reference range, affects up to 1.7% of pregnant women. This condition has not been found to be associated with adverse outcomes and doesn't require ATD therapy [31].

5.3 Laboratory

The usual findings from the laboratory studies show low, below the trimester-specific 95% lower confidence limit, TSH level together with elevated serum thyroid hormone (FT4 and FT3) concentrations. We should always consider the fact that up to 50% of women with hyperemesis gravidarum may have similar changes of theh hormonal levels (suppressed serum TSH level and/or elevated FT4) [52]. An elevated free T3 index or free T3 level may be the most clinically useful test to distinguish hyperthyroid patients from those with hyperemesis gravidarum as less than 15% of hyperemetic women have elevations in these measures. TSH receptor antibodies are usually detectable and may also be of diagnostic utility. High levels of TRAb cross placental barrier [53]. and the risk of fetal and neonatal thyrotoxicosis increases with TSRAb values 3–5 times above normal [54, 55].

5.4 Pregnancy outcomes

Maternal hyperthyroidism is associated with increased morbidity for both mother and fetus. Prior to the development of ATD, only about 50% of hyperthyroid women were be able to conceive. About in half of those who conceived, spontaneous miscarriage and premature delivery occurred [56]. The degree and duration of hyperthyroidism strongly correlate with pregnancy outcomes for both mother and fetus. The highest risk was reported in those with uncontrolled or poorly controlled disease and a decreased risk in those appropriately treated with ATD. Established thyrotoxicosis during gestation or before a planned pregnancy, requires appropriate treatment, because in cases with uncontrolled maternal hyperthyroidism in the first trimester, the period of embryogenesis, there is an increased risk for congenital malformations (imperforate anus, polydactyly, harelip) [57]. The use of ATD during this period itself is not associated with a higher incidence of structural anomalies. For optimal pregnancy outcomes it is very important to keep maternal hyperthyroidism under control, avoiding the development of drug induced hypothyroidism, understanding the crucial significance of thyroid hormones for the normal embryogenesis. Significantly, subclinical hyperthyroidism, has not been found to be associated with adverse pregnancy outcomes and doesn't require antithyroid therapy [22]. Pregnancy complications reported in hyperthyroid women vary in frequency in different studies and include: miscarriage from 8 to 10–21% [58, 59], preterm delivery [58, 60, 61] from 3 to 14% to 21–88%, preeclampsia [60] from 2–11%, heart failure [61] from 3–63%, stillbirth [58, 61] from 0% -7 to 50%, small for gestational age [59, 62] and thyroid storm during delivery.

5.5 Treatment

Unfortunately, because the cause of the immune dysregulation in Graves' Disease remains unclear, the available treatments are directed at the thyroid gland rather than the underlying autoimmunity. In general, the available therapies include: Antithyroid drugs, surgery and radioiodine, with predominant use of ATD in pregnancy hyperthyroidism, surgery in exception, during the second trimester and iodine ablation being absolutely contraindicated. Because the degree of hyperthyroidism can vary from patient to patient, those who are relatively asymptomatic may remain undiagnosed and untreated till the delivery, when usually aggravation of thyrotoxicosis is observed. Even when they had been properly diagnosed, they may do not want to accept the diagnosis and ask whether specific treatment is really necessary, fearing of possible side effects of the drugs both for them and for their developing fetuses. Usually they consider their complaints to be related with the pregnancy itself. Those with overt hyperthyroidism require restoration of a euthyroid state because of potentially negative outcomes, both for the mother and the fetus. Fully controlled hyperthyroidism substantially decrease the potential risk for these negative outcomes and at the same time is not a reason for recommending abortion.

Therapeutic approaches differ from case to case. In the *first* scenario, when GD is preceding pregnancy, the woman will be advised to conceive after restoration of euthyroidism. Taking into account patent's plan for the time of the future pregnancy, treatment with thionamide drugs is started, and the treatment continues throughout the whole pregnancy. In this case, the patient should be fully aware of the possible side effects of ATD, both for the mother and fetus and of the need for frequent monitoring of thyroid hormones levels. To avoid this an if the woman with GD is willing to postpone her future pregnancy, than alternatively radioiodine ablation can be offered. Pregnancy should be delayed for at least 4 months after radioiodine therapy, but a longer period, 6 months or even a year, is usually required for restoring euthyroid state and establishing the necessary stable dose of the inevitable postablational replacement therapy with thyroid hormones. Surgery may also be considered as an alternative because of more rapid restoration of euthyroidism.

In the *second* scenario, if GD is diagnosed during pregnancy, ATD are almost the only therapeutic option. Radioiodine is absolutely contraindicated, because it may result in congenital hypothyroidism and may cause malformations. Thyroidectomy is restricted to exceptional cases.

In the *third* scenario, if GD is established after delivery and when the possibility of transient, self-limiting destructive thyrotoxicosis has been excluded, it is prudent to start thionamide treatment. In this case breast feeding should be stopped, because of the risk for development of neonatal hypothyroidism (see below). Radioiodine ablation with its delayed effect of achieving euthyroidism, the need for concomitant use of ATD to control symptoms in some cases and the need for isolation for several days, usually is not well accepted by the mothers. Surgery is an option in patients who experienced side effects of ATD use, or found it difficult to adhere to the prescribed drugs, either due to the number of pills or to the frequency of their intake.

Decision to initiate ATD treatment depends on the severity of the clinical symptoms and the pretreatment levels of FT4, FT3 and TSH. In mild cases with Graves' Disease, when FT4 values are at or slightly above the reference range, treatment may be withheld with a subsequent monitoring of the thyroid status as long as there is a satisfactory clinical progression of pregnancy. In other words, the pregnant woman with Graves' Disease should be kept in slight *subclinical hyperthyroidism*, because there are no reported gestational adverse effects of maternal subclinical hyperthyroidism [63]. The goal of treatment is to keep the patient euthyroid, using the lowest possible dose of antithyroid drugs necessary to maintain FT4 levels in the upper one-third of the normal non pregnant range or up to 10% above the normal range [64]. This level will ensure fetal euthyroidism, because FT4 in the mother's serum correlates with fetal FT4 levels in cord blood [65]. Maternal serum T3 levels may not be as helpful because there is no correlation with fetal thyroid function [66] The dose should be adjusted every 2–4 weeks to maintain a serum FT4 of 1.7 to 2.0 ng/L and TSH at or just below at the 95% confidence interval trimester-specific lower limit [67]. The presence of detectable TSH is an indication to decrease ATD dose [60]. A low TSH level is not a reliable index to judge the adequacy of treatment, because it doesn't promptly reflect the changes in thyroid function like FT4. It is important to monitor TSH level, because a high level always indicates over dosage of ATD and the need for proper dosage correction of the drugs. Because of the expected immunosuppression during the second and third trimester, a partial and transient remission of Graves' Disease may occur and appropriate reduction of the dose or even discontinuation of ATD could be done. Otherwise excessive doses of ATDs, indeed, may affect fetal thyroid function, with the development of hypothyroidism and/or goiter [68, 69]. Relapse of the hyperthyroidism is frequent in postpartum period [70].

5.5.1 Antithyroid drugs

ATD are the first choice for treatment of Graves' Disease during pregnancy. Propylthiouracil (PTU) and methimazole (MMI) are equally effective in the management of hyperthyroidism during pregnancy. Propylthiouracil and methimazole inhibit thyroid hormone synthesis by interfering with intrathyroidal iodine utilization and the iodotyrosine coupling reaction, both of which are catalyzed by thyroid peroxidase. Antithyroid drugs do not directly affect iodine uptake or hormone release by the thyroid. Because of this, the clinical and hormonal improvement is delayed for 10-14 days after their implementation in the therapeutic regimen. PTU, but not methimazole, inhibits the conversion of T4 to T3 in peripheral tissues, thus theoretically it can ensure faster alleviation of the symptoms and reaching the desired levels of FT4. In clinical practice this is not considered relevant. Comparative study showed that methimazole generally normalizes serum T4 and T3 levels faster than PTU [71]. Both antithyroid agents are well absorbed from the gastrointestinal tract. They differ in their ability to bind to proteins in circulation, with PTU being strongly protein-bound, mainly to albumin, at physiologic pH, while methimazole binding to proteins is negligible [72]. Other studies have found that both drugs readily cross the placenta [73, 74]. The serum half-lives of PTU and methimazole are 1 and 4 to 6 hours, respectively. The intrathyroidal duration of action of both drugs is longer than that. Both drugs are metabolized in the liver and their metabolites are excreted by the kidney. However, so far there are no data, that the doses used to treat hyperthyroidism generally need to be altered in patients with liver or kidney disease. This characteristic, apart from their side effects, may determine the choice of the antithyroid drug in pregnancy and lactation, since PTU crosses the placenta and breast epithelium less readily than methimazole. So it is reasonable to begin therapy with PTU because there are no reported cases of PTU-associated aplasia cutis. However, if a woman cannot tolerate PTU for any reason, experience side effects does not want to take the prescribed number of pills (PTU usually requires multiple daily dosages, whereas MMI can often be given once daily), MMI may be substituted. The initial dose rarely exceeds more than 450 mg of PTU or 30 mg of MMI daily in order to achieve the predefined levels of FT4 and TSH. The median time, usually seven to eight weeks, to normalization of the maternal FT4 index for both PTU and MMI is equal [75], but improvement in these parameters may be seen earlier at three to four weeks. This fact, makes clinically relevant to reassess maternal FT4 or total T4 at an interval of three to four weeks and to adjust ATD dosage appropriately based upon the current levels of thyroid hormones. We should keep in mind, that maternal serum TSH levels may remain suppressed for several weeks after normalization of thyroid hormone levels. So measuring TSH level is not helpful early in treatment, and may mislead us to continue with the unnecessary high dose of ATD, causing drug induced hypothyroidism and thus depriving the developing fetus from crucially important maternal T4 delivery. As was discussed above, due to the changes of the activity of Graves' Disease throughout pregnancy, determined by fluctuations of TRAbs concentrations, in the late second and third trimesters the dose of ATD can be reduced or even stopped by 32 to 34 weeks of gestation in 30% of women [76]. Of course, the same spectrum of adverse effects related to ATD therapy in the nonpregnant state applies to use during gestation.

Both drugs are showing similar fetal outcomes, in terms of thyroid function. The risk for congenital abnormalities had been considered to be higher in MMI than in PTU.

Aplasia cutis and also other malformations have been reported in the offspring of mothers who had taken methimazole during pregnancy [67, 77]. Aplasia cutis is a congenital localized absence of skin that occurs spontaneously in approximately 1 in 2000 births [78]. Many years, the fear from the possible development of this complication had restricted the use of methimazole during pregnancy, nevertheless, there is no definitive proof that MMI is actually responsible for the condition. Additional possible congenital malformation in children exposed to MMI during the first trimester of pregnancy are choanal and esophageal atresia, minor facial abnormalities and psychomotor delay, which either isolated or associated with aplasia cutis define the so called methimazole embryopathy [67, 77].

Because there are no reports of aplasia cutis in association with PTU, this drug is preferred by some physicians. Growing data from the literature for the causative roll of PTU for acute liver injury, had limited the use of the drug only during the first trimester of the pregnancy due to its lower risk for congenital malformations. Before pregnancy and during the second and third trimester methimazole is preferred, considered to be less hepatotoxic. Pregnancy itself does not appear to alter the maternal pharmacokinetics of MMI, although serum PTU levels may be lower in the latter part of gestation compared to the first and second trimesters [71].

The treatment of Graves' Disease during pregnancy should aim to achieve normalization of FT4 and FT3 levels with strict monitoring of maternal thyroid function at an appropriate intervals. Careful surveillance of fetal development to optimize fetal outcomes is also important, and this makes the team approach with a close collaboration between endocrinologist and obstetrician crucial. Apart from monitoring the laboratory parameters, there are clinical signs of improvement, that include maternal weight gain, decrease in pulse rate and appropriate fetal growth, that should be followed up. Clinical signs and laboratory values must always be considered together when a therapeutic decision is necessary, and if for example, there is a detected lack of maternal weight gain in conjunction with mild elevations in thyroid hormone levels, the initiation of a low dose of ATD should be considered.

5.5.1.1 Antithyroid drugs: effect on the Fetus

In pregnancies complicated with concomitant Graves' Disease, fetal thyroid status is influenced by two maternal factors, both of which cross the placenta: maternal ATD dosage and maternal TRAb activity. There are two potentially opposing influences on fetal thyroid function by maternal TRAb, because they can be with either stimulating or blocking effect on the developing fetal thyroid gland. Different assays for maternal TRAb exist. Some, like one of the most commonly used radioreceptor assay does not distinguish between blocking and stimulating antibodies, so their peripheral effect can be estimated only by assessing the thyroid function [79]. The currently available bioassay is the thyroid stimulating immunoglobulin (TSI), which measures the generation of cyclic adenosine monophosphate by cells that express TSH receptor when incubated with the patient's serum [66].

Because both PTU and MMI can cross the placenta and they may decrease fetal thyroid hormone production The dose–response relationship between maternal ATD dose and neonatal thyroid function is controversial, as some studies have reported a direct correlation [66, 69, 80] and others have not demonstrated this [64, 69, 73]. There are data showing that ATD drugs even at low daily dosages (PTU ≤ 100 mg, MMI ≤ 10 mg) at term may affect the fetal thyroid function. An elevated cord TSH level was found in 23% of babies born to such PTU-treated mothers and in 14% of those treated MMI [81]. There is an individual variability in serum PTU and MMI levels after a standard oral dose and that could partly explain the observed lack of correlation between maternal dosage and fetal thyroid function [81, 82]. Transplacental passage of maternal TRAb resulting in excessive fetal thyroid stimulation is the second factor that can influence fetal thyroid function. Usually, this becomes clinically relevant at 24 to 26 weeks, of gestation. Maternal levels reflect the degree of fetal exposure [83]. At term there is a strong correlation between maternal and cord TRAb levels with development of neonatal hyperthyroidism. Clinically relevant is to measure the maternal TRAb levels at term, because the combination of continued use of maternal ATD therapy with low maternal TRAb levels may lead to elevated serum TSH levels in approximately 50–60% of infants [80]. This shows how important is to adjust appropriately the maternal ATD dosage during pregnancy especially when maternal immune thyroid stimulation is low. In nonimmune types of thyrotoxicosis, like toxic adenoma for example, dose relationship between ATD and the risk of suppression of the fetal thyroid function is more profound, since there is no contribution of fetal thyroid stimulation by the maternal immune system. Therefore, it is not surprising that fetal thyroid status is not strictly correlated with maternal ATD dosage. Inappropriately high doses of ATD may result in development of fetal or neonatal goiter, which in the most severe cases if markedly enlarged at birth may cause respiratory distress. In the past, due to the concomitant iodide therapy and ATD, goiter occurred more frequently. The combined inhibitory effect on the fatal thyroid gland of iodide and ATD resulted in the development of goiter. One clinical approach is to perform a fetal utrasound in all women who are still taking relatively high ATD doses at 26 to 28 weeks (PTU ≥450 mg/day, MMI ≥30 mg/day) [84]. If a fetal goiter is detected this could be due to either fetal hyperthyroidism, transplacental passage of stimulating TRAbs, or to fetal hypothyroidism caused by transplacental passage of maternal ATD therapy. In both situations intrauterine growth retardation may occur. The presence of fetal tachycardia (160–180 beats per minute) and advanced fetal bone age is highly suggestive of hyperthyroidism [85, 86]. When caused by maternal ATD use, a quick resolution within two weeks after birth of the neonatal goiter is observed, reflecting the discontinuation of drug exposure [69]. Therefore, stopping maternal ATD therapy and monitoring the fetal goiter by ultrasound is advisable. Other therapeutic approach for treatment of the fetal goiter due to maternal ATD exposure includes intra-amniotic levothyroxine injections [87, 88], but because it was done concomitantly with lowering of the maternal PTU dose, it is difficult to estimate the relative importance of each factor on the resolution of the fetal goiter. The cessation of maternal ATD therapy alone may result in decrease in the fetal goiter assessed ultrasonographically [89]. Discontinuation or decreasing the dose of ATD therapy is crucial in cases where hypothyroidism is suspected because of transplacental ATD passage. Fetal goiter must be followed with sequential ultrasounds and if no reduction in size, within two to three weeks, occurs, fetal thyroid function should be determined by performing periumbilical blood sampling, and intra-amniotic levothyroxine therapy should considered if necessary. Several studies have reported no cognitive and somatic defects in development of children exposed to maternal ATD in utero [90–93] and this was so even after accounting for higher dosage or first trimester exposure. These were cross sectional studies that measured cognitive development by intelligence quotient. Therefore, it is unknown if transient, or more subtle developmental changes might have been present.

5.5.2 Beta-adrenergic blockers

Considering the relation between thyroid hormones and sympathetic nervous system, beta-adrenergic blocking agents may be used transiently to control adrenergic symptoms, while waiting for ATD therapy to decrease thyroid hormone levels. The fact, that combined use of ATD and propranolol in comparison with ATD alone was related with a higher rate of spontaneous first trimester miscarriages, although the similar levels of thyroid hormone [94], beta-blockers should be used for short period and with caution.

5.5.3 Iodides

As was previously discussed, chronic use of iodides during pregnancy has been associated with hypothyroidism and goiter in neonates, sometimes in severe cases resulting in asphyxiation because of tracheal obstruction [95]. Iodides should not be used as a first line therapy in women with Grave's because of the well-known dual effect of iodine upon the thyroid function and the risk for provocation of a latent autoimmune disorder and also for aggravation of the thyrotoxicosis increasing the iodine store in an already hyperfunctioning thyroid gland. Iodides could be used transiently if needed in preparation for thyroidectomy.

5.5.4 Surgery

Subtotal thyroidectomy for Graves' Disease is rarely considered during pregnancy. The reasons for such treatment could be the need to use high levels of ATD (PTU 450 mg/day, MMI 40 mg/day) to control the clinical symptoms and thyroid hormonal levels, if compressive symptoms due to goiter size develop or if a patient is allergic to ATD therapy or noncompliant to the therapeutic regiment. The surgery is usually performed in latter half of the second trimester. The surgery in the first trimester is relatively contraindicated, because that this is the time of the highest spontaneous abortion rate and surgery and anesthesia could possibly further increase the risk, but if clinically indicated subtotal thyroidectomy may be done in some specific cases [96].

5.5.5 131I therapy

The use of 131I therapy is completely contraindicated in pregnancy. The most vulnerable for the fetus period to 131I therapy is that after 12 weeks gestation, because at this period the fetal thyroid begins to concentrate radioiodine at higher rate than the maternal thyroid and other fetal tissues are generally more radiosensitive [97]. It is essentially important to exclude pregnancy in all women prior to radioiodine therapy. The therapeutic administration of 131I to a nursing mother is contraindicated and lactation should be stopped immediately if this occurs.

5.6 Lactation

Because the ATD present in breast milk in sufficient concentrations that can influence infant's thyroid, their use in breast-feeding women was considered contraindicated. Due to the ability of PTU to bind more tightly with protein than MMI, less amount of PTU is available in the milk. The ratio of milk to serum levels is found to be lower for PTU (0.67) [98] than for MMI (1.0) [99], moreover the amount of ingested drug secreted in breast milk is approximately six times higher for MMI than for PTU (0.14 vs. 0.025% of the ingested dose) [99]. Despite this, the fetal thyroid function assessed in newborns breast-fed by mothers treated with ATD with daily doses of PTU (50–300 mg), MMI (5–20 mg), or carbimazole (5–15 mg) for periods ranging from three weeks to eight months, remained normal, even in overtreated women with elevated serum TSH levels [100]. Data from the literature show that ATD therapy (PTU 300 mg/day, MMI 20 mg/day) may be considered relatively safe during lactation [100]. Generally, PTU would be preferred than MMI, because of its less availability in breast milk. It is wise the drug to be taken by the mother after a feeding. So far, there are no reports of the development of ATD side-effects in an infant breast fed by a mother treated with ATD [101].

Abbreviations

GD	Graves' Disease
TSH	Thyroid-stimulating hormone
TSHR	Thyroid-stimulating hormone receptor
GTT	Gestational transient thyrotoxicosis
ATD	Antithyroid drugs
hCG	Chorionic gonadotropin
TBG	Thyroid-binding globulin
TT4	Total thyroxine
TT3	Total triiodothyronine
FT4	Free thyroxine
FT3	Free triiodothyronine
rT3	Reverse triiodothyronine
NIS	Sodium Iodine symporter
TRAb	TSH receptor antibody
PPT	Postpartum thyroiditis
PTU	Propylthiouracil
MMI	Methimazole
HG	Hyperemesis gravidarum

Author details

Nikolay Petrov Botushanov[1*], Aleksandar Nikolaev Botushanov[2] and Albena Dimitrova Botushanova[3]

1 Department of Endocrinology and Metabolic Diseases, Medical University, Plovdiv, Bulgaria

2 Department of Propaedeutics of Internal Diseases, Medical University, Plovdiv, Bulgaria

3 Department of Clinical Oncology, Medical University, Plovdiv, Bulgaria

*Address all correspondence to: nbotush@gmail.com

References

[1] Lauberg P, Pedersen KM, Vestergaard H, et al. High incidence of multinodular toxic goiter in the elderly population in a low iodine intake area vs high incidence of Graves' disease in the young in a high iodine intake area: comparative surveys of thyrotoxicosis epidemiology in East-Jutland Denmark and Iceland. J Intern Med 1991;229:415-420.

[2] Aghini-Lombardi F,Antonangeli L, Martino E, et al. The spectrum of thyroid disorders in an iodine-deficient community: the Pescopagno survev. J Clin Endocrinol Metab 1999;84: 561-566.

[3] Tunbridge W, Evered DC, Hall R, et al. The spectrum of thyroid disease in a community: the Whickham survey. Clin Endocrinol (Oxf) 1977;7: 481-493.

[4] Zandman-Goddard G, Peeva E, Schoenfeld Y. Gender and autoimmunity. Autoimmunity Rev 2007. 2007;6:366-372.

[5] Chiovato L, Lapi P, Fiore E, et al. Thyroid autoimmunity and female gender. J Endocrinol Invest 1993; 16:384-391.

[6] Chiovato L, Larizza D, Bendinelli G,et al. Autoimmune hypothyroidism and hyperthyroidism in patients with Turner's syndrome. Eur J Endocrinol 1996;134:568-575.

[7] Jacobson EM, Tomer Y. The genetic basis of thyroid autoimmunity. Thyroid 2007;17:949-961.

[8] Yin X, Latif R, Tomer Y, et al. Thyroid epigenetics: X chromosome inactivation in patients with autoimmune thyroid disease. Ann N Y Acad Sci 2007;1110:193-200.

[9] Amino N, Tada H, Hidaka Y. Postpartum autoimmune thyroid syndrome: a model of aggravation of autoimmune disease. Thyroid 1999; 9:705-713.

[10] Davies TF. The thyroid immunology of the postpartum period. Thyroid 1999;9:675-684.

[11] Negro R, Mestman JH. Thyroid disease in pregnancy. Best Pract Res Clin Endocrinol Metab 2011; 25: 927-943.

[12] Klein RZ, Haddow JE, Falx JD, et al. Prevalence of thyroid deficiency in pregnant women. Clin Endocrinol 1991; 35: 41-46.

[13] Soldin OP. Guidelines of the American Thyroid Association for the diagnosis and management of thyroid disease during pregnancy and postpartum. Clin Chem 2011; 21: 1081-1125.

[14] Hershman JM. Physiological and pathological aspects of the effect of human chorionic gonadotropin on the thyroid. Best Practice & Research: Clinical Endocrinology & Metabolism 2004 ;vol.18:249-265.

[15] Soldin OP, Tractenberg RE, Hollowell JG, Jonklaas J, Janicic N, Soldin SJ. Trimester-specific changes in maternal thyroid hormone, thyrotropin, and thyroglobulin concentrations during gestation: trends and associations across trimesters in iodine sufficiency. Thyroid 2004 ;14:1084-1090.

[16] Kahric-Janicic N, Soldin SJ, Soldin OP, West T, Gu J, Jonklaas J Tandem mass spectrometry improves the accuracy of free thyroxine measurements during pregnancy. Thyroid 2007;17:303-311.

[17] Glinoer D. The regulation of thyroid function in pregnancy: pathways of endocrine adaptation from physiology

to pathology. Endocr Rev 1997;18:404-433.

[18] Li C, Shan Z, Mao J, Wang W, Xie, et al. Assessment of thyroid function during first-trimester pregnancy: what is the rational upper limit of serum TSH during the first trimester in Chinese pregnant women? J Clin Endocrinol Metab 2014; 99:73-79.

[19] Cooper DS, Laurberg P. Hyperthyroidism in pregnancy. Lancet Diabetes Endocrinol 2013;1:238-249.

[20] Sapin R, D'Herbomez M, Schlienger JL Free thyroxine measured with equilibrium dialysis and nine immunoassays decreases in late pregnancy. Clin Lab 2004;50:581-584.

[21] Soldin OP, Tractenberg RE, Hollowell JG, et al. Trimester-specific changes in maternal thyroid hormone, thyrotropin, and thyroglobulin concentrations during gestation: trends and associations across trimesters in iodine sufficiency. Thyroid. 2004;14:1084-1090.

[22] Casey BM, Dashe JS, Wells CE, ,et al. Subclinical hyperthyroidism and pregnancy outcomes. Obstet Gynecol 2006; 107:337-341.

[23] Skjoldebrand L, Brundin J, Carlstrom A, Pettersson T. Thyroid associated components in serum during normal pregnancy. Acta Endocrinol. 1982;100(4):504-511

[24] Kurtz A, Dwyer K, Ekins R. Serum free thyroxine in pregnancy. Br Med J. 1979;2(6189):550-551.

[25] Boss AM, Kingstone D. Further observations on serum free thyroxine concentrations during pregnancy. Br Med J (Clin Res Ed) 1981;283:584

[26] Hopton MR, Ashwell K, Scott IV, Harrop JS. Serum free thyroxine concentration and free thyroid hormone indices in normal pregnancy. Clin Endocrinol. 1983;18:431-437

[27] Roti E, Fang SL, Emerson CH, Braverman LE. Placental inner ring iodothyronine deiodination: a mechanism for decreased passage of T4 and T3 from mother to fetus. Transactions of the Association of American Physicians 1981;vol. 94:183-189.

[28] Dafnis E, Sabatini S. The effect of pregnancy on renal function: physiology and pathophysiology. Am Journal of the Medical Sciences 1992 ;303: 184-205.

[29] Glinoer D. Pregnancy and iodine. Thyroid 2001 ;11: 471-48.

[30] De Escobar GM, Obregón MJ, Del Rey FE. Iodine deficiency and brain development in the first half of pregnancy. Public Health Nutrition 2007 ;10(2): 1554-1570.

[31] Casey B, Leveno K. Thyroid disease in pregnancy. Obstet Gynecol. 2006;108(5):1283-1292.

[32] Stagnaro-Green A, Roman SH, Cobin RH, et al. Detection of at-risk pregnancy by means of highly sensitive assays for thyroid autoantibodies. Journal of the American Medical Association. 1990;264:1422-1425.

[33] Thangaratinam S, Tan A, Knox E, et al. Thyroid autoantibodies are strongly associated with miscarriage and preterm birth: a meta-analysis of evidence. British Medical Journal. 2011;342:d2616.

[34] Glinoer D, Riahi M, Grun JP, Kinthaert J. Risk of subclinical hypothyroidism in pregnant women with asymptomatic autoimmune thyroid disorders. J Clin Endocrinol Metab. 1994;79:197-204.

[35] Ghafoor F, Mansoor M, Malik T, et al. Role of thyroid peroxidase antibodies in the outcome of pregnancy. Journal of

College of Physicians and Surgeons Pakistan. 2006;16:468-471.

[36] Haddow JE, Cleary-Goldman J, McClain MR, et al. First- and Second-Trimester Risk of Aneuploidy (FaSTER) Research Consortium. Thyroperoxidase and thyroglobulin antibodies in early pregnancy and preterm delivery. Obstetrics & Gynecology. 2010;116:58-62.

[37] Ijima T, Tada H, Hidaka Y, et al. Effects of autoantibodies on the course of pregnancy and fetal growth. Obstetrics & Gynecology. 1997;90:364-369.

[38] Luton D, Le Gac I, Vuillard E, et al. Management of Graves' disease during pregnancy:The key role of fetal thyroid gland monitoring. J Clin Endocrinol Metab 2005; 90(11):6093-6098.

[39] Amino N, Izumi Y, Hidaka Y, et al. No increase of blocking type anti-thyrotropin receptor antibodies during pregnancy in patients with Graves' disease. J Clin Endocrinol Metab 2003; 88(12):5871-5874.

[40] Zakarija M, McKenzie JM. Pregnancy-associated changes in the thyroid-stimulating antibody of Graves' disease and the relationship to neonatal hyperthyroidism. J Clin Endocrinol Metab 1983; 57(5):1036-1040.

[41] Amino N, Tanizawa O, Mori H, et al. Aggravation of thyrotoxicosis in early pregnancy and after delivery in Graves' disease. J Clin Endocrinol Metab 1982; 55(1):108-112.

[42] Jacobson DL, Gange SJ, Rose NR, et al. Epidemiology and estimated population burden of selected autoimmune diseases in the United States. Clin Immunol Immunopathol 1997;84:223-243.

[43] Mestman JH. Hyperthyroidism in pregnancy. Curr Opin Endocrinol Diabetes Obes. 2012;19:394-401.

[44] Cooper DS, Laurberg P. Hyperthyroidism in pregnancy. Lancet Diabetes Endocrinol 2013;1:238-249.

[45] Casey B, De Veciana M. Thyroid screening in pregnancy. Am J Obstet Gynecol 2014; 211: 351-353

[46] Chan GW, Mandel SJ. Therapy insight: Management of Graves' disease during pregnancy. Nat Clin Pract Endocrinol Metab 2007; 3(6):470-478.

[47] Momotani N, Noh J, Ishikawa N, et al. Relationship between silent thyroiditis and recurrent Graves' disease in the postpartum period. J Clin Endocrinol Metab 1994;79(1):285-289.

[48] Glinoer D, Spencer CA. Serum TSH determinations in pregnancy: how, when and why? Nature Reviews Endocrinology. 2010;6:526-529.

[49] Nguyen CT, Sasso EB, Barton L, et al. Graves' hyperthyroidism in pregnancy: a clinical review. Clin Diabetes Endocrinol 2018; 4: 4.

[50] Tan JY, Loh KC, Yeo GS, et al. Transient hyperthyroidism of hyperemesis gravidarum. British Journal of Obstetrics and Gynaecology. 2002;109:683-688. Alexander EK. 2017 guidelines of the American Thyroid Association for the diagnosis and management of thyroid disease during pregnancy and the postpartum. Thyroid 2017; 27: 315-389.

[51] Yoshihara A, Noh JY, Mukasa K, et al. Serum human chorionic gonadotropin levels and thyroid hormone levels in gestational transient thyrotoxicosis: is the serum hCG level useful for differentiating between active Graves' disease and GTT? Endocr J 2015; 62: 557-560.

[52] Goodwin TM, Montoro M, Mestman JH, et al. The role of chorionic gonadotropinin transient hyperthyroidism of hyperemesis

gravidarum. J Clin Endocrinol Metab 1992; 75(5):1333-1337.

[53] Lee RH, Spencer CA, Mestman JH, et al. Free T4 immunoassays are flawed during pregnancy. American Journal of Obstetrics and Gynecology. 2009;200:260-267.

[54] Peleg D, Cada S, Peleg A, et al. The relationship between maternal serum Thyroid-stimulating immunoglobulin and fetal and neonatal thyrotoxicosis. Obstetrics & Gynecology. 2002;99:1040-1043.

[55] Polak M, Le Gac I, Vuillard E, et al. Fetal and neonatal thyroid function in relation to maternal Graves' disease. Best Practice & Research Clinical Endocrinology & Metabolism. 2004;18:289-302.

[56] Gardiner-Hill H. Pregnancy complicating simple goitre and Graves' disease. Lancet 1929; 1:120-12

[57] Momotani N, Ito K, Hamada N, et al. Maternal hyperthyroidism and congenital malformation in the offspring. Clin Endocrinol (Oxf) 1984; 20(6):695-700.

[58] Mestman JH, Manning PR, Hodgman J. Hyperthyroidism and pregnancy. Arch InternMed 1974; 134(3):434-439.

[59] Sugrue D, Drury MI. Hyperthyroidism complicating pregnancy: Results of treatment by antithyroid drugs in 77 pregnancies. Br J Obstet Gynaecol 1980; 87(11):970-975.

[60] Millar LK, Wing DA, Leung AS, et al. Low birth weight and preeclampsia in pregnancies complicated by hyperthyroidism. Obstet Gynecol 1994; 84(6):946-949.

[61] Davis LE, Lucas MJ, Hankins GD, et al. Thyrotoxicosis complicating pregnancy. Am J Obstet Gynecol 1989; 160(1):63-70.

[62] Mitsuda N, Tamaki H, Amino N, et al. Risk factors for developmental disorders in infants born to women with Graves disease. Obstet Gynecol 1992; 80(3 Pt 1):359-364.

[63] Casey BM. Subclinical hypothyroidism and pregnancy. Obstet Gynecol Surv 2006; 61(6):415-420; quiz 23.

[64] Momotani N, Noh J, Oyangi H, et al. Antithyroid drug therapy for Graves' disease during pregnancy: optimal regimen for fetal thyroid status. The New England Journal of Medicine. 1986;315:24-28.

[65] Santini F, Chiovato L,Ghirri P, et al. Serum iodothyronines in the human fetus and the newborn: evidence for an important role of placenta in the fetal thyroid hormone homeostasis. J Clin Endocrinol Metab 1999;84:493-498.

[66] Mortimer RH, Tyack SA, Galligan JP, et al. Graves' disease in pregnancy: TSH receptor binding inhibiting immunoglobulins and maternal and neonatal thyroid function. Clin Endocrinol (Oxf) 1990; 32(2):141-1452.

[67] Abalovich M, Amino N, Barbour LA, et al: Management of thyroid dysfunction during pregnancy and postpartum: an Endocrine Society Clinical Practice Guideline. J Clin Endocrinol Metab 2007;92 (8 Suppl):S1-47.

[68] Burrow GN. Neonatal goiter after maternal propylthiouracil therapy. J Clin Endocrinol Metab. 1965;25:403-408.

[69] Cheron RG, Kaplan MM, Larsen PR, et al. Neonatal thyroid function after propylthiouracil therapy for maternal

Graves' disease. The New England Journal of Medicine. 1981;304:525-528.

[70] Rotondi M, Cappeli C, Pirali B, et al. The effect of pregnancy on subsequent relapse from Graves' disease following a successful course of ant-thyroid drug therapy. J Clin Endocrinol Metab 2008 (in press).

[71] Mandel SJ, Brent GA, Larsen PR. Review of antithyroid drug use during pregnancy and report of a case of aplasia cutis. Thyroid 1994; 4(1):129-133.

[72] Marchant B, Brownlie BE, Hart DM, et al. The placental transfer of propylthiouracil, methimazole and carbimazole. J Clin Endocrinol Metab 1977; 45(6):1187-1193

[73] Gardner DF, Cruikshank DP, Hays PM, et al. Pharmacology of propylthiouracil (PTU) in pregnant hyperthyroidwomen: Correlation of maternal PTU concentrations with cord serum thyroid function tests. J Clin Endocrinol Metab 1986; 62(1):217-220.

[74] Mortimer RH, Cannell GR, Addison RS, et al. Methimazole and propylthiouracil equally cross the perfused human term placental lobule. J Clin Endocrinol Metab 1997; 82(9):3099-3102.

[75] Wing DA, Millar LK, Koonings PP, et al. A comparison of propylthiouracil versus methimazole in the treatment of hyperthyroidism in pregnancy.AmJ Obstet Gynecol 1994; 170(1 Pt 1):90-95.

[76] Mestman JH. Hyperthyroidism in pregnancy. Clin Obstet Gynecol 1997; 40(1):45-64.

[77] Cooper DS. Antithyroid drugs. N Eng J Med 2005; 352:905-917.

[78] Ribuffo D, Costantini M, Gullo P, et al. Aplasia cutis congenitaof the scalp, the skull, and the dura. Scand J Plast Reconstr Surg Hand Surg 2003;37:176-180

[79] Davies TF, Roti E, Braverman LE, et al. Thyroid controversy–stimulating antibodies. J Clin Endocrinol Metab 1998; 83(11):3777-3785.

[80] Davis LE, Lucas MJ, Hankins GD, et al. Thyrotoxicosis complicating pregnancy. Am J Obstet Gynecol 1989; 160(1):63-70.

[81] Momotani N, Noh JY, Ishikawa N, et al. Effects of propylthiouracil and methimazole on fetal thyroid status in mothers with Graves' hyperthyroidism. J Clin Endocrinol Metab 1997; 82(11):3633-3636.

[82] Cooper DS, Saxe VC, Meskell M, et al. Acute effects of propylthiouracil (PTU) on thyroidal iodide organification and peripheral iodothyronine deiodination: Correlation with serum PTU levels measured by radioimmunoassay. J Clin Endocrinol Metab 1982; 54(1):101-107.

[83] Fisher DA. Fetal thyroid function: Diagnosis and management of fetal thyroid disorders. Clin Obstet Gynecol 1997; 40(1):16-31.

[84] Momotani N, Iwama S, Noh J, et al. Anti-thyroid drug therapy for Graves' disease during pregnancy: Mildest thyrotoxic maternal free thyroxine concentrations to avoid fetal hypothyroidism. In: 77th Annual Meeting of the American Thyroid Association.; 2006; Phoenix, AZ.

[85] Chopra IJ. Fetal and neonatal hyperthyroidism. Thyroid 1992; 2(2):161-163.

[86] Nachum Z, Rakover Y, Weiner E, et al. Graves' disease in pregnancy: Prospective evaluation of a selective invasive treatment protocol. Am J Obstet Gynecol 2003;189(1):159-165.

[87] Davidson KM, Richards DS, Schatz DA, et al. Successful in utero treatment of fetal goiter and hypothyroidism. N Engl J Med 1991; 324(8):543-546.

[88] Van Loon AJ, Derksen JT, Bos AF, et al. In utero diagnosis and treatment of fetal goitrous hypothyroidism, caused by maternal use of propylthiouracil. Prenat Diagn 1995; 15(7):599-604.

[89] Ochoa-Maya MR, Frates MC, Lee-Parritz A, et al. Resolution of fetal goiter after discontinuation of propylthiouracil in a pregnant woman with Graves' hyperthyroidism. Thyroid 1999; 9(11):1111-1114.

[90] McCarroll AM, Hutchinson M, McAuley R, et al. Long-term assessment of children exposed in utero to carbimazole. Arch Dis Child 1976; 51(7):532-536.

[91] Burrow GN, Klatskin EH, Genel M. Intellectual development in children whose mothers received propylthiouracil during pregnancy. Yale J Biol Med 1978; 51(2):151-156.

[92] Messer PM, Hauffa BP, Olbricht T, et al. Antithyroid drug treatment of Graves' disease in pregnancy: Long-term effects on somatic growth, intellectual development and thyroid function of the offspring. Acta Endocrinol (Copenh) 1990; 123(3):311-316.

[93] Eisenstein Z, Weiss M, Katz Y, et al. Intellectual capacity of subjects exposed to methimazole or propylthiouracil in utero. Eur J Pediatr 1992; 151(8):558-559.

[94] Sherif IH, Oyan WT, Bosairi S, et al. Treatment of hyperthyroidism in pregnancy. Acta Obstet Gynecol Scand 1991; 70(6):461-463.

[95] Momotani N, Hisaoka T, Noh J, et al. Effects of iodine on thyroid status of fetus versus mother in treatment of Graves' disease complicated by pregnancy. J Clin Endocrinol Metab 1992; 75(3):738-744.

[96] Brodsky JB, Cohen EN, Brown BW Jr, et al. Surgery during pregnancy and fetal outcome. Am J Obstet Gynecol 1980; 138(8):1165-1167.

[97] Stoffer SS, Hamburger JI. Inadvertent 131I therapy for hyperthyroidism in the first trimester of pregnancy. J Nucl Med 1976; 17(02):146-149.

[98] Kampmann JP, Johansen K, Hansen JM, et al. Propylthiouracil in human milk. Revision of a dogma. Lancet 1980; 1(8171):736-737.

[99] Johansen K, Andersen AN, Kampmann JP, et al. Excretion of methimazole in human milk. Eur J Clin Pharmacol 1982; 23(4):339-341.

[100] Azizi F, Khoshniat M, Bahrainian M, et al. Thyroid function and intellectual development of infants nursed by mothers taking methimazole. J Clin Endocrinol Metab 2000; 85(9):3233-3238.

[101] Mandel SJ, Cooper DS. The use of antithyroid drugs in pregnancy and lactation. J Clin Endocrinol Metab 2001; 86(6):2354-2359.

Chapter 14

Pregnancy in Women with Graves' Disease: Focus on Fetal Surveillance

Anca Maria Panaitescu

Abstract

Graves' Disease (GD) is one of the most common autoimmune conditions in women of reproductive age. The disorder is characterized by the presence of pathogenic immunoglobulins that bind the TSH receptors (TRAbs) and stimulate the production of thyroid hormones leading to hyperthyroidism (the occurrence of inhibiting or neutral antibodies being rare). Affected individuals can be treated by radioiodine therapy, surgical removal of the gland or by antithyroid drugs (ATDs). Thyroid stimulating immunoglobulins may persist for years after medical treatment, radioiodine therapy or surgical removal of the gland in those affected by GD and during pregnancy can cross the placenta and can act on the fetal thyroid gland resulting in the development of fetal and neonatal hyperthyroidism and sometimes to goiter. Antithyroid drugs used during pregnancy can also cross the placenta and may be teratogenic and act on the fetal thyroid gland, leading to fetal and neonatal hypothyroidism and goiter. This chapter will discuss specific aspects of GD during pregnancy and postpartum focusing on fetal and neonatal consequences related to this disorder.

Keywords: pregnancy, Graves' Disease, TRAb, anti-thyroid drugs, fetal goiter, fetal hypothyroidism, fetal hyperthyroidism

1. Introduction

Graves' Disease (GD) is one of the most common autoimmune conditions in women of reproductive age. Pathogenic immunoglobulins that bind the TSH receptors (TRAbs) are the hallmark of GD and stimulate the production of thyroid hormones leading to hyperthyroidism (the occurrence of inhibiting or neutral antibodies being exceptional). Treatment for affected individuals is either by radioiodine therapy, surgical removal of the gland or by antithyroid drugs (ATDs). TRAbs may persist for years after medical treatment, radioiodine therapy or surgical removal of the gland in those affected by Graves' Disease and during pregnancy can cross the placenta by hijacking the physiological maternal-fetal antibody transfer pathways [1] and can act on the fetal thyroid gland resulting in the development of fetal hyperthyroidism and sometimes to fetal goiter. Antithyroid drugs used during pregnancy can also cross the placenta and may be teratogenic and act on the fetal thyroid gland, leading to hypothyroidism and fetal goiter.

The maternal thyroid gland undergoes extensive changes during pregnancy and postpartum. These changes are supported by the interaction between the fetal-placental unit and the maternal endocrine system and are reflected in the thyroid

 IntechOpen

function tests, which differ from outside pregnancy as early as first trimester. Normal fetal development depends on maternally derived thyroid hormones (TH) at least until 16–18 weeks' gestation when the fetal thyroid starts to function [2].

This chapter will discuss specific aspects of Graves' Disease during pregnancy and postpartum with focus on its fetal and neonatal consequences.

2. Physiological changes of the thyroid gland and the thyroid hormone metabolism during pregnancy

The maternal thyroid gland and thyroid hormone metabolism undergo significant changes in pregnancy. The volume of the gland and its blood supply increase in pregnancy [3]. Plasma volume expands thus increasing total T4 and T3 pool size (T4 - thyroxine and T3 - tri-iodothyronine). The placenta produces estrogen that induces hepatic synthesis of thyroid-binding globulin (TBG), the main protein involved in serum transport of TH, thus increasing levels of total T4 (TT4) and T3 (TT3) in the maternal plasma. Thyroid hormone production is dependent of iodine supply so iodine metabolism needs to keep up with these changes, hence, there is an increase in iodine requirements during pregnancy to both meet the maternal and fetal demands and to overcome the increased clearance by the kidneys. The placenta also produces HCG (human chorionic gonadotropin), a glycoprotein hormone with molecular similarity of its α-subunit with TSH (thyroid stimulating hormone) which acts as an agonist of TSH raising transiently free T4 levels and decreasing serum TSH levels. These changes are more relevant to the first trimester, and, beyond it, maternal thyroid hormone levels gradually return to those seen in the nonpregnant state [4].

Thyroid hormones are essential for normal development of the fetus and particularly of the fetal brain. The fetal thyroid gland only starts to produce adequate amounts of thyroid hormones in the second trimester; the first trimester fetus relies on maternal delivery of thyroid hormones to develop [2]. In the first part of pregnancy, before the fetal thyroid starts to work, T4 can be detected in fetal blood and brain, indicating that there is relevant transfer of maternal thyroid hormones to the fetus. The way maternal thyroid hormones are transferred across the placenta and in the fetal brain is not completely understood. Even though thyroid hormones are lipophilic, they can not passively cross the placenta nor the fetal blood–brain barrier because they are charged and thus can not cross a phospholipid bilayer [5]. Passage across the placenta and into the fetal brain is thought to be dependent on the function of several mechanisms [6] including: the existence of a specific transportation system, the function and expression of iodothyronine deiodinases (D) (enzymes that TH) in the placenta and fetal brain, and proteins within trophoblast and fetal brain which specifically bind TH. At the level of the placenta specific transporters capable of transporting maternal TH like monocarboxylate transporters MCT8 and MCT10 have been identified [6, 7]. Deiodinases found in the placenta in high concentration are D3, the main inactivating enzyme that catalyze monodiodination of T4 to reverse T3 and of T3 to T2, but also, D2, which the primary activating enzyme in tissues and locally catalyzes the monodeiodination of T4 to T3 [8]. The iodine released by this process might be used as a substrate by the fetus for the synthesis of its own thyroid hormones. D2 has been identified in the fetal brain [9] converting T4 to active T3, thus making it readily available. In the serum, TH are bound to liver-synthetized transportation proteins mainly TBG but also albumin and transthyretin. Transthyretin has been identified in the placenta and fetal choroid plexuses and is thought to play a role in transporting TH into the cells [10]. TSH does not cross the placenta and TSH in the fetal blood remains relatively constant throughout pregnancy between 4–8 mU/L [11]. The coordination and interplay between these systems ensures adequate availability of maternal TH to the fetus in a critical period of development (**Figure 1**).

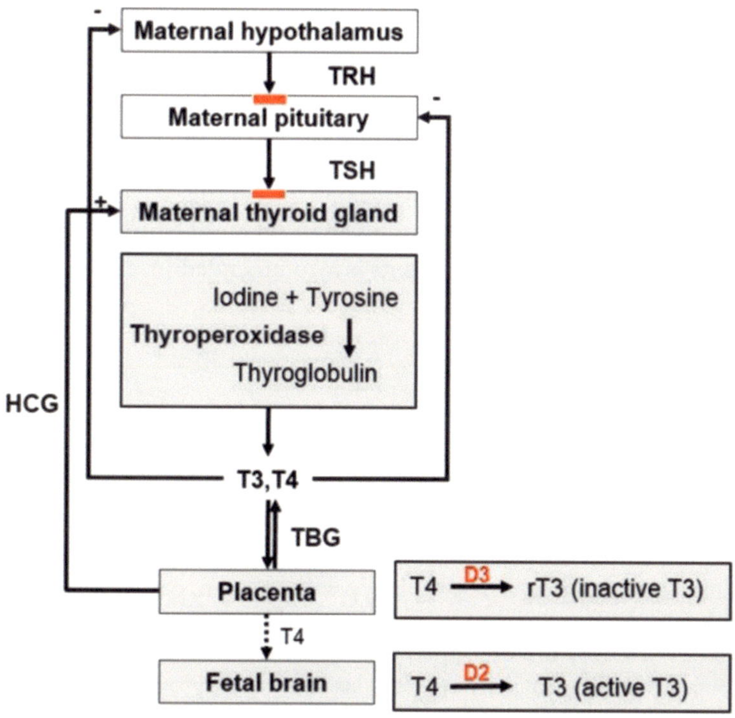

Figure 1.
The interaction between the fetal-placental unit and the maternal endocrine system during pregnancy. TRH – Thyrotropin releasing hormone; TSH – Thyroid stimulating hormone; T3 - tri-iodothyronine; T4 – Thyroxine; HCG - human chorionic gonadotrophin; TBG - thyroid hormone binding globulin; D3 - type 3 iodothyronine deiodinase; D2 - type 2 iodothyronine deiodinase; rT3 – Reverse T3.

3. Thyroid function tests in pregnancy

The physiological changes occurring in the thyroid gland from the beginning of pregnancy reflect in changes of the thyroid function tests. International guidelines recommend that ideally, for each population, there should be available trimester specific normal ranges for TSH and maternal TH [4]. These data should be derived from studies in healthy pregnant women with no known thyroid disease, with no evidence of thyroid autoimmunity and with an adequate amount of iodine intake for each trimester of pregnancy. In the absence of such data, which in many clinical settings can be difficult to obtain, in order to determine normal first-trimester reference ranges for TSH it has been suggested that the lower limit of its reference interval used in the non-pregnant state can be reduced by 0.4 mU/L and the upper limit by 0.5 mU/L [4]. For a healthy young pregnant woman the upper limit of TSH would therefore correspond to a value of 4.0 mU/L in the first trimester. This downshifting of the normal TSH reference interval only applies to the first trimester values, between 7 and 12 weeks of pregnancy since in the second and third trimesters, TSH levels recover and intervals valid outside pregnancy could be used.

The second most common test used to investigate thyroid function outside as well as in pregnancy is free T4 (FT4). FT4 represents the thyroxin that is not bound to plasmatic proteins; it constitutes less then 0.1% of total T4 (TT4) but is the active form that is up taken by cells. Precise measurement of FT4 is difficult in pregnancy in part because of the limitation of the widely used commercial immunoassays to account for thyroid hormone concentration changes that occur under the influence of increased levels of TBG, nonesteryfied fatty acids and decreased albumin.

Therefore, it has been suggested that TT4 and the index of T4 are more accurate in determining shifts in thyroid hormone levels in pregnancy. With TT4 it is important to acknowledge that its level increases by 50% during weeks 7 to 16 and remain high thereafter throughout pregnancy. When the level of TT4 is determined before 16 weeks, an adjustment to the upper limit of the non-pregnancy interval by 5% per week between weeks 7 to 16 could be made. A TT4 measurement with reference value 1.5 times the non-pregnancy range may be used in second and third trimesters as discussed above. When trimester-specific FT4 values are not available, use of the reference range for non-pregnant patients is recommended [4, 12–14].

4. Graves' Disease in pregnancy

4.1 Incidence and pathophysiology

Graves' Disease is one of the most common causes of thyrotoxicosis in women of reproductive age. It has been reported in as much as 1 in 500 pregnancies [15] but is more frequent in the years prior and after conception. GD presents clinically in pregnancy as outside pregnancy with hyperthyroidism, goiter, ophthalmopathy. The condition is autoimmune and is characterized by the presence of abnormal autoantibodies (TRAbs) directed against the TSH receptor in the thyroid gland. These antibodies, unlike anti-thyroperoxidase and anti-tyroglobulin antibodies, do have a pathogenic role in the thyroid-related and extra-thyroidal manifestation of GD and in pregnancy can cross the placenta and act on the fetal thyroid gland [16]. TRAbs are the pathogenic hallmark of GD and are measurable in around 95% of patients with active Graves' hyperthyroidism but can also be found, sometimes in high levels, in patients with a history of treated GD [17]. TRAbs are usually of the stimulating type, but blocking or neutral autoantibodies have been described [18]. TRAbs can cross the placenta by hijacking normal physiological mechanisms of antibody transfer that become functional after 16 weeks of pregnancy and can get into the fetal blood and act on the fetal TSH receptor, therefore they also have a pathogenic role in the fetal consequences of maternal GD, especially when in high titers (> 2 to 3 times the upper limit of normal [4].

The types of assays used in clinical settings for TRAb determination are relevant to pregnancy. There are two major methods to assess TRAbs in maternal blood: by using "receptor assays" and the newer "bioassays". Receptor or TSH Binding Inhibitory Immunoglobulin (TBII) assays detect serum autoantibodies that can block the binding of THS to an in vitro prepared receptor. They are of three generations, with the third-generation TRAbs assays reaching very high sensitivity and specificity [19]. They do not measure antibodies' activity and can not distinguish between stimulating or blocking TRAbs types, hence they do not predict the phenotype of maternal or fetal GD and do not correlate well with the clinical and biochemical severity of the disease in neither mother nor the fetus [20]. The new bioassays are functional tests that characterize the biological properties of TRAbs – stimulating (TSAbs) or blocking (TBAbs). New bioassays are commercially available to measure either TSAbs or TBAbs [21–23]. The functional activity of TRAbs relevant in pregnancy since, depending on their type, they can cause either hyperthyroidism or hypothyroidism in the fetus, for whom we do not readily have access to blood to assess fetal thyroid function as for the mother. Moreover, many women with a history of GD enter pregnancy in a euthyroid state either by taking medication (ATDs) or after undergoing surgery/radioiodine therapy, however, TSAbs and TBAbs can stay elevated for years after these procedures. As stated by international guideline [4]. TRAbs should be determined during pregnancy for the following categories:

1. Pregnant women with recently diagnosed GD

2. Pregnant women known with GD and treated with ATDs

3. Women with a previous history of GD with past treatment by radioiodine or thyroidectomy

4. A previous history of delivering an infant with hyperthyroidism

5. Known history of thyroidectomy for treatment of hyperthyroidism in pregnancy

Fetal and neonatal hyperthyroidism has been reported in 1–5% of infants of mothers with GD [24]. In a follow-up study of 47 newborns of mothers with TRAbs during pregnancy, 9 infants developed hyperthyroidism and 5 required ATD medication [25]. A maternal TRAb serum concentration approximately 3 times the upper limit of normal for the assay in the second and third trimesters predicted neonatal hyperthyroidism with 100% sensitivity and 43% specificity [25]. A similar risk cut-off for TRAb level was also found in other studies [26]. It is therefore recommended to take into consideration determining TRAb levels at the initial thyroid function assessment during early pregnancy for those with a history of GD and maybe even in those that present for the preconceptional visit. TRAbs should definitely be measured at the first visit in pregnant women with previous GD that underwent radioiodine or surgery, in those requiring ATDs and in those that are first diagnosed with GD in pregnancy. If maternal TRAb is undetectable or low in early pregnancy, no further testing could be proposed. However, for those with elevated levels, repeated testing should occur at 18–22 weeks to guide fetal follow-up. If levels are persistently high at 18–22 weeks, repeat testing at 30–34 weeks guides neonatal monitoring [4].

4.2 Differential diagnosis

Graves' Disease can rarely first manifest in the first trimester of pregnancy when it is important to be distinguished from gestational transient thyrotoxicosis (GTT) or in the postpartum when it should not be confused with the thyrotoxicosis phase of the postpartum thyroiditis (PPT). Gestational transient thyrotoxicosis is defined as hyperthyroidism of new-onset in the first trimester of pregnancy; it is usually associated with hyperemesis gravidarum and is mediated by the interaction of high level of HCG with the TSH receptor, hence it is expected to be more common with multiple gestation, hydatidiform mole and choriocarcinoma, where HCG levels are higher, but it can occur in any pregnant woman. In GTT there are no previous signs or symptoms of GD and importantly, TRAbs are not detectable. The condition is self-limiting and improves in the second trimester of pregnancy, therefore ATDs, which are known teratogenic, should be avoided. Supportive treatment with hydration, antiemetics, electrolyte replacement and occasionally a short-course of beta-blockers is sufficient [27]. Postpartum thyroiditis is characterized by inflammation secondary to autoimmunity (antithyroid peroxidase antibodies [TPO], anti-thyroglobulin antibodies) against the thyroid gland that manifests as new-onset thyroid dysfunction specifically developing in the first 12 months after a pregnancy in a previously euthyroid woman [28]. The condition typically ensues with a hyperthyroid state where the reservoir of thyroid hormones stored in the gland is released consequent to inflammation, followed by a hypothyroid state. The thyrotoxicosis state is more common in the first 6 months after delivery and again is different from GD because it lacks the presence of TRAbs and is generally characterized by milder symptoms: palpitations, heat intolerance, fatigue and irritability. PPT is encountered in women with known TPO antibodies in the first trimester or in those with a personal or familial history of thyroid disease or other autoimmune conditions. It tends to recur after each pregnancy and in most cases the affected women recover their euthyroid function within 12 months, however, some of them may be persistently hypothyroid. PPT has a prevalence of about 5% [29]. Complete and partial hydatidiform moles as in gestational trophoblastic disease can sometimes present with thyrotoxicosis in pregnancy. This is more rare than previously believed. In a recent cohort-study, completed by a systematic review and meta-analysis of cases of hydatidiform moles in missed-miscarriages, in 295 women with a confirmed histological diagnosis of hydatidiform mole in the first trimester there were no cases of thyrotoxicosis [30]. However, in a review of 196 patients treated for gestational trophoblastic disease over a 5-years period at a major specialized center, 7% (14/196) patients had biochemical hyperthyroidism and 4 had clinical signs and symptoms of hyperthyroidism [31]. Causes of thyrotoxicosis in pregnancy are described in **Table 1** [27, 28, 32–36].

4.3 Clinical scenarios with Graves' Disease in pregnancy

There are several clinical scenarios related to pregnancy in women with Graves' Disease and they will be discussed in detail further.

4.3.1 Preparing for pregnancy in women with known Graves' Disease

Graves' Disease is common in women of reproductive age. Pregnancy should be carefully planned because both the characteristic pathogenic antibodies and the treatment of GD may be deleterious to the fetus. Also, uncontrolled GD may lead to unfavorable outcomes of pregnancy such as miscarriage, gestational hypertension, preeclampsia, preterm birth, fetal growth restriction, fetal intrauterine death, fetal and neonatal goiter, neonatal abnormal thyroid function with potential life-long disability for the infant. Contraception is strongly advised in women with newly diagnosed GD or in those with uncontrolled GD until euthyroidism is reached by treatment. Many patients will first be prescribed ATDs, however options of ablative therapy with I131 or surgery (total thyroidectomy) are also considered. These options should be discussed with women with GD in relation to how they may interfere with a potential pregnancy. Benefits and risks of options used for management of GD in women of reproductive age desiring a pregnancy are given in **Table 2** [4].

Gestational transient thyrotoxicosis
Hyperthyroid phase of postpartum thyroiditis
Graves' Disease
Toxic nodular goiter
Toxic adenoma
Thyroiditis
Excessive thyroid hormone drugs intake, factitious thyrotoxicosis
Gestational trophoblastic disease
Familial nonautoimmune hyperthyroidism

Table 1.
Causes of thyrotoxicosis in pregnancy and postpartum [27, 28, 32–36].

Approach	Benefits	Risks
ATDs	Euthyroidism in 1–2 months Gradual decrease of TRAb Easy to take, inexpensive Easy to discontinue or modify	Mild adverse effects: 5%, Severe adverse effects: 0.2% Birth defects (see below) Relapse after discontinuation: 50%–70%
Ablative therapy (I131)	Oral administration Reduction in goiter size Relapse rare	Repeat therapy at times Increase in TRAb for months to years – risk for the fetus Conception delayed for at least 6 months Worsening of orbitopathy Lifelong dependence of substitution with exogenous levothyroxine
Total thyroidectomy	Definitive treatment Autoimmunity gradually resolves Removal of the goiter	Surgical site complications: 5% Chronic hypoparathyroidism Permanent neck scar Life-long dependence of substitution with exogenous levothyroxine

Table 2.
Benefits and risks of the options for management of GD in women desiring a pregnancy. Adapted and modified from [4]; TRAb – TSH receptor antibodies.

Antithyroid drugs, thionamides propylthiouracil (PTU), carbimazol and methimazole (MMI) have been the traditional mode of treating GD. These drugs inhibit the enzyme thyroperoxidase which facilitates the addition of iodine to tyrosine in the production of thyroglobulin (**Figure 1**), an essential step in the formation of thyroid hormones. ATDs have their advantages, however, when it comes to preparing for pregnancy, counseling on the continuation of treatment and on what drugs should be preferred is of great use. ATDs can have adverse effects to the mother, but during pregnancy, they can cross the placenta and affect the fetus. Use of ATDs in the first trimester of pregnancy has been linked with congenital malformations. Later usage may lead to fetal/neonatal hypothyroidism and goiter. Carbimazol and methimazole administration during the first trimester and especially between 6 to 10 weeks has been associated in epidemiological and case-report studies with a pattern of anomalies (carbimazole/methimazole embryopathy) characterized by dysmorphic facies, choanal atresia, aplasia cutis congenita and other skin defects, heart and gastrointestinal abnormalities and abdominal wall defects [37]. Prudently, many authorities recommend for pregnant women with GD on ATDs, that PTU should be used in the first trimester and MMI thereafter. While PTU has a very small risk of maternal liver toxicity, it could be preferred in the first trimester, however, switching from one ATD to another at the beginning of pregnancy is not an easy process and it may lead to worsening in control of the thyroid function which in itself may increase the chance of congenital anomalies [37]. Recent reports show that PTU also is not devoid of the risk of congenital anomalies. In a Danish study, 2–3% of children exposed to PTU presented facial anomalies, necks cysts and urinary tract abnormalities, often requiring surgery in later life [38].

Women with GD treated with I131 before at least six months prior to conception who are in an euthyroid state had similar outcomes of their pregnancies as healthy controls in a retrospective study [39]. Obviously, I131 is contraindicated in pregnancy and women undertaking this treatment should prove a negative pregnancy test 48 hours prior to it [4].

Total thyroidectomy is the definitive treatment for GD but it can lead to surgical complications such as recurrent laryngeal nerve paralysis and hypoparathyroidism.

Hypoparathyroidism is the most common complication after total thyroidectomy and is usually underrecognized. In a recent retrospective study of patients undergoing total thyroidectomy for benign thyroid conditions, the incidence of transient hypoparathyroidism was 43.3% and permanent was 13.4%. In patients with GD chronic hypoparathyroidism developed in 27.3% [40]. Entering pregnancy with hypoparathyroidism has its own potential risks for both mother and the fetus [41].

A preconceptional visit should ideally be planned for women with known GD of reproductive age that are considering pregnancy. This consultation should be given by a team of physicians that includes an endocrinologist and a maternal-fetal medicine specialist/obstetrician with experience in dealing with GD during pregnancy. Women with GD seeking pregnancy should be euthyroid – exhibit normal levels of thyroid hormones for at least 1–2 months successively. It may be sensible that in patients who underwent thyroidectomy but especially in those previously treated with I131 ablative therapy, TRAb titers be assessed at the preconceptional visit, since the level of these antibodies could interfere with fetal thyroid development in the second half of pregnancy and they can remain increased many months even years. Pregnancy could be postponed if the levels are very high. For those with a total thyroidectomy, parathyroid function should be checked if not assessed before. For women with GD, other autoimmune conditions should be looked for and a thorough clinical exam complemented in specific cases with targeted tests should be prescribed. A recent systematic review and meta-analysis found overt polyautoimmunity in 14% of patients with autoimmune thyroid disease. Most common autoimmune conditions associated with GD were type 1 diabetes mellitus and autoimmune gastritis, but rheumatological, dermatological and neurological autoimmune disorders could also be found in GD affected patients [42]. Folic acid is usually recommended to these women in the preparation of pregnancy.

4.3.2 Pregnancy in women with Graves' Disease on anti-thyroid drugs

For many women with Graves' Disease ATDs are a good choice of treatment gradually inducing remission of autoimmunity. Drugs can be stopped after 1–2 years of trail, and even though, hyperthyroidism will eventually develop in almost 50% of these patients, reactivation of TRAb positivity is not usually expected. In a prospective study on 218 patients with GD treated for 12 months with ATDs, only 5% of those that were TRAb-negative with treatment became hyperthyroid within 8 weeks after stopping the medication [43]. It has therefore been suggested that, under good clinical judgment, in women with GD on ATDs that become pregnant and that are considered in remission, drugs could be stopped at least during the first trimester of pregnancy, especially between weeks 6 to 10, the major teratogenic period [4]. This approach is very different from what is recommended for other autoimmune conditions in early pregnancy where discontinuation of the chronic medication is strongly discouraged. Clinical assessment and thyroid function tests are recommended frequently in these patients and if relapse is diagnosed and ATD therapy is required, PTU is the preferred drug during the first trimester. The risk of rapid relapse of hyperthyroidism after stopping ATDs during early pregnancy is higher in women that were treated less then 6 months, in those that required more then 5 mg MMI per day to remain euthyroid, in those with suppressed or low levels of TSH, in those with large goiters, with orbitopathy and those with high levels of TRAbs [44].

In women where ATDs can not be discontinued during pregnancy, MMI is usually changed with PTU for the first trimester and reintroduced thereafter. Some women will have a worsening of their symptoms with GD in the first trimester and improvement later in pregnancy. Many pregnant women will not require ATDs by the third trimester as autoimmunity subsides characteristically in pregnancy. Normal THS levels and disappearance of maternal TRAb guide the decision to stop ATDs. If this is not done, there is a risk of overtreatment that can lead to hypothyroidism in the fetus (see below).

4.3.3 When Graves' Disease is first diagnosed in pregnancy

Uncontrolled maternal hyperthyroidism is associated with adverse maternal, fetal and neonatal outcomes [4]. When GD is first diagnosed during pregnancy, thionamides are the mainstay of treatment and they should be prescribed to achieve an euthyroid state. Beta-adrenergic blockers, which are generally considered safe in pregnancy, are also prescribed to control the hypermetabolic state until patients become euthyroid on ATDs. I131 is contraindicated in pregnancy and thyroidectomy, if required should ideally be performed in the second trimester. Thyroidectomy is considered for those women that have contraindications to ATDs, are not compliant with drug therapy, and in women where euthyroidism is not achieved despite large doses of ATDs. Preparation for surgery with beta-blockers and a short course of potassium iodide solution (50–100 mg/day) is permitted during pregnancy [4]. TRAb levels decrease slowly after surgery, therefore, continuation of monitoring should be in place for the remainder of pregnancy, since these antibodies can cross the placenta when in high titers (> 3 times the upper reference for the assay) and render the fetus hyperthyroid despite euthyroidism in the mother. Initial doses of ATDs for GD diagnosed in pregnancy depend on the severity of the symptoms and the degree of hyperthyroxinemia. During pregnancy MMI is prescribed at doses between 5–30 mg/d, typically in an average patient about 10–20 mg; CMZ at 10–40 mg/d and PTU at 100–600 mg/d (typically the average dose for PTU in an average patient is 200–400 mg/d). The beneficial effects of the drugs are seen gradually over weeks as the reservoir of hormones stored in the thyroid gland is consumed. The risk of maternal side effects from ATDs is not increased during pregnancy and is similar with one would expect in the non-pregnant state. Allergic skin reactions are the most common side effects while severe agranulocytosis and liver failure are rarely expected. Because of its potential risk of liver hepatotoxicity and liver transplant, some authorities recommend that the use of PTU should be limited to the first trimester of pregnancy and considered for use thereafter for those with MMI allergy and for those in thyroid storm [4]. The greatest concern however, with ATDs use in pregnancy remains their potential teratogenic effect and their risk of inducing fetal and neonatal hypothyroidism by crossing the placenta. Beta-blockers are considered safe in pregnancy even in the first trimester [45]. Usual doses for pregnancy are 10 to 40 mg of propranolol every 6 to 8 hours for several weeks. There is a concern related to fetal growth, fetal bradycardia and neonatal hypoglycemia with long term use of some beta-blockers [46], however propranolol and metoprolol have a more favorable safety profile then other beta-blockers during pregnancy [47].

Thyroid function tests could be carried out every 2 to 4 weeks in these patients at the beginng of the ATDs course and every 5 to 6 weeks after reaching and euthyroid state. When specific population lab values for pregnancy by trimester are not available, it is recommended to use the reference ranges for nonpregnant patients [4]. [See Thyroid function tests in pregnancy above]. The aim of GD treatment is to maintain maternal TT4/FT4 values at or just above the pregnancy specific upper limit of normal on the lowest effective dose of ATDs, to avoid potential harm to the fetus. Worthy of mentioning, ATDs are considered more potent in the fetus then in the mother, hence, in a well controlled mother, we could expect hypothyroidism in the fetus.

4.4 Fetal and neonatal consequences

Fetal and neonatal outcomes of GD are related to the control of the maternal hyperthyroid state, the presence or absence of TRAbs and the effect of ATDs. Uncontrolled maternal thyrotoxicosis can negatively influence how pregnancy progresses. TRAbs, when in high levels can cross the placenta and lead to fetal hyperthyroidism and goiter and ATDs, by also crossing the placenta, can lead to fetal hypothyroidism and goiter. When assessing a fetus in a mother with GD, a maternal-fetal specialist checks with the use of ultrasound the fetal neck in both gray-scale and color doppler, looking for signs of fetal goiter. Assessment of fetal growth, Doppler studies for assessment of fetal oxygenation, bones, heart rate, amniotic fluid volume are also performed. The exact incidence of fetal goiter is not known but it may be up to 1 in 5,000 births, usually, but not exclusively, in association with maternal Graves' Disease [48]. It has been estimated form different studies that the incidence of fetal goiter with either hypo- or hyperthyroidism in mothers with treated or untreated Graves' Disease is about 10% [49–53]. Fetal hypothyroidism is found more frequently than fetal hyperthyroidism in mothers with GD because of the inadequate use of ATDs [50, 51]. Fetal goiter can be diagnosed prenatally by ultrasound with the demonstration of an anterior cervical echogenic mass of variable size. (**Figure 2**) Large fetal goiters may lead to obstruction of fetal swallowing with consequent polyhydramnios and an increased risk of preterm birth; the neck may be hyperextended. As with other causes of obstructive polyhydramnios (duodenal stenosis, esophageal atresia) this becomes evident usually after 24 weeks' gestation. With fetal goiter there may also be a higher risk of birth dystocia because of the inadequate head flexion during labor and increased incidence of neonatal breathing problems and difficulties in intubation. Fetal goiter harbors thyroid dysfunction. Ultrasound is not a reliable tool to distinguish between fetal hyper- and hypothyroidism. In some cases of fetal hyperthyroidism there can be associated intrauterine growth restriction with accelerated bone maturation, tachycardia, intrauterine death by cardiac failure or thyrotoxicosis and craniosynostosis [54, 55]. In severe fetal hypothyroidism there can be a delay in bone maturation [56] and there may be impaired growth and bradycardia. There are usually no other associated structural anomalies and the incidence of chromosomal or genetic anomalies is not increased in fetal goiters in maternal Graves' Disease. In terms of management, in most cases of fetal goiter, assessment of the maternal condition can help decide whether the cause is fetal hypothyroidism or hyperthyroidism. In uncertain cases,

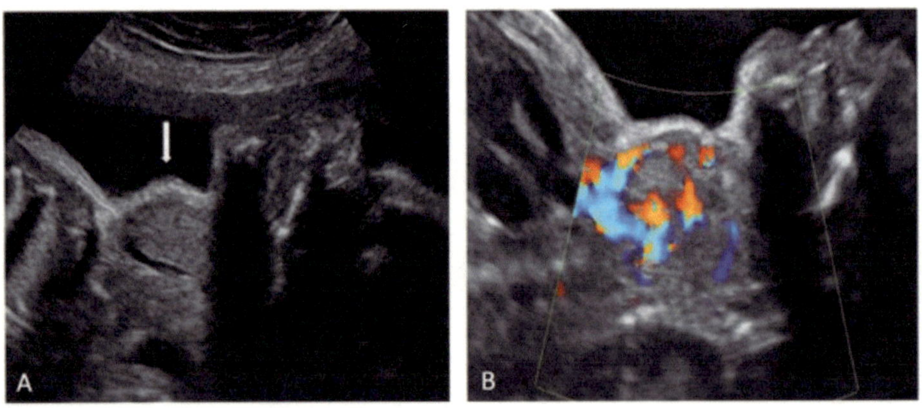

Figure 2.
Ultrasound imaging of a fetal thyroid goiter (A in gray scale, B with color doppler). Courtesy of the Fetal Medicine Foundation, reproduced with permission.

cordocentesis and measurement of fetal blood thyroid hormones and TSH can help distinguish between hypothyroidism, with low thyroid hormones and high TSH, due to ATDs and hyperthyroidism, with high thyroid hormones and low TSH, due to TRAbs [49, 57]. Normal ranges for the thyroid hormones level in the fetal blood have been previously reported [58, 59].

In fetal hypothyroid goiter the first-line of treatment is to reduce or even discontinue maternal ATD medication aiming to maintain maternal blood thyroxine in the upper level of the gestational age-specific normal range. As noted before, GD, similar to other autoimmune conditions, improves during pregnancy and consequently requires less medication. The second-line of treatment is intra-amniotic injection of levothyroxine (100 μg/kg) every 1–2 weeks until delivery at term [49, 60]. The goiter usually decreases in size within a few days to weeks after the first course of treatment. Subsequent injections are given depending on sonographic evidence of re-enlargement of the gland or serial measurements of levels of thyroid hormones in amniotic fluid or fetal blood [49, 61, 62].

In fetal hyperthyroid goiter the treatment is administration of ATDs to the mother [63]. Occasionally, the mother should also be given levothyroxine, as the dose of ATDs can be appropriate for the fetus but could lead to hypothyroidism in the mother (one of the few occasions block and replace therapy is used) [4]. The fetal goiter usually decreases in size after initiation of the treatment, but if this does not occur measurement of levels of thyroid hormones in fetal blood [24] may be needed and the dose of ATDs adjusted. Follow-up should be arranged depending on the clinical context, but generally at every 2–4 weeks to monitor fetal growth, size of the tumor, fetal heart rate, amniotic fluid volume and cervical length (for the prediction of risk of preterm birth). Delivery in the case of fetal goiter should take place in a hospital with neonatal intensive care capacities and pediatric surgery facilities, ideally around 38 weeks. With large goiters, where there is hyperextension of the neck, cesarean section is preferred for delivery. An EXIT (ex utero intrapartum treatment) procedure may be required to access and stabilize neonatal breathing while maintaining placental flow through the umbilical cord from the mother [24]. Adequately treated fetal thyroid goiters generally have good prognosis. However, fetal hyperthyroidism may lead to neonatal thyrotoxicosis [64] and, to long term intellectual impairment [65] while fetal hypothyroidism may result in long term abnormal psychomotor development [66].

Neonatal thyroid function abnormalities are frequent in newborns of mothers with GD. In a recent study in 32 newborns from mothers with GD, 3 cases had hypothyroidism and 2 had hyperthyroidism despite not showing a goiter. These affected babies all had higher levels of TRAbs in their cord blood at delivery and in the follow-up tests [67]. Newborns of mothers with GD can present with hyperthyroidism but also with central or primary hypothyroidism. There are no clear guidelines as to how these neonates should be followed, but most authorities do recommend testing for TRAbs in the cord blood/blood with subsequent discharge of negative testing newborns. FT4 and TSH can be performed at 3 to 5 days of life and repeated at 10 to 14 days. For hyperthyroid newborns MMI and beta-blockers can be used [68]. Maternal TRAbs passed to the newborn will be cleared from the neonates' serum within weeks to months as in the case of other maternal autoimmune conditions [48].

4.5 The postpartum in women with GD

Worsening of GD, relapse or need for increased medication do occur after delivery even in mothers that were previously under remission [69, 70] and women should be counseled and informed about this. Pregnant women with positive TRAbs in early pregnancy are at high-risk of developing postpartum GD. Postpartum GD usually occurs after 3 months from delivery and this helps in differentiating it from other forms of thyrotoxicosis specific to this period that tend to develop earlier. Women with known GD before or during pregnancy should be regularly checked with thyroid function tests in the postpartum. Treatment options for postpartum GD are the same as for any GD patient. ATDs are an initial good choice since in many instances GD postpartum can be transient and mothers can continue breastfeeding on them. Both MMI (up to maximal recommended dose of 20 mg/d) and PTU (up to maximal dose of 450 mg/d) can be safely administered in breastfeeding mothers [4]. Monitoring the infants for appropriate growth and development routinely is advised [4]. It may be necessary to check the infants' thyroid function when antithyroid drugs are administered at higher doses. Medication should be taken just after breastfeeding, which should provide a 3 to 4 hours lactating free interval [71]. Considering the possibility of side effects of severe hepatic injury of PTU in mothers and infants [72], and high incidence of general side effects with PTU [73], MMI is the preferred drug in the treatment of breastfeeding women. The use of I131 is strictly contraindicated during lactation. If circumstances require it I123, when available can be used in lactating women. The half-life of 123I is 13 hours so breast milk should be pumped and discarded for 3–4 days until the radioactive iodine has cleared from the body [74]. Similarly, Tc-99 m pertechnetate administration requires breast milk to be pumped and discarded during the day of testing [4].

5. Conclusions

Graves' Disease is frequent in women of reproductive age and in pregnancy. It can lead to maternal, fetal and neonatal complications with potential long-term sequels. For those with known GD before pregnancy a preconception plan should be made to ensure optimal timing for pregnancy when GD is well under control. Management options for GD and their implications to pregnancy should be discussed. TRAbs are the pathogenic hallmark of GD and they can cause harm to the fetus and the neonate by crossing the placenta. Antithyroid drugs are traditionally used to treat GD, however in pregnancy they can be teratogenic and they can induce fetal and neonatal hypothyroidism by placental passage. Fetal ultrasound during pregnancy is helpful for fetal assessment and for diagnosing fetal goiter. The type of fetal thyroid disfunction when goiter is associated can be usually deduced by assessing the maternal state. Fetal treatment is in most cases achieved by treating the mother – increasing or decreasing ATDs. Neonatal assessment in newborns of mothers with known GD is recommended. Maternal GD, like other autoimmune conditions can flare in the postpartum, therefore, the mother should also be under supervision. Breastfeeding is allowed in women on regular doses of ATDs.

Conflict of interest

The author declares no conflict of interest.

Author details

Anca Maria Panaitescu
Carol Davila University of Medicine and Pharmacy, Bucharest, Romania

*Address all correspondence to: anca.panaitescu@umfcd.ro

References

[1] Ciobanu AM, Dumitru AE, Gica N, Botezatu R, Peltecu G, Panaitescu AM. Benefits and Risks of IgG Transplacental Transfer. Diagnostics (Basel). 2020 Aug 12;10(8):583. doi: 10.3390/diagnostics10080583.

[2] Patel J, Landers K, Li H, Mortimer RH, Richard K. Thyroid hormones and fetal neurological development. J Endocrinol 2011; 209(1):1-8.

[3] Vannucchi G, Covelli D, Vigo B, Perrino M, Mondina L, Fugazzola L. Thyroid volume and serum calcitoninchanges during pregnancy. J Endocrinol Invest 2017;40:727-32.

[4] Alexander EK, Pearce EN, Brent GA, Brown RS, Chen H, Dosiou C, et al. 2017 guidelines of the American Thyroid Association for the diagnosis and management of thyroid disease during pregnancy and the postpartum Thyroid 2017;27:315-89.

[5] Schweizer U, Köhrle J. Function of thyroid hormone transporters in the central nervous system. Biochim Biophys Acta. 2013 Jul;1830(7):3965-73.

[6] Chan, S., Vasilopoulou, E. & Kilby, M. The role of the placenta in thyroid hormone delivery to the fetus. Nat Rev Endocrinol 2009;5:45-54.

[7] Friesema EC, Ganguly S, Abdalla A, Manning Fox JE, Halestrap AP, Visser TJ. Identification of monocarboxylate transporter 8 as a specific thyroid hormone transporter. J Biol Chem. 2003 Oct 10;278(41):40128-35.

[8] S. Chan, S. Kachilele, E. Hobbs, J. N. Bulmer, K. Boelaert, C. J. McCabe, P. M. Driver, A. R. Bradwell, M. Kester, T. J. Visser, J. A. Franklyn, M. D. Kilby, Placental Iodothyronine Deiodinase Expression in Normal and Growth-Restricted Human Pregnancies, The Journal of Clinical Endocrinology & Metabolism 2003;88(9):4488-4495.

[9] Obregon MJ, Calvo RM, Del Rey FE, de Escobar GM. Ontogenesis of thyroid function and interactions with maternal function. Endocr Dev 2007; 10:86-98.

[10] Landers, K., Richard, K., Traversing barriers – How thyroid hormones pass placental, blood-brain and blood-cerebrospinal fluid barriers, Molecular and Cellular Endocrinology (2017), doi: 10.1016/j.mce.2017.01.041.

[11] Grüters A, Krude H. Detection and treatment of congenital hypothyroidism. Nat Rev Endocrinol. 2011 Oct 18;8(2):104-13

[12] Arash Derakhshan, Huan Shu, Maarten A C Broeren, Ralph A de Poortere, Sverre Wikström, Robin P Peeters, Barbara Demeneix, Carl-Gustaf Bornehag, Tim I M Korevaar. Reference Ranges and Determinants of Thyroid Function During Early Pregnancy: The SELMA Study. The Journal of Clinical Endocrinology & Metabolism 2018;103(9): 3548-3556.

[13] Xiaotong Gao, Yongze Li, Jiashu Li, Aihua Liu, Wei Sun, Weiping Teng, Zhongyan Shan. 2018. Gestational TSH and FT4 Reference Intervals in Chinese Women: A Systematic Review and Meta-Analysis. Frontiers in Endocrinology 9.

[14] Victor Pop, Maarten Broeren, Hennie Wijnen, Joyce Endendijk, Anneloes van Baar, Wilmar Wiersinga, Graham R Williams. 2018. Longitudinal Trajectories of Gestational Thyroid Function: A New Approach to Better Understand Changes in Thyroid Function. The Journal of Clinical Endocrinology & Metabolism 103:8, 2889-2900

[15] Cooper DS, Laurberg P. Hyperthyroidism in pregnancy. Lancet Diabetes Endocrinol 2013; 1: 238-249.

[16] Michalek K, Morshed SA, Latif R, Davies TF. TSH receptor autoantibodies. Autoimmun Rev; 2009(9):113-6. doi:10.1016/j.autrev.2009.03.012.

[17] Laurberg P, Wallin G, Tallstedt L, Abraham-Nordling M, Lundell G, Tørring O 2008 TSH-receptor autoimmunity in Graves' disease after therapy with anti-thyroid drugs, surgery, or radioiodine: a 5-year prospective randomized study. Eur J Endocrinol 158:69-75.

[18] McLachlan SM, Rapoport B. Thyrotropin-blocking autoantibodies and thyroid-stimulating autoantibodies: potential mechanisms involved in the pendulum swinging from hypothyroidism to hyperthyroidism or vice versa. Thyroid (2013) 23:14-24. doi:10.1089/thy.2012.0374.

[19] Giuliani C, Saji M, Bucci I, Napolitano G. Bioassays for TSH receptor autoantibodies, from FRTL-5 cells to TSH receptor-LH/CG receptor chimeras: the contribution of Leonard D. Kohn. Front Endocrinol (2016) 7:103. doi:10.3389/fendo.2016.00103

[20] Bucci I, Giuliani C and Napolitano G(2017) Thyroid-Stimulating Hormone Receptor Antibodies in Pregnancy: Clinical Relevance. Front. Endocrinol. 8:137.doi: 10.3389/fendo.2017.00137.

[21] Giuliani C, Cerrone D, Harii N, Thornton M, Kohn LD, Dagia NM, et al. A TSHr-LH/CGr chimera that measures functional TSAb in Graves' disease. J Clin Endocrinol Metab (2012) 97:E1106-15. doi:10.1210/jc.2011-2893

[22] Giuliani C, Cerrone D, Harii N, Thornton M, Kohn LD, Dagia NM, et al. A TSHr-LH/CGr chimera that measures functional thyroid-stimulating autoantibodies (TSAb) can predict remission or recurrence in Graves' patients undergoing antithyroid drug (ATD) treatment. J Clin Endocrinol Metab (2012) 97:E1080-7. doi:10.1210/jc.2011-2897

[23] Li Y, Kim J, Diana T, Klasen R, Olivo PD, Kahaly GJ. A novel bioassay for anti-thyrotrophin receptor autoantibodies detects both thyroid-blocking and stimulating activity. Clin Exp Immunol (2013) 173:390-7. doi:10.1111/ cei.12129.

[24] Panaitescu AM, Nicolaides K. Fetal goitre in maternal Graves' disease. Acta Endocrinol (Buchar). 2018 Jan-Mar;14(1):85-89.

[25] Abeillon-du Payrat J, Chikh K, Bossard N, Bretones P, Gaucherand P, Claris O, Charrie´ A, Raverot V, Orgiazzi J, Borson-Chazot F, Bournaud C 2014 Predictive value of maternal second-generation thyroid-binding inhibitory immunoglobulin assay for neonatal autoimmune hyperthyroidism. Eur J Endocrinol 171:451-460.

[26] Besancon A, Beltrand J, Le Gac I, Luton D, Polak M 2014 Management of neonates born to women with Graves' disease: a cohort study. Eur J Endocrinol 170:855-862.

[27] Pearce EN. Management of thyrotoxicosis: preconception, pregnancy, and the postpartum period. Endocr Pract. 2019 Jan;25(1):62-68.

[28] Amino N, Mori H, Iwatani Y, et al. High prevalence of transient post-partum thyrotoxicosis and hypothyroidism. N Engl J Med. 1982;306:849-852.

[29] Stagnaro-Green A. Approach to the patient with postpartum thyroiditis. J Clin Endocrinol Metab. 2012;97:334-342.

[30] Memtsa M, Johns J, Jurkovic D, Ross JA, Sebire NJ, Jauniaux E. Diagnosis and outcome of hydatidiform moles in missed-miscarriage: a cohort-study, systematic review and meta-analysis. Eur J Obstet Gynecol Reprod Biol. 2020 Oct;253:206-212

[31] Walkington L, Webster J, Hancock BW, Everard J, Coleman RE. Hyperthyroidism and human chorionic gonadotrophin production in gestational trophoblastic disease. Br J Cancer. 2011 May 24;104(11):1665-9. doi: 10.1038/bjc.2011.139.

[32] Amino N, Arata N. Thyroid dysfunction following pregnancy and implications for breastfeeding. Best Pract Res Clin Endocrinol Metab. 2020 Jul;34(4):101438. doi: 10.1016/j.beem.2020.101438.

[33] Labadzhyan A, Brent GA, Hershman JM, Leung AM. Thyrotoxicosis of Pregnancy. J Clin Transl Endocrinol. 2014;1(4):140-144. doi:10.1016/j.jcte.2014.07.008.

[34] Notsu M, Yamauchi M, Sugimoto T, Kanasaki K. A pregnant woman with an autonomously functioning thyroid nodule: a case report. Gynecol Endocrinol. 2020 Dec;36(12):1140-1143. doi: 10.1080/09513590.2020.1822798.

[35] Düğeroğlu H, Özgenoğlu M. Thyroid function among women with gestational trophoblastic diseases. A cross-sectional study. Sao Paulo Med J. 2019 Aug 8;137(3):278-283. doi: 10.1590/1516-3180.2018.0481090519.

[36] Okazaki Y, Arata N, Umehara N, Yamauchi T, Tajiri J, Hishinuma A, Kogai T, Idegami T, Murashima A, Sago H. A case of familial nonautoimmune hyperthyroidism during pregnancy. AACE Clin Case Rep. 2020 Jan 22;6(2):e94-e97. doi: 10.4158/ACCR-2019-0361.

[37] Romeo AN, Običan SG. Teratogen update: Antithyroid medications. Birth Defects Res. 2020 Sep;112(15):1150-1170. doi: 10.1002/bdr2.1771.

[38] Andersen SL, Olsen J, Wu CS, Laurberg P 2013 Birth defects after early pregnancy use of antithyroid drugs: a Danish nationwide study. J Clin Endocrinol Metab 98:4373-4381.

[39] Zhang LH, Li JY, Tian Q, et al. Follow-up and evaluation of the pregnancy outcome in women of reproductive age with Graves' disease after 131Iodine treatment. J Radiat Res. 2016;57(6):702-708. doi:10.1093/jrr/rrw049

[40] Jørgensen CU, Homøe P, Dahl M, Hitz MF. High incidence of chronic hypoparathyroidism secondary to total thyroidectomy. Dan Med J. 2020 May 1;67(5):A11190647.

[41] Sullivan SA. Parathyroid Diseases. Clin Obstet Gynecol. 2019 Jun;62(2):347-358.

[42] Botello A, Herrán M, Salcedo V, Rodríguez Y, Anaya JM, Rojas M. Prevalence of latent and overt polyautoimmunity in autoimmune thyroid disease: A systematic review and meta-analysis. Clin Endocrinol (Oxf). 2020 Oct;93(4):375-389. doi: 10.1111/cen.14304.

[43] Nedrebo BG, Holm PI, Uhlving S, Sorheim JI, Skeie S, Eide GE, Husebye ES, Lien EA, Aanderud S 2002 Predictors of outcome and comparison of different drug regimens for the prevention of relapse in patients with Graves' disease. Eur J Endocrinol 147:583-589.

[44] Laurberg P, Krejbjerg A, Andersen SL 2014 Relapse following antithyroid drug therapy for Graves' hyperthyroidism. Curr Opin Endocrinol Diabetes Obes 21:415-421.

[45] Wu Y, Yao JW, Xu LJ, Chen M, Wan L. Risk of congenital

malformations in offspring of women using β-blockers during early pregnancy: An updated meta-analysis of observational studies. Br J Clin Pharmacol. 2020 Sep 25. doi: 10.1111/bcp.14561.

[46] Tanaka K, Tanaka H, Kamiya C, Katsuragi S, Sawada M, Tsuritani M, Yoshida M, Iwanaga N, Yoshimatsu J, Ikeda T. Beta-Blockers and Fetal Growth Restriction in Pregnant Women With Cardiovascular Disease. Circ J. 2016 Sep 23;80(10):2221-6.

[47] Duan L, Ng A, Chen W, Spencer HT, Lee MS. Beta-blocker subtypes and risk of low birth weight in newborns. J Clin Hypertens (Greenwich). 2018 Nov;20(11):1603-1609.

[48] Panaitescu AM, Nicolaides K. Maternal autoimmune disorders and fetal defects. J Matern Fetal Neonatal Med 2017; 18:1-9.

[49] Bliddal S, Rasmussen AK, Sundberg K, Brocks V, Feldt-Rasmussen U. Antithyroid drug-induced fetal goitrous hypothyroidism. Nat Rev Endocrinol 2011; 7:396-406.

[50] Burrow GN. Neonatal goiter after maternal propylthiouracil therapy. J Clin Endocrinol Metab 1965; 25:403-408.

[51] Volumenie JL, Polak M, Guibourdenche J, Oury JF, Vuillard E, Sibony O. Management of fetal thyroid goitres: a report of 11 cases in a single perinatal unit. Prenat Diagn 2000; 20:799-806.

[52] Luton D, Le Gac I, Vuillard E, Castanet M, Guibourdenche J, Noel M, Toubert ME, Léger J, Boissinot C, Schlageter MH, Garel C, Tébeka B, Oury JF, Czernichow P, Polak M: Management of Graves' disease during pregnancy: the key role of fetal thyroid gland monitoring. J Clin Endocrinol Metab 2005; 90:6093-6098.

[53] Rosenfeld H, Ornoy A, Shechtman S, Diav-Citrin O. Pregnancy outcome, thyroid dysfunction and fetal goitre after in utero exposure to propylthiouracil: a controlled cohort study. Br J Clin Pharmacol 2009; 68: 609-617.

[54] Daneman D, Howard NJ. Neonatal thyrotoxicosis: intellectual impairment and craniosynostosis in later years. J Pediatr 1980; 97:257-259.

[55] Heckel S, Favre R, Schlienger JL, Soskin P. Diagnosis and successful in utero treatment of a fetal goitrous hyperthyroidism caused by maternal Graves' disease. A case report. Fetal Diagn Ther 1997; 12:54-58

[56] Avni EF, Rodesch F, Vandemerckt C, Vermeylen D. Detection and evaluation of fetal goitre by ultrasound. Br J Radiol 1992; 65:302-305

[57] Kilpatrick S. Umbilical blood sampling in women with thyroid disease in pregnancy: Is it necessary? Am J Obstet Gynecol 2003; 189:1-2.

[58] Thorpe-Beeston JG, Nicolaides KH, Felton CV, Butler J, McGregor AM. Maturation of the secretion of thyroid hormone and thyroid-stimulating hormone in the fetus. N Engl J Med. 1991; 324(8):532-6.

[59] Thorpe-Beeston JG, Nicolaides KH. Fetal thyroid function. Fetal Diagn Ther. 1993; 8(1):60-72.

[60] Bliddal S, Rasmussen ÅK, Sundberg K, Brocks V, Skovbo P, Feldt-Rasmussen U. Graves' disease in two pregnancies complicated by fetal goitrous hypothyroidism: successful in utero treatment with levothyroxine. Thyroid 2011; 21:75-81

[61] Munoz JL, Kessler AA, Felig P, Curtis J, Evans MI. Sequential Amniotic Fluid Thyroid Hormone Changes Correlate with Goiter Shrinkage

following in utero Thyroxine Therapy. Fetal Diagn Ther 2016; 39:222-227.

[62] Nachum Z, Rakover Y, Weiner E, Shalev E. Graves' disease in pregnancy: prospective evaluation of a selective invasive treatment protocol. Am J Obstet Gynecol 2003; 189:159-165.

[63] Polak M. Thyroid disorders during pregnancy: impact on the fetus. Horm Res Paediatr 2011; 76 Suppl 1:97-101.

[64] Bruinse HW, Vermeulen-Meiners C, Wit JM. Fetal treatment for thyrotoxicosis in non-thyrotoxic pregnant women. Fetal Ther 1988; 3:152-157

[65] Daneman D, Howard NJ. Neonatal thyrotoxicosis: intellectual impairment and craniosynostosis in later years. J Pediatr 1980; 97:257-259.

[66] Rovet J, Ehrlich R, Sorbara D. Intellectual outcome in children with fetal hypothyroidism. J Pediatr 1987; 110:700-704.

[67] Luz IR, Martins JR, Jerónimo M, Caetano JS, Cardoso R, Dinis I, Mirante A. Neonates Born to Mothers with Graves' Disease: 15 Year Experience of a Pediatric Endocrinology Department. Acta Med Port. 2020 Jul 1;33(7-8):483-490.

[68] van der Kaay DC, Wasserman JD, Palmert MR. Management of Neonates Born to Mothers With Graves' Disease. Pediatrics. 2016 Apr;137(4):e20151878.

[69] Amino N, Tanizawa O, Mori H, Iwatani Y, Yamada T, Kurachi K, Kumahara Y, Miyai K 1982 Aggravation of thyrotoxicosis in early pregnancy and after delivery in Graves' disease. J Clin Endocrinol Metab 55:108-112

[70] Andersen SL, Olsen J, Carle A, Laurberg P 2015 Hyperthyroidism incidence fluctuates widely in and around pregnancy and is at variance with some other autoimmune diseases: a Danish population-based study. J Clin Endocrinol Metab 100:1164-1171

[71] Mandel SJ, Cooper DS. The use of antithyroid drugs in pregnancy and lactation. J Clin Endocrinol Metab, 2001;86: 2354-9.

[72] Bahn RS, et al. The role of propylthiouracil in the management of Graves' disease in adults: report of a meeting jointly sponsored by the American Thyroid Association and the Food and Drug Administration. Thyroid, 2009;19: 673-4

[73] Nakamura H, Noh JY, Itoh K, Fukata S, Miyauchi A, Hamada N. Comparison of methimazole and propylthiouracil in patients with hyperthyroidism caused by Graves' disease. J Clin Endocrinol Metab, 2007;92: 2157-62.

[74] Howe DB, Beardsley M, Bakhsh S 2008 Appendix U. Model procedure for release of patients or human research subjects administered radioactive materials. In Consolidated Guidance About Materials Licenses. Program-Specific Guidance About Medical Use Licenses. Final Report. U.S. Nuclear Regulatory Commission Office of Nuclear Material Safety and Safeguards. NUREG-1556, vol. 9, rev. 2.

Section 5

Graves' Disease in Children

Chapter 15

Graves' Disease in Childhood

Madhukar Mittal and Vanishri Ganakumar

Abstract

Graves' Disease (GD) is an autoimmune disease caused by autoantibodies against thyroid stimulating hormone receptor (TSH-R), resulting in stimulation of thyroid gland and overproduction of thyroid hormones resulting in clinical manifestations. It is uncommon in children and is 6 times more prevalent in females. The symptomatology, clinical and biochemical severity are a function of age of onset of disease. Prepubertal children tend to present with weight loss and bowel frequency, associated with accelerated growth and bone maturation. Older children are more likely to present with the classical symptoms of thyrotoxicosis like palpitations, tremors and heat intolerance. Prepubertal children tend to have a more severe disease, longer duration of complaints and higher thyroid hormone levels at presentation than the pubertal and postpubertal children. The non-specificity of some of the symptoms in pediatric age group can lead to children being initially seen by other specialities before being referred to endocrinology. Management issues are decided based on patient's priorities and shared decision making between patient and treating physician. Radioactive Iodine Ablation is preferred when there is relatively higher value placed on Definitive control of hyperthyroidism, Avoidance of surgery, and potential side effects of ATDs. Similarly Antithyroid drugs are chosen when a relatively higher value is placed on possibility of remission and avoidance of lifelong thyroid hormone treatment, Avoidance of surgery, Avoidance of exposure to radioactivity. Surgery is preferred when access to a high-volume thyroid surgeon is available and a relatively higher value is on prompt and definitive control of hyperthyroidism, avoidance of exposure to radioactivity and avoidance of potential side effects of ATDs. Continental differences with regards to management do exist; radio-iodine ablation being preferred in North America while Anti-thyroid drug treatment remains the initial standard care in Europe.

Keywords: Graves, hyperthyroidism, radioactive iodine, antithyroid, thyrotoxicosis, children

1. Introduction

Graves' Disease (GD) is an autoimmune disease caused by autoantibodies against thyroid stimulating hormone receptor (TSH-R), resulting in stimulation of thyroid gland and overproduction of thyroid hormones resulting in clinical manifestations. GD is a relatively uncommon entity in pediatric age group, in contrast to adults, where prevalence ranges from 0.5–1%. Pediatric GD in the age group 0–15 years comprises of only 5–6% of the total number of Graves' thyrotoxic patients. It usually occurs in the context of a family history of autoimmune thyroid disease or in association with other autoimmune diseases like type 1 diabetes, Hashimoto's thyroiditis, rheumatoid arthritis or adrenal insufficiency. It is also found in association with genetic syndromes like Down's syndrome and Turner's syndrome. However, GD is the most common cause of thyrotoxicosis in children, accounting for atleast 95% cases of hyperthyroidism and 10–15% of all childhood thyroid disorders [1]. Other rare causes of juvenile thyrotoxicosis include toxic adenoma (TA), toxic multinodular goitre (TMNG), McCune Albright syndrome (MAS), Hashimoto's thyroiditis and iatrogenic causes. In children, GD can occur at any age, but is most often diagnosed in adolescent age group, occurring more frequently in females than in males [2, 3].

The eye changes accompanying GD are termed thyroid-associated ophthalmopathy (TAO) or Graves' ophthalmopathy (GO). The symptoms of GO can run an independent course from the clinical course of thyrotoxicosis and often require specific treatment. Clinical characteristics of GO are often milder in children than in adults, nevertheless adversely affecting quality of life.

2. Epidemiology

Very few epidemiological studies are available to document the incidence of pediatric Graves' Disease in different populations, mostly involving Northern Europe and Hongkong. These have resulted in widely variable incidence rates, ranging from 0.79 to 6.5/100000 patient-years [4–9]. Iodine intake in populations could be one of the factors for differences observed in different populations, with higher incidence rates being observed in populations with higher iodine intake, particularly in studies from Hong-Kong compared to Caucasian children [7, 8].

GD, in concordance with other autoimmune disorders, is more common in females, particularly after 4 years of age. Female to male ratio has varied from 2.37–9.7 in various studies, depending on the age groups included [9]. The female preponderance becomes particularly marked in adolescent years, merging into the adult trends.

In one of the earliest nation-wide comprehensive studies, the incidence ratio of thyrotoxicosis was 0.79/100 000 person-years in Danish children under the age of 15 years between 1982 and 1988. The incidence was very low in age < 4 years, gradually increasing in both genders to peak incidence at 10–14 years of age. As with other autoimmune disorders, there was a female preponderance of 6.7: 1, but this difference was virtually non-existent in age group 0–4 years. The gender disparity widened gradually after early childhood to reach the maximum in the 10–14 year age group. Diffuse toxic goitre accounted for 96% of the cases, toxic adenoma and toxic multi-nodular goitre (MNG) were rare entities [4].

However, a more recent study in the Danish population spanning between 1998 and 2012 revealed a higher incidence rate of 1.58/100000 person-years [6], GD accounting for 86.8% of the cases. This increasing trend was consistent with rising incidences of other autoimmune disorders like type 1 diabetes and celiac disease. The authors postulated that environmental factors, including hygiene hypothesis, could play a key role in explaining the increasing trends in autoimmune disorders [6].

Similar trends of rising incidence rates have also been documented in studies from Hong-Kong as well. This could not be explained by the slight advancement in pubertal age or increasing disease awareness. The trends were primarily ascribed to the increasing iodine intake in the population, reflected by high urinary iodine concentration in the population [7, 8].

Similar to GD, GO is rare in pediatric age group. One of the earliest data about the incidence of pediatric GO came from the Olmsted County cohort study from Minnesota, USA. The study identified 120 incident cases of GO from 1976 to 1990. Peak incidence of GO had a bimodal distribution in the age groups 40–49 year and 60–69 years in both females and males, with a 5 year later presentation in males. The overall age-adjusted incidence rates per 100000 population were 16 and 2.9

cases in females and males respectively. On the other hand, GO was much less frequent in the pediatric age group. Incidence rates per 100000 population per year in the age groups 5–9, 10–14, and 15–19 years were 3.5, 1.8 and 3.3 and 0, 1.7 and 0, for females and males respectively. Only 6 out of the 120 incident cases of GO observed in this cohort study were in patients below the age of 20 years [10]. The prevalence of GO in different countries has also been seen to be directly related to the prevalence of smoking in teenage population in the respective countries, emphasising the importance of smoking as risk factor for development of GO [11].

3. Pathogenesis

GD is a classical autoimmune disorder, characterised by a complex interplay of genetic susceptibility and environmental factors. GD had long been recognized as having a genetic background in view of clustering of cases in families. Family H/O autoimmune thyroid disease (AITD) is apparent in nearly half of the affected patients. AITD also tends to occur in more than a third of siblings and thyroid autoantibodies occur in over half of asymptomatic children of affected patients. This was further confirmed by twin studies where concordance of AITD in monozygotic twins was 30–40%, as compared to less than 5% concordance in dizygotic twins. It has also been proposed that genetic anticipation may occur in successive generations leading to younger ages at onset of disease [12, 13].

The genetic predisposition to GD is polygenic in origin, with each individual gene conferring a modest increase in risk. The most commonly implicated genes are located in the HLA region in the short arm of chromosome 6, the odds ratio (OR) for GD ranging from 2 to 4. HLA DRB1*03 and DQA1*05 in Caucasian patients, and HLA DPB1*05:01 allele in Han Chinese populations have been found to confer 2–3 times increased risk of GD. Similarly HLA class I alleles C*07 and B*08 have also been implicated as risk factors, and DRB1*07, DRB1*12:02, DQB1*03:02, B*44, C*03, C*16 have been observed to have a protective effect in various populations.

Some of the other genes which confer a modest increase in risk of GD (OR ranging from 1.1–2) are Protein Tyrosine Phosphatase-22 (PTPN22), Cluster of Differentiation 40 (CD40), Cytotoxic T-lymphocyte-associated factor 4 (CTLA4), TSH-R, Thyroglobulin (Tg), FC-Receptor Like-3 (FCRL3), Secretoglobin 3A2 (SCGB3A2), Interleukin-2 receptor alpha (IL2RA) etc. Possible mechanisms postulated are variation in binding of self-antigens, defective regulation of thymic selection of autoreactive clones, regulation of T cell responses and effect of HLA class I molecules on natural killer cells.

Some studies have also observed genotype phenotype correlation. For example, several genes like interferon γ (IFN γ, TNF, IL-1A, IL-23R, IL-5, CTLA4, PTPN-12, ICAM-1 have been associated with development of Graves ophthalmopathy (GO). Similarly several candidate genes have been associated with clinical course of GD, including age of onset (HLA, ICAM-1, PTPN22, NFKB1, CD40), severity and remission/relapse rates of GD (CTLA4, CXCL10) [14].

With the concordance rate in monozygotic twins being clearly less than 100%, it highlights the importance of environmental factors for predisposing an individual for developing GD. Analysis of Danish twin studies in GD attributed 79% of liability to develop GD on genetic factors, whereas 21% could be explained by environmental factors not shared by the twins [15].

Stressful life events and post-partum periods can result in a dysregulated immune response, predisposing to autoimmunity. Smoking, radiation, excess iodine intake, dietary selenium deficiency, drugs like amiodarone, interferons, alemtuzumab have been associated with development of AITD. Recent evidence has brought into light the role of Endocrine disrupting chemicals (EDCs), which are environmental toxicants that interfere with thyroid hormone production, metabolism and action. Most widely studied EDCs are polychlorinated biphenyls (PCBs), which have thyroid-disrupting effects and can have intrinsic thyroid hormone agonist action. Others chemicals like bisphenol A, phthalates, perflourinated chemicals and brominated flame retardants have also been shown to have thyroid-disrupting effects, predisposing to AITD [16, 17].

The thyroid gland typically demonstrates a non-homogenous lymphocytic infiltration and absence of follicular destruction. T-lymphocytes can cause local inflammation and cytokine release resulting in dysregulation of B- cells and production of autoantibodies. These TSH-R auto antibodies (TRAb) can bind to the TSH-R on thyroid follicular cells. These are of the IgG1 subclass and can have different functional implications of stimulation, blockade or neutral effects on the TSH-R. Thyroid stimulating antibodies (TSIs) act via G proteins like Gs and Gq to cause increased thyroid hormone production, secretion and modulation of cell proliferation respectively [2, 18].

Graves ophthalmopathy is a distinct pathological process that may precede or follow the hyperthyroid phase. Orbital fibroblasts are the target cells in the pathology. Plausible explanation for this cellular origin include antigen sharing with the TSH-R, enhanced expression of Thy-1 (CD90) and IGF-1 receptor, exaggerated inflammatory response to cytokines and hyaluronan synthesis. Environmental factors like smoking and radioiodine therapy play a major role in development of ophthalmopathy [19].

4. Clinical features

GD can present at any age, with peak prevalence occurring in adolescent years. Around 10% of cases can present in very young children less than 5 years of age. GD is clinically characterized by the triad of thyrotoxicosis, ophthalmopathy and dermopathy. GD in children often presents with classical symptoms and signs of thyrotoxicosis like in adults.

The frequency of the symptomatology, however, is variable across literature. Major presenting symptoms symptoms include goitre (19–99%), excessive sweating and heat intolerance (28–53%), fatigue or weakness (10–54%), irritability, nervousness or restlessness (17–47%), tremors (17–58%), ocular symptoms, ophthalmopathy or exophthalmos (10–43%), weight loss or no weight gain (28–63%), tachycardia (34–45%). Decreased academic performance can be seen in 1–24% of patients, whereas decreased athletic performance can be seen in upto 15% of patients. Other common complaints included behavioural changes (50%), headache (1–22%), increased bowel frequency (11–16%) and slight fever (10.5%) [5, 20–22]. Children can also present with ocular complaints like pain, foreign body sensation and grittiness, tearing, redness, photosensitivity, and rarely diplopia [23].

Children, like adults, can have low bone mass for age and increased fracture risk in the presence of untreated thyrotoxicosis, but this is often reversible once euthyroidism is restored for 2 years with treatment. Thyrotoxicosis may rarely be associated with choreiform movements in childhood and adolescence. This may manifest as involuntary, coordinated, rapid spastic movements like flexion and extension of fingers, raising and lowering of shoulders and grimacing. Thyrotoxicosis can also result in proximal muscle weakness and wasting syndrome, termed the thyrotoxic myopathy, which can mimic limb girdle muscular dystrophy. Importantly, these symptoms can even precede the more typical thyrotoxic symptoms. Another type of muscular weakness associated with thyrotoxicosis is thyrotoxic periodic paralysis, characterized by recurrent transient episodes of muscular weakness, usually precipitated by a stressor event like exposure to cold, high carbohydrate meal, infections and stress. This phenomenon has been more commonly described in Asian populations in middle aged males. It is rare in pediatric age groups, and is virtually not reported in very young populations [24].

The symptomatology, clinical and biochemical severity are also a function of age of onset of disease. Prepubertal children tend to have a more severe disease, longer duration of complaints and higher thyroid hormone levels at presentation than the pubertal and postpubertal children. Prepubertal children tend to present with weight loss and bowel frequency, associated with accelerated growth and bone maturation. Older children are more likely to present with the classical symptoms of thyrotoxicosis like palpitations, tremors and heat intolerance [25].

The risk of developing GO in pediatric GD appears to be to be similar to or slightly higher than the risk in adult patients with GD. Female preponderance (87%) is also similar to that observed in adult patients (83%). However, pediatric GO tends to be less severe and debilitating as compared to adult manifestations. Soft tissue involvement, lid lag, proptosis and punctate corneal epithelial erosions are more commonly seen with pediatric GO, whereas the more severe manifestations like restricted ocular motility, severe strabismus and optic nerve affection are virtually never seen in pediatric GO. This has been attributed to the lower prevalence of smoking in children as compared to adults. Manifestations of GO tended to become similar to adults as adolescence approached in pediatric patients with GO in another study, likely due to increased prevalence of smoking in adolescent ages. Hence active or passive smoking seems to increase the risk and severity of GO in children as well as adults [11, 26, 27].

The non-specificity of some of the symptoms in pediatric age group can lead to children being initially seen by psychologists, gastroenterologists, neurologists, cardiologists and ophthalmologists, before being referred to endocrinology.

Examination may reveal tachycardia, increased blood pressure for age and raised pulse pressure. Skin may be warm and moist, thinning of hair, onycholysis and softening of nails can be present.Vitiligo and alopecia areata can be seen in patients with associated autoimmune disorders. Precordial pulsations may be prominent, accompanied by a apical systolic regurgitant murmur due to functional mitral insufficiency secondary to papillary muscle dysfunction. Tremors may be present, along with hyperactive deep tendon reflexes. Musculoskeletal examination may reveal proximal muscle weakness and wasting.

On local examination, size of the gland can be variable, with a large proportion of patients having none to small or moderate sized goitre, which may escape patient's and family's attention [28]. The thyroid gland is usually symmetrically enlarged, non-tender, smooth and having firm consistency, and may be associated with a palpable thrill and a thyroid bruit in upto one fourth of patients due to increased vascularity. A large goitre can cause tracheal compression and other compressive symptoms.

Lid retraction, especially of the upper eyelid, and a staring appearance may be evident in upto one-third of the cases. Lid retraction is a sign of adrenergic overactivity, and is not considered a sign of GO per se. Other common signs in pediatric GO are lagophthalmos or von Graefe's sign (9–74%), proptosis (4–91%), signs of soft tissue involvement (19–26%), including conjunctival injection (8–49%), chemosis (1–23%) and lid edema in around 10% of the patients. Corneal involvement can occur in the form of corneal punctate staining (12–34%), exposure keratitis and superior limbic keratitis. Extraocular muscle motility defects has been described in relatively fewer number of patients (2–11%), except in a study by Eha et al., where it was observed in 36% of the patients [23] (**Table 1**). Similarly, dysthyroid optic neuropathy (DON) can be seen very rarely in pediatric age groups.

Differences	Pediatric Graves	Adult Graves
Symptoms	Classic symptoms less common (Tachycardia is a reliable sign than blood pressure changes)	Classic
Ophthalmopathy	Less common Less severe	More common
Pretibial Myxedema	Rare	5% (15% in Graves' Disease with ophthalmopathy)
Thyroid storm	Rare	1–2%
Atrial fibrillation	Rare	10–15% (25% in age > 60 years)
Remission rate with ATD	<30% (Higher in Koreans) (Lower rates in prepubertal children ~17%)	40–60%
Surgery	Higher complication rates Requires experienced high-volume thyroid surgeon	Relatively safe and easy surgery
Cosmesis	Greater concern	Lesser concern
RAIA	Increased sensitivity to radiation Increased susceptibility to carcinogenic effects of radiation	Lesser sensitivity Negligible carcinogenic effects

Table 1.
Differences in Pediatric vs. Adult Graves' Disease.

Some of the key differences in the presentation of pediatric GD vis-à-vis adult GD are as follows:

- Weight loss is less common in children. Increased appetite with/without weight loss, or absence of weight gain during pubertal years can be an indicator of thyrotoxicosis. Growth charts can be pivotal in identifying trends for early detection. BMI SD scores have been reported to be particularly lower in younger children as compared to older children in few studies.

- Early symptoms like behavioural changes, emotional lability, fatigue, nervousness, palpitations, sleep disturbances with insomnia are particularly subtle and difficult to identify.

- Difficulty in concentrating, restlessness, hyperactivity, impaired scholastic performance can be the presenting complaints, especially in younger children. These can be commonly mistaken to be Attention deficit hyperactivity disorder (ADHD), leading to a delay in diagnosis and treatment.

- Untreated thyrotoxicosis can lead to increases in height velocity and advancement of skeletal age, which can be apparent as an increased height SDS in growth charts. Increase in height SDS is seen more commonly in prepubertal children than pubertal and post-pubertal children. This may be explained by the fact that prepubertal bone maturation is driven by growth hormone (GH) and thyroid hormones, whereas pubertal bone growth is driven primarily by estradiol. Another plausible reason could be the delay in diagnosis in younger children. The effect on final height, however is variable across literature, where some studies show achievement of a normal height within target range, some showing increased final height [25, 29]

- Ophthalmic abnormalities are less severe. Soft tissue involvement, lagophthalmos, proptosis and punctate corneal erosions more common, extraocular muscle restriction and optic neuropathy are rare

- Pretibial myxedema is rare (0.9%)

- Atrial fibrillation is rare

- Thyroid storm is rare in children

Pediatric GD can commonly be associated with other conditions as follows [2, 30].

5. Differential diagnosis

GD is the most common cause of thyrotoxicosis in children. However, it has to be clinically differentiated from other causes of thyrotoxicosis in childhood. These include hyperthyroid disorders, associated with increased secretion of the thyroid hormones from the thyroid gland, or cases of thyroiditis, where symptoms occur due to thyroid follicular disruption leading to release of preformed causes. Some of the common differential diagnostic causes have been summarized in **Tables 2–4**.

Consumption of biotin as a part of management of metabolic or dermatological diseases can lead to surreptitious laboratory results of elevated thyroid hormones, suppressed TSH and positive thyroid receptor autoantibodies with immunoassays utilizing the streptavidin-biotin platforms. Hence, laboratory results must be reconsidered and rechecked in the absence of supportive clinical features of thyrotoxicosis [31].

Endocrine autoimmune disorders	Non-endocrine autoimmune disorders	Syndromic disorders
• Hashimoto's thyroiditis • Celiac disease • Type 1 diabetes • Primary adrenal insufficiency	• Vitiligo • Systemic lupus erythematosus (SLE) • Rheumatoid arthritis (RA) • Myasthenia gravis	• Down syndrome • Turner syndrome

Table 2.
Common associations of pediatric GD.

Differential diagnosis of GD	Remarks
TA	• Focal increase in uptake on nuclear scans with suppressed uptake in rest of the gland • Surgical excision preferred therapy
TMNG	• Multiple foci of increased uptake with suppressed uptake in remainder of the gland on nuclear scan • Surgery preferred modality
Germline activating mutations of TSH-R	• Familial or denovo forms • Can lead to simple or multinodular goitre
McCune Albright syndrome	• One-third can develop hyperthyroidism • Polyostotic fibrous dysplasia, café-au-lait spots, precocious puberty
TSH producing pituitary adenoma	• Rare • Elevated T4 with an inappropriately normal TSH • High serum alpha subunit concentration and alpha subunit to TSH ratio, little to no response to thyrotropin releasing hormone (TRH)
Resistance to thyroid hormone	• Autosomal dominant • Elevated T4 with a normal or elevated TSH • Generally euthyroid, clinical manifestations depend on the site of the defect in thyroid hormone receptor

Table 3.
Differential diagnosis of GD: Hyperthyroid disorders.

Acute suppurative thyroiditis	• Bacterial infection: Haemophilus influenza, Group A streptococci • Painful thyroid, fever, fistula can be present • Transient thyrotoxicosis • Associated with elevated ESR and WBC count, decreased uptake on nuclear scan (Tc-99 m or radioiodine)
Subacute granulomatous thyroiditis/ de Quervain disease	• Viral infection • Fever, painful thyroid, symptoms less severe than bacterial thyroiditis
Hashimoto's thyroiditis	• 5–10% of children can present with "Hashitoxicosis" • Transient thyrotoxicosis • Low or absent uptake in thyroid on nuclear scans
Thyroid injury	• H/O significant neck trauma or exposure to radiation
Thyrotoxicosis factitia	• Exogenous ingestion of thyroid hormones, particularly in the setting of adolescents trying to lose weight • Low or absent thyroid uptake in nuclear scans • Low serum thyroglobulin is diagnostic

Table 4.
Differential diagnosis of GD: Thyrotoxic disorders without hyperthyroidism.

6. Diagnosis

6.1 Biochemical diagnosis

6.1.1 Thyroid function tests

All patients with suspected thyrotoxicosis should undergo detailed thyroid function tests, including TSH, free thyroxine (FT4) and preferably total triiodothyronine (T3). Measurement of total T3 is preferred over free T3 (FT3) as the FT3 assays are less robust and less validated as compared to the FT4 assays. Measurement of free hormones makes the assay reports more reliable in the presence of conditions affecting the concentrations of thyroid binding globulin (TBG) like liver disease, nephrotic syndrome. Serum TSH is more sensitive the changes in thyroid hormone levels due to the log-linear relationship of TSH with the free thyroid hormone levels.

Assays have been constantly evolving from the older manual radioimmunoassays (RIA) to the modern day fully automated chemiluminescent immunoassay (CLIA) and electrochemiluminescent immunoassay (ECLIA) platforms. Results have to interpreted in the light of age and assay-specific reference ranges. Lack of consistency between biochemical reports and clinical presentation should alert the physician to consider assay interferences like presence of heterophile antibodies and excess biotin consumption.

Thyroid function tests typically reveal elevated free thyroxine (FT4) and T3 with a suppressed TSH in overt thyrotoxicosis. Patients with milder thyrotoxicosis may exhibit only elevated T3 values and suppressed TSH with normal T4 values, a state known as T3 toxicosis, a common presentation in pediatric age groups. Higher T3 values have been noted in prepubertal children as compared to post-pubertal children, and have been observed to be a negative predictor of the likelihood of remission in pediatric GD [25, 32].

6.1.2 Markers of thyroid autoimmunity

TRAbs are specific for GD, and are found in majority of the patients at diagnosis, with a reported prevalence of >70% in pediatric GD in some studies [33, 34]. TRAb levels can be higher in younger patients <5 years of age and in clinically severe disease [2].

Traditionally, TRAb concentrations were measured using either bioassays or receptor assays. Estimation of TRAb levels by bioassays was based on the ability of TRAbs to increase cyclic adenosine monophosphate (cAMP) production either directly from thyroid follicular cells in vitro, or indirectly via TSH-R transfected Chinese hamster ovary (CHO) cells. These also enabled detection of functional subtypes of TRAbs, including inhibitory TRAb antibodies. Receptor assays, on the other hand, provide an estimate of TRAb levels by measuring the ability of TRAb to inhibit the binding of labelled TSH to thyroid membranes, and provided enhanced sensitivity [1].

TRAb assays subsequently evolved with the advancements in immunoassays techniques. The "liquid phase" first generation immunoassays were competitive immunoassays based on inhibition of binding of radionuclide or enzyme labelled TSH. These provided excellent specificity of 97.5–100%, but suffered from a suboptimal sensitivity ranging from 52 to 94%. Subsequently, 2nd generation "solid phase" immunoassays utilized monoclonal antibodies and human or porcine TSH-R immobilized on a solid surface, improving the sensitivity to 87–100%. The 3rd generation immunoassays utilized a stimulating biotinylated monoclonal antibody

(M22) to bind to immobilized TSH-R. In recent years, fully automated platforms have been developed using the ECLIA and fluoroenzymatic immunoassay principles, with excellent sensitivity of 95–100% and specificity of 97–100% [35].

GD may also be associated with other anti-thyroid antibodies like thyroid peroxidase (TPO) autoantibodies, anti-thyroglobulin antibodies, as well as other autoantibodies like antimicrosomal antibodies (AMA) and antinuclear antibodies (ANA) [33].

6.2 Thyroid imaging

6.2.1 Thyroid scintigraphy

Thyroid scans utilize a gamma camera to provide a planar image, which provides anatomical information in addition to the functional status, whereas uptake scans are used to measure the % radioiodine uptake (RAIU), typically measured by placing a non-imaging gamma scintillation probe detector over the neck. Most commonly used radiopharmaceuticals for nuclear thyroid imaging are iodine-123 (I-123) and 99 m-technetium (Tc99m-pertechnetate). Drugs which can potentially interfere the tracer uptake like thionamides and sources of excess iodine have to be stopped atleast 3–7 days and 2–4 weeks prior to the study respectively. The doses for diagnostic imaging should be weight-based rather than fixed doses especially in children. The scintigraphic images and uptake studies are typically performed around 4 hours after I-123 intake, or 20 minutes after the iv injection of Tc-99 m pertechnetate. While technetium scans result in a low radiation exposure, they result in a high background noise and a low range of normal uptake in the thyroid gland [36].

GD is characterized by a homogenous increase in tracer uptake in the thyroid scans and an increased %RAIU on uptake studies. These studies are not done routinely for diagnosis in pediatric GD. Their primary role is in differential diagnosis of thyrotoxicosis in cases with inconclusive clinical and biochemical findings, and in assessing the radioiodine uptake in order to calculate the dose of therapeutic I-131 when radioiodine ablation is planned as therapy. However, germline TSH-R activating mutations can also give rise to a diffuse and homogenously increased uptake in the thyroid gland. On the other hand, McCune Albright syndrome, TA and TMNG are typically associated with focal increases in uptake with suppressed uptake in the remainder of the gland, whereas autoimmune thyroiditis, iodine excess and thyrotoxicosis factitia are associated with decreased to absent uptake in the thyroid gland [22, 37].

6.2.2 Thyroid ultrasonography

A thyroid ultrasound and doppler study provides a safe and non-invasive modality for differential diagnosis of thyrotoxicosis. Thyroid gland is classically diffusely enlarged in GD, and may display normal echogenicity or hypoechogenicity like in thyroiditis. GD is characterized by a diffuse increase in parenchymal vascularization, often referred to as a "thyroid inferno". Autoimmune thyroiditis may be associated with a lesser degree of increase in parenchymal vascularity as well. Quantitative measurements of the thyroidal blood flow can also be vital in diagnosing GD, with superior and inferior thyroidal artery's mean peak systolic velocities of more than 45–50 cm/second suggestive of a diagnosis of GD, providing a sensitivity and specificity of 81–83% and 92–96% respectively.

Ultrasound should also be performed in the case of thyroid asymmetry or a palpable nodule [2, 18, 38–40].

7. Management

The three cornerstones of management of pediatric GD are antithyroid drugs (ATDs), radioiodine (RAI) therapy and surgical management. Age of the patient, likelihood of remission, availability of expertise and facilities, patient preferences determine the choice of modality. The choice of initial therapy also depends on the prevailing practices in different geographic regions of the world. For instance, antithyroid drug therapy remains overwhelmingly the most popular choice in Japan, with >90% of children with newly diagnosed GD being instituted on ATDs, whereas the proportion is >80% in Europe, Asia, Oceania and South America. RAI therapy is more commonly used in the United States of America, with >70% of newly diagnosed pediatric GD patients being treated with I-131 previously. However, the use has been declining, with current estimates of 40% of patients being instituted on ATDs [22].

7.1 Medical management

Antithyroid medications still remain the modality of choice in most pediatric patients with GD, despite lower remission rates as compared to adults. Methimazole (MMI) or carbimazole (CBZ) are the drugs of choice, with the former used commonly in the United States and Japan, and the latter being used in Europe.

All the drugs act by inhibition of the critical enzyme thyroid peroxidase, effectively inhibiting the organification of iodine by inhibiting its binding to the tyrosyl residues on thyroglobulin. They also inhibit thyroglobulin synthesis, coupling of iodotyrosine residues, and secretion of thyroid hormones. PTU additionally inhibits type 1 deiodinase enzyme, decreasing the conversion of T4 to the peripherally active T3. Carbimazole is a prodrug and it get converted to methimazole completely after hepatic metabolism. 10 mg CBZ is equivalent to 7.5 mg MMI and 100 mg PTU. Besides the differences in potencies, the drugs differ in their pharmacokinetics, with MMI having a half-life of 6–8 hours, whereas PTU has a much shorter half-life of 30 minutes, necessitating 3 times a day dosing [22].

7.1.1 Dosing considerations

The starting dose of MMI is typically 0.2–0.5 mg/kg/day, ranging from 0.1-1 mg/kg/day. French guidelines suggest a dose of 0.4 mg/kg/day in moderate thyrotoxicosis (FT4 < 50 pmol/L), and doses of 0.8 mg/kg/day in severe thyrotoxicosis (FT > 70 pmol/L). As MMI is usually available in the form of 5 or 10 mg tablets, ATA guidelines also put forth a simplified guideline to ease administration, suggesting doses of 1.25 mg/day, 2.5–5 mg/day, 5–10 mg/day and 10–20 mg/day in the age groups of infancy, 1–5 years, 5–10 years and 10–18 years respectively, with dose escalation of 50–100% above the suggested doses in cases of severe hyperthyroidism. The doses are typically administered in a single dose or divided into two or three doses a day in the initial stages. Single dose therapy may result in better patient compliance.

PTU may be considered in doses of 2–7.5 mg/kg/day in three divided doses. But it is strictly avoided in pediatric patients due to concerns of severe hepatotoxicity, except in cases of thyroid storm and patients with adverse reactions to MMI requiring short-term control of thyrotoxicosis prior to definitive therapy. French guidelines contraindicate PTU use in children, and Japanese guidelines advocate caution with PTU use [22, 31, 36].

Symptoms of sympathetic overactivity including tremors, tachycardia, muscle weakness, neuropsychological disturbances are treated with beta blockers, propranolol at 1–2 mg/kg/day in 2–3 divided doses, or atenolol at 0.5–1.2 mg/kg/day as a once daily dose. Selective beta blockers like atenolol and metoprolol are preferred in children with reactive airway disease [22, 31, 36].

7.1.2 Adverse effects

Most adverse reactions to antithyroid drugs emerge within 3 months of initiating treatment. PTU was widely used for medical management of pediatric GD until it fell out of favour in early 2000s, due to multiple reports of serious hepatotoxicity. PTU is associated with idiosyncratic hepatocellular necrosis, leading to hepatic dysfunction ranging from reversible injury to acute liver failure requiring transplantation, and rarely leading to death. PTU was the third most common cause of drug-induced liver failure, accounting for approximately 10% of drug-related liver transplantations in the United States [41].

The risk of hepatotoxicity is considerably higher in children than in adults, with children accounting for almost half of the patients in case reports of PTU-induced liver failure. Rivkees et al. estimated that the risk of reversible liver injury in children taking PTU was atleast 1 in 200, and the risk of liver failure requiring transplantation was atleast 1 in 2000–4000. It was also noted that PTU-induced liver failure was rapidly progressive and with low chances of reversibility, and there were no meaningful biochemical markers to predict the risk of hepatotoxicity [42]. FDA issued a boxed warning for PTU use in 2010, noting that 22 adult and 10 pediatric cases of serious liver injury were associated with PTU use, and limited its use to patients intolerant to other modalities and in first trimester of pregnancy [43].

MMI can also be associated with hepatotoxicity, although it is typically milder and of the cholestatic pattern. No cases of liver failure or transplantation have been reported in association with MMI use in children, in contrast to adults in whom hepatocellular toxicity has been described.

PTU is also associated with a 40 times higher risk of antineutrophil cytoplasmic antibody (ANCA) vasculitis than with MMI use. The positivity rate of ANCA in pediatric users is higher, approximately 64%, approximately 20% of whom can develop vasculitis. The antibodies tend to develop at or after 1 year of treatment. Usually asymptomatic, it can occasionally manifest as polyarthritis, dermatologic involvement in the form of purpuric skin lesions, pulmonary and renal involvement. There exist few case reports of renal failure in children due to vasculitis. Majority of the cases resolve with discontinuation of the offending medication, but severe involvement may require glucocorticoid and other immunosuppressive therapy.

MMI is more commonly associated with minor adverse events in upto 25% of the children being treated with MMI, most commonly involving mucocutaneous adverse events like urticaria, rash, oral ulcers and arthralgias, myalgias. The risk of agranulocytosis appears to be similar for MMI and PTU, affecting 0.3% of treated adults, with possibly lower prevalence in children. The risk appears to be dose-dependent with MMI use, with most of the cases occurring with daily MMI doses exceeding 20 mg/day.

Minor allergic reactions are usually managed with antihistamines, while continuing the drug under watchful guidance. On the other hand, occurrence of serious adverse reactions warrant drug discontinuation and consideration of alternative therapies. PTU and MMI exhibit significant cross-reactivity, hence use of either drugs should be avoided with the occurrence of a serious adverse reaction to the other drug [22, 31, 36].

7.1.3 Monitoring and dose titration

Patients should be monitored clinically for symptoms and signs of thyrotoxicosis. Weight and height should be checked periodically during clinic visits and charted in appropriate growth charts. Parents should also be counselled about possible weight gain in the first few months of therapy, which can persist.

ATA guidelines suggest a complete hemogram and liver function testing prior to initiating ATDs. Routine monitoring of WBC counts and liver function tests is not advocated due to sudden onset of agranulocytosis and rapidly progressive nature of PTU-related hepatotoxicity. WBC counts should be ordered in the presence of febrile illnesses or pharyngitis. Similarly, liver functions should be obtained when patients develop symptoms of hepatotoxicity like jaundice, pruritus, anorexia, light-coloured stools or dark urine, drug should be discontinued if transaminases are elevated upto 2–3 times the upper limit of normal. Subsequently, liver function tests should be monitored till normalization. Japanese guidelines also advocate annual urinalysis and MPO-ANCA measurement for early detection of ANCA-associated vasculitis in children on PTU [22, 36].

Thyroid function tests should first be obtained after 2–6 weeks of initiation of therapy, every 4–6 weeks till dose is stabilized and every 3 months thereafter. MMI dose can be reduced by 50% once thyroid hormones normalize. The usual maintenance doses range from 5 mg every alternate day to 10 mg a day [22, 36].

Alternatively, "block and replace" strategy has been used, where replacement levothyroxine is added so that ATDs can be continued at higher doses. A 2010 metanalysis by Abraham et al. showed that block and replace regimens had similar efficacy to titration regimens, but had higher risk of treatment withdrawal due to adverse effects [44]. This is especially true for MMI as most adverse effects of MMI are dose-related. However, some authors attributed these findings to the unconventionally higher doses of MMI in the studies using block-and-replace regimens in the meta-analysis, and hence maintain that block-and-replace can be a worthwhile strategy, especially in patients who are sensitive to minor increases in doses of MMI and become hypothyroid [36, 45].

7.1.4 Duration of therapy

Multiple prognostic factors determine the response to antithyroid drugs. It is usually assessed by remission rates, defined as the proportion of patients who remain euthyroid 1 year after cessation of ATD. Remission rates in children after 1–2 years of ATD therapy are typically 20–30%, lower than in adults.

In contrast to older studies which suggested a 25% chance of remission for every 2 years of continued treatment, longer duration of therapy has not translated into significant improvements in remission rates in more recent studies. For example, treatment beyond 2 years has been seen to associated with remission rates of 23–37% after 4 years, and only 15% after 4–10 years of therapy. Relapse can occur in as many as 36–47% of patients after initial remission. Additionally, longer treatment durations carry the risk of non-compliance and drug toxicities. However, more recent studies have shown encouraging data on relapse rates. In a retrospective study involving 1138 pediatric GD patients by Ohye et al., remission rate was 46% after a median duration of 3.8 years of ATD therapy, with no significant predictors for remission identified. The cumulative rates of remission increased with duration of anti-thyroid medication till 5 years of therapy. Similar findings were seen in the prospective study by Leger et al., in which remission rates were 20, 37, 45 and 49% after 4, 6, 8 and 10 year of ATD therapy respectively, suggesting a plateau of remission after 8–10 years of ATD therapy [36, 46, 47].

Evidence for prognostic factors predicting remission and relapse in pediatric GD have been mostly derived from many retrospective and few prospective studies. Older age and pubertal onset of disease, higher BMI, lower levels of thyroid hormone levels at presentation, early achievement of euthyroidism within 3 months of institution of ATDs and smaller goitres, have all been associated with early remission. Pre-pubertal children also tend to require longer duration of therapy to achieve remission vis-à-vis pubertal children [25, 32, 33, 48]. Non-Caucasian origin, higher TRAb levels additionally have also been associated with increased risk of relapse in treated patients [49]. In a study by Smith et al., TRAb antibodies decreased with duration of antithyroid therapy, but normalized only in 18% of children even after 24 months of therapy, with no further significant decreases with prolonged therapy. This points to a persistence of autoimmunity in pediatric age groups in contrast to adults, in whom TRAb levels tend to decline with anti-thyroid therapy, and may be used to guide decision-making for stopping anti-thyroid medication [50].

ATA guidelines suggest 1–2 years of ATD therapy before considering definitive modalities of RAI or surgery, depending on age of the child. Japanese guidelines suggest a duration of atleast 18–24 months, extending upto 5–10 years for better remission rates. They also suggest utility of TRAb assays in deciding duration of therapy.

7.1.5 Other drug therapies

Patients of thyrotoxicosis intolerant to MMI, awaiting surgery can be treated with inorganic iodine, either with 3–7 drops thrice a day of saturated solution of potassium iodide (SSKI) containing 50 mg iodide per drop, or 3–4 drops a day of Lugol's solution, containing 6.3 mg of iodine per drop, for 10 days prior to surgery. Inorganic iodine can also be used in the management of thyroid storm. It acts by inhibiting organification of iodine and thyroid hormone release, termed the "Wolff-Chaikoff effect". Caution has to be exercised for potential development of escape phenomenon, or exacerbation of thyrotoxicosis after drug withdrawal.

Alternatively, other drugs like lithium carbonate can be used, which acts by inhibiting the synthesis and release of thyroid hormones, but needs watchful care for any adverse effects. Some of the other medications that have been used are perchlorate, cholestyramine, corticosteroids and rituximab [22, 36].

7.2 Radioiodine therapy

The target of I-131 therapy is to achieve hypothyroidism by thyroid ablation with a single optimal dose of I-131 rather than euthyroidism. This is particularly relevant in pediatric age groups due to sensitivity of the thyroid gland to radiation.

The concerns over increased risk of malignancy with radioiodine were born after the Chernobyl incident, where increased risk of thyroid malignancies was attributed to low doses of I-131 and other radionuclides, in the presence of a dietary iodine deficiency in the population. Importantly, the maximum risk appeared to occur in children less than 5–6 years of age, decreasing gradually through 12 years of age. However, the highest risk of thyroid malignancy is seen with low levels of radiation exposure of about 0.09–30 μCi/g, and not with the higher activities administered in treatment of GD.

In a retrospective study by Read et al. involving 36 years follow up of 116 patients who had received RAI therapy between the ages of 3–19 years, there were no cases of thyroid malignancy or leukemia. There was also no increase in congenital anomalies in the offspring or rate of spontaneous abortions in the cohort [51]. Similarly, no significant increase in risk of non-thyroid malignancies has been observed in recipients of I-131 treatment.

Hence, ATA guidelines suggest avoiding RAI therapy in children less than 5 years of age, and considering RAI therapy in children between 5 and 10 years of age when the required activity for treatment is <10 mCi, while emphasizing that these restrictions are based on theoretical concerns of malignancy [18, 22, 31, 36].

7.2.1 Preparation

ATA guidelines suggest achieving euthyroidism with anti-thyroid drugs and beta blockers in patients with total T4 > 20 μg/dl, and free T4 > 5 ng/dl prior to RAI therapy. Iodine intake has to be restricted atleast 1 week prior to I-131 therapy. Anti-thyroid medications are typically stopped 2–3 days prior to administering I-131. This is associated with potential risk of worsening thyrotoxicosis and precipitating thyroid storm after radioiodine therapy. Alternatively, 20% higher dose can be administered while patient is on anti-thyroid medication, minimizing the risk of thyroid storm. Either of these approaches have not been well studied in pediatric age groups.

ATDs are restarted only 1 week after RAI therapy to optimize the likelihood of successful ablation, although this is seldom required in children as thyroid hormone levels begin to decrease within one week after RAI treatment [18, 22, 31, 36].

7.2.2 Dosing considerations

The activity to be administered as fixed doses of about 15 mCi or calculated using the Quimby-Marinelli formula, or the modified version based on the 24-hour uptake values on RAIU scan. Estimation of total gland size can be done by physical examination or by ultrasound dimensions of the gland, and is particularly challenging in pediatric patients. In general, the total dose of I-131 should be atleast 150 μCi/g of thyroid tissue, resulting in hypothyroidism in >95% of cases. Increased doses of 200–300 μCi/g may be required in patients with large goitres and lower radioiodine uptake. There are no studies available to compare the two methods in children.

Radioiodine is retained in the thyroid for several days, and is also excreted in body fluids like saliva, tears, sweat, stool and urine. Appropriate local radiation safety precautions have to be observed by the patient and family members after RAI treatment [18, 22, 31, 36].

7.2.3 Complications

Pain in the gland can develop in the week after I-131 therapy in less than 10% of the patients. It can be managed by symptomatic treatment with analgesics for 1–2 days. There may be temporary exacerbation of thyrotoxicosis, requiring treatment with ATDs, glucocorticoids and iodine preparations. Long-term risks include the theoretical risk of secondary malignancies following radiation [36].

7.2.4 Monitoring

Patient has to be clinically monitored for signs and symptoms of hyperthyroidism as well as for development of hypothyroidism. Patients can experience an exacerbation in ophthalmopathy, which may require treatment with glucocorticoids.

Hypothyroidism is usually achieved at 1–3 months after an optimal dose of I-131, with occasional patients taking upto 6 months to achieve hypothyroidism. Thyroid function tests should be obtained 4 weeks after I-131, followed by periodic testing at 4–6 weeks till hypothyroidism is achieved, when thyroid hormone replacement can be initiated [22, 36].

7.2.5 Contraindications

RAI therapy is an absolute contraindication in children less than 5 years of age as per AT and French guidelines. The latter also mention it as a relative contraindication in pre-pubertal children. Japanese guidelines advocate "careful administration" in children younger than 18 years of age on account of risk of thyroid malignancy and gonadal injury post radiation.

RAI therapy can be considered in pediatric patients with GO in non-severe cases. The NO-SPEC severity classification and clinical activity score (CAS) have not been validated in pediatric population. RAI therapy may still be considered in the presence of more severe manifestations like corneal involvement, persistent lid retraction and chemosis with concomitant oral glucocorticoid therapy, beginning a day after RAI, and tapered over 1–3 months [22, 31, 36].

7.3 Surgery

Surgery should be considered in patients with large goitres, presence of compressive symptoms, coexisting differentiated thyroid cancer (DTC), patients wishing to achieve faster remission, patients who do not wish to use ATDs or have adverse effects or contraindications to use of ATDs. ATA guidelines recommend thyroidectomy in children younger than 5 years of age, in whom definitive therapy is indicated and have accessibility to surgical expertise.

The major limiting factor for choice of surgery as the modality is the access to a high volume thyroid surgeon, defined as performing more than 30 cervical endocrine procedures in a year. The surgical complication rates are inversely related to the annual number of procedures by the operating surgeon, rather than the training or surgical specialty per se. The centre should be capable of handling pediatric anesthestic challenges and post-operative intensive care requirements. In the presence of availability of expertise and infrastructure, surgery can be offered as equivalent to RAI therapy to the parents [18].

7.3.1 Preparation

Patient should be rendered euthyroid with medications prior to surgery (thionamides, inorganic iodide and beta blockers). Potassium iodide, containing 50 mg iodide/drop can be administered as 1–2 drops thrice a day, 7–10 days prior to surgery can alleviate thyrotoxicosis as well as decrease vascularity of the gland. Dexamethasone can also help in rapid control of thyrotoxicosis [22, 36].

7.3.2 Procedure

Total or a near-total thyroidectomy (with <3 g of residual thyroid tissue) are the procedures of choice for management of GD. Partial or subtotal thyroidectomies may result in recurrence rates of 10–15%. Intra-operative PTH monitoring can be valuable in predicting the occurrence of post-operative hypocalcemia.

7.3.3 Complications

Most common post-operative complications include transient hypoparathyroidism and recurrent laryngeal nerve palsy. These complications tend to occur at the rate of 10–20%, more frequent than in adults, and are particularly more common in younger children. Other severe complications like permanent hypoparathyroidism, hematoma, infection, recurrent laryngeal nerve palsy occur less frequently. Significant bleeding occurs more frequently with large goitres, necessitating blood transfusions in children. Caution has to be exercised in handling of recurrent laryngeal nerves as they are thinner in children. Growth-related bone metabolism may make the patient prone for transient hypoparathyroidism post-operatively. Post-operative hypocalcemia requiring intravenous calcium correction occurs more frequently in children. Its risk can be decreased by preoperative calcitriol, usually started 3 days before surgery and weaned off over the first 2 weeks post-operatively.

Surgery offers the advantages of definitive therapy. This has to be weighed against the risks associated with an invasive procedure, and the requirement of life-long thyroxine replacement with appropriate monitoring after surgery [22, 31, 36].

7.4 Choice of modality

Anti-thyroid drugs are usually the first line of management, typically administered for atleast 1–2 years. Definitive therapy with RAI therapy or surgery should be considered if remission is not attained after 1–2 years of ATD therapy. Continued medical management with periodic biochemical monitoring is a viable option in patients who are not candidates for either of the two definitive modalities. They offer the advantages of ease of administration, availability, reasonable safety and avoidance of exposure to radioactivity and surgical procedure. These have to be weighed against long duration of therapy and associated followup, lower rates of remission, low rates of compliance, higher frequency of adverse effects.

Radioiodine therapy in sufficient doses results in achievement of hypothyroidism in majority of patients, and should be considered as the modality of choice for definitive therapy in children >10 years of age, and in children 5–10 years of age with calculated dose requirements of less than 10 mCi. This has to be balanced against the risks of temporary flare, radiation thyroiditis and concerns of malignancy, even if theoretical as per most studies.

Medical management	RAI therapy	Surgery

• First line of therapy in most patients
• Lack of access to definitive therapies
• Good compliance to medication and periodic followup
	• Risk factors for poor response to ATDs:
	  ○ Prepubertal
	  ○ Severe biochemical thyrotoxicosis and elevated TRAb at presentation
	  ○ Prolonged time to achieve euthyroidism
	  ○ Persistently elevated TRAb
	  ○ Large goitre
	• Adverse effects and poor compliance to ATDs
	• Contraindications or unwilling for surgery
	• Relapse after medical and surgical management
	• Avoidance of surgical scar and risks associated with surgery
		• Risk factors for poor response to ATDs as described
		• Children younger than 5 years of age
		• Large goitres more than twice the normal size for age or > 80 g
		• Compressive symptoms
		• Nodular goitre, suspicion of malignancy
		• Inability to comply with precautions and follow-up instructions after RAI therapy
		• Severe eye disease
		• Post-pubertal patients considering pregnancy

Table 5.
Clinical factors influencing choice of modality in pediatric GD.

Surgery offers immediate and definitive therapy. However, the need for hospitalization, associated complications, surgical scarring preclude its use as a first line therapy. It can be considered in patients requiring definitive therapy and not being suitable candidates for RAI ablation.

Clinical factors that can influence the choice of modality are summarized in **Table 5**.

8. Special considerations

8.1 Thyroid storm

Encephalopathy can occur in association with thyroid storm. Initial presentation can include mental status changes including behavioural abnormalities, agitation, confusion, anxiety and emotional lability. Patients can also present with seizures, which can range from generalized tonic clonic to complex partial to more focal seizures.

8.2 Neonatal GD

Neonatal GD, though rare, can be life-threatening with significant morbidity and mortality. Maternal transfer of thyroid-stimulating immunoglobulins (TSIs) to the fetus, can occur in 1 in 80 cases of maternal GD. The risk of neonatal GD is directly proportional to the magnitude of elevation of TSI levels, typically increased at levels 2–4 times the upper limit of normal. The fetal thyroid can respond to TSIs resulting in excessive production of thyroid hormones.

This can manifest as fetal thyrotoxicosis, especially in second half of gestation. The condition should be suspected in the presence of fetal tachycardia (heart rate > 160/min after 20 weeks of gestation), goitre on antenatal ultrasound. Uncontrolled fetal thyrotoxicosis can result in intrauterine growth retardation (IUGR), premature fusion of cranial sutures, advanced skeletal age, accelerated maturation of femoral ossification centre, learning disabilities and mental retardation.

Management consists of adequate control of maternal thyrotoxicosis with anti-thyroid drugs. Propylthiouracil (PTU) is often the first choice at the time of organogenesis. Methimazole (MMI) is avoided in first trimester due to risk of methimazole embryopathy (Odds ratio of 1.66 for developing birth defects). This can manifest as aplasia cutis congenita, omphalocele, choanal and esophageal atresia and other omphalomesenteric duct anomalies in the newborn [52, 53].

The condition usually resolves by 3–6 months of age, due to clearance of TSIs from the infant's circulation. Infants may meanwhile require medical management of thyrotoxicosis. This entails treatment with antithyroid medications (PTU 5–10 mg/kg/day or MMI 0.5–1 mg/kg/day) and propranolol (1 mg/kg/day). Rapid biochemical control may require administration of Lugol's solution or saturated solution of potassium iodide (SSKI) for 7–10 days. Thyroid hormones typically normalize after 2 weeks of medical therapy, and may necessitate addition of levothyroxine to prevent hypothyroidism. Anti-thyroid medication can usually be weaned by 3 months, guided by monitoring of infant's serum TSI levels.

9. Summary

Graves' Disease in children is a classic example of children not being small adults. There are differences in management and response to treatment in children with Graves' Disease. Nuances exist for the various modalities for children and requires specialist pediatric endocrinology care. Therapeutic options need to be discussed with parents before deciding on choice of definitive therapy. Smooth transitioning to adult endocrinology clinic is important to continue quality medical care.

Abbreviations

EDCs	Endocrine-disrupting chemicals
GD	Graves' Disease
MAS	McCune Albright syndrome
TA	Toxic adenoma
TMNG	Toxic multinodular goitre

Author details

Madhukar Mittal* and Vanishri Ganakumar
Department of Endocrinology and Metabolism, All India Institute of Medical Sciences Jodhpur, India

*Address all correspondence to: mittalspace@gmail.com

References

[1] Zimmerman D, Lteif AN. THYROTOXICOSIS IN CHILDREN. Endocrinol Metab Clin. 1998 Mar 1;27(1):109-26.

[2] Léger J, Kaguelidou F, Alberti C, Carel JC. Graves' disease in children. Best Pract Res Clin Endocrinol Metab. 2014 Mar 1;28(2):233-43.

[3] Krassas GE, Segni M, Wiersinga WM. Childhood Graves' ophthalmopathy: results of a European questionnaire study. Eur J Endocrinol. 2005 Oct 1;153(4):515-21.

[4] Lavard L, Ranløv I, Perrild H, Andersen O, Jacobsen BB. Incidence of juvenile thyrotoxicosis in Denmark, 1982-1988. A nationwide study. Eur J Endocrinol. 1994 Jun;130(6):565-8.

[5] Williamson S, Greene SA. Incidence of thyrotoxicosis in childhood: a national population based study in the UK and Ireland. Clin Endocrinol (Oxf). 2010 Mar;72(3):358-63.

[6] Kjær RH, Andersen MS, Hansen D. Increasing Incidence of Juvenile Thyrotoxicosis in Denmark: A Nationwide Study, 1998-2012. Horm Res Paediatr. 2015;84(2):102-7.

[7] Wong GW, Kwok MY, Ou Y. High incidence of juvenile Graves' disease in Hong Kong. Clin Endocrinol (Oxf). 1995 Dec;43(6):697-700.

[8] Wong GWK, Cheng PS. Increasing incidence of childhood Graves' disease in Hong Kong: A follow-up study. Clin Endocrinol (Oxf). 2001;54(4):547-50.

[9] Simon M, Rigou A, Le Moal J, Zeghnoun A, Le Tertre A, De Crouy-Chanel P, et al. Epidemiology of Childhood Hyperthyroidism in France: A Nationwide Population-Based Study. J Clin Endocrinol Metab. 2018 01;103(8):2980-7.

[10] Bartley GB, Fatourechi V, Kadrmas EF, Jacobsen SJ, Ilstrup DM, Garrity JA, et al. The Incidence of Graves' Ophthalmopathy in Olmsted County, Minnesota. Am J Ophthalmol. 1995 Oct 1;120(4):511-7.

[11] Krassas GE, Gogakos A. Thyroid-associated ophthalmopathy in juvenile Graves' disease--clinical, endocrine and therapeutic aspects. J Pediatr Endocrinol Metab JPEM. 2006 Oct;19(10):1193-206.

[12] Vos XG, Smit N, Endert E, Tijssen JGP, Wiersinga WM. Variation in phenotypic appearance of Graves' disease: effect of genetic anticipation and duration of complaints. Eur J Endocrinol. 2009 Jul;161(1):113-8.

[13] Manji N, Carr-Smith JD, Boelaert K, Allahabadia A, Armitage M, Chatterjee VK, et al. Influences of Age, Gender, Smoking, and Family History on Autoimmune Thyroid Disease Phenotype. J Clin Endocrinol Metab. 2006 Dec 1;91(12):4873-80.

[14] Płoski R, Szymański K, Bednarczuk T. The Genetic Basis of Graves' Disease. Curr Genomics. 2011 Dec;12(8):542-63.

[15] Brix TH, Kyvik KO, Christensen K, Hegedüs L. Evidence for a major role of heredity in Graves' disease: a population-based study of two Danish twin cohorts. J Clin Endocrinol Metab. 2001 Feb;86(2):930-4.

[16] Brent GA. Environmental Exposures and Autoimmune Thyroid Disease. Thyroid. 2010 Jul;20(7):755-61.

[17] Ferrari SM, Fallahi P, Antonelli A, Benvenga S. Environmental Issues in Thyroid Diseases. Front Endocrinol [Internet]. 2017 [cited 2020 Nov 30];8. Available from: https://www.frontiersin.org/articles/10.3389/fendo.2017.00050/full

[18] Bauer AJ. Approach to the pediatric patient with Graves' disease: when is definitive therapy warranted? J Clin Endocrinol Metab. 2011 Mar;96(3):580-8.

[19] Bahn RS. Graves' Ophthalmopathy. N Engl J Med. 2010 Feb 25;362(8):726-38.

[20] Azizi F, Amouzegar A. Management of thyrotoxicosis in children and adolescents: 35 years' experience in 304 patients. J Pediatr Endocrinol Metab. 2018 Jan 26;31(2):159-65.

[21] Esen İ, Bayramoğlu E, Yıldız M, Aydın M, Karakılıç Özturhan E, Aycan Z, et al. Management of Thyrotoxicosis in Children and Adolescents: A Turkish Multi-center Experience. J Clin Res Pediatr Endocrinol. 2019 Jun;11(2): 164-72.

[22] Affairs TC on P, Pediatric-Endocrinology JS for, Committee and the PTD, Disease) JTA (Taskforce for the R of the G for the T of C-OG, Minamitani K, Sato H, et al. Guidelines for the treatment of childhood-onset Graves' disease in Japan, 2016. Clin Pediatr Endocrinol. 2017;26(2):29.

[23] Szczapa-Jagustyn J, Gotz-Więckowska A, Kocięcki J. An update on thyroid-associated ophthalmopathy in children and adolescents. J Pediatr Endocrinol Metab. 2016 Oct 1;29(10):1115-22.

[24] Nandi-Munshi D, Taplin CE. Thyroid-Related Neurological Disorders and Complications in Children. Pediatr Neurol. 2015 Apr 1;52(4):373-82.

[25] Lazar L, Kalter-Leibovici O, Pertzelan A, Weintrob N, Josefsberg Z, Phillip M. Thyrotoxicosis in Prepubertal Children Compared with Pubertal and Postpubertal Patients. J Clin Endocrinol Metab. 2000 Oct 1;85(10):3678-82.

[26] Chan W, Wong GWK, Fan DSP, Cheng ACK, Lam DSC, Ng JSK. Ophthalmopathy in childhood Graves' disease. Br J Ophthalmol. 2002 Jul 1;86(7):740-2.

[27] Gogakos AI, Boboridis K, Krassas GE. Pediatric aspects in Graves' orbitopathy. Pediatr Endocrinol Rev PER. 2010 Mar;7 Suppl 2:234-44.

[28] Kourime M, McGowan S, Towati MA, Ahmed SF, Stewart G, Williamson S, et al. Long-term outcome of thyrotoxicosis in childhood and adolescence in the west of Scotland: the case for long-term antithyroid treatment and the importance of initial counselling. Arch Dis Child. 2018 Jul 1;103(7):637-42.

[29] Sato H, Minamitani K, Minagawa M, Kazukawa I, Sugihara S, Wataki K, et al. Clinical features at diagnosis and responses to antithyroid drugs in younger children with Graves' disease compared with adolescent patients. J Pediatr Endocrinol Metab JPEM. 2014 Jul;27(7-8):677-83.

[30] Gastaldi R, Poggi E, Mussa A, Weber G, Vigone MC, Salerno M, et al. Graves Disease in Children: Thyroid-Stimulating Hormone Receptor Antibodies as Remission Markers. J Pediatr. 2014 May 1;164(5):1189-1194.e1.

[31] Léger J, Oliver I, Rodrigue D, Lambert A-S, Coutant R. Graves' disease in children. Ann Endocrinol. 2018 Dec;79(6):647-55.

[32] Shulman DI, Muhar I, Jorgensen EV, Diamond FB, Bercu BB, Root AW. Autoimmune Hyperthyroidism in Prepubertal Children and Adolescents: Comparison of Clinical and Biochemical Features at Diagnosis and Responses to Medical Therapy. Thyroid. 1997 Oct 1;7(5):755-60.

[33] Glaser NS, Styne DM. Predictors of Early Remission of Hyperthyroidism in Children1. J Clin Endocrinol Metab. 1997 Jun 1;82(6):1719-26.

[34] Foley TP, White C, New A. 8 THYROTROPIN RECEPTOR

ANTIBODIES (TRAb) IN PATIENTS WITH JUVENILE GRAVES DISEASE (JGD). Pediatr Res. 1985 Jun;19(6): 604-604.

[35] Tozzoli R, Bagnasco M, Giavarina D, Bizzaro N. TSH receptor autoantibody immunoassay in patients with Graves' disease: Improvement of diagnostic accuracy over different generations of methods. Systematic review and meta-analysis. Autoimmun Rev. 2012 Dec 1;12(2):107-13.

[36] Ross DS, Burch HB, Cooper DS, Greenlee MC, Laurberg P, Maia AL, et al. 2016 American Thyroid Association Guidelines for Diagnosis and Management of Hyperthyroidism and Other Causes of Thyrotoxicosis. Thyroid Off J Am Thyroid Assoc. 2016;26(10): 1343-421.

[37] Clerc J, Monpeyssen H, Chevalier A, Amegassi F, Rodrigue D, Leger FA, et al. Scintigraphic Imaging of Paediatric Thyroid Dysfunction. Horm Res Paediatr. 2008;70(1):1-13.

[38] Uchida T, Takeno K, Goto M, Kanno R, Kubo S, Takahashi S, et al. Superior thyroid artery mean peak systolic velocity for the diagnosis of thyrotoxicosis in Japanese patients. Endocr J. 2010;57(5):439-43.

[39] Zhao X, Chen L, Li L, Wang Y, Wang Y, Zhou L, et al. Peak systolic velocity of superior thyroid artery for the differential diagnosis of thyrotoxicosis. PloS One. 2012;7(11):e50051.

[40] Chung J, Lee YJ, Choi YJ, Ha EJ, Suh CH, Choi M, et al. Clinical applications of Doppler ultrasonography for thyroid disease: consensus statement by the Korean Society of Thyroid Radiology. Ultrasonography. 2020 Aug 25;39(4):315-30.

[41] Russo MW, Galanko JA, Shrestha R, Fried MW, Watkins P. Liver transplantation for acute liver failure from drug induced liver injury in the United States. Liver Transplant Off Publ Am Assoc Study Liver Dis Int Liver Transplant Soc. 2004 Aug;10(8):1018-23.

[42] Rivkees SA, Mattison DR. Propylthiouracil (PTU) Hepatoxicity in Children and Recommendations for Discontinuation of Use. Int J Pediatr Endocrinol. 2009 Dec;2009(1):1-8.

[43] Research C for DE and. FDA Drug Safety Communication: New Boxed Warning on severe liver injury with propylthiouracil. FDA [Internet]. 2019 Jun 28 [cited 2020 Dec 11]; Available from: https://www.fda.gov/drugs/postmarket-drug-safety-information-patients-and-providers/fda-drug-safety-communication-new-boxed-warning-severe-liver-injury-propylthiouracil

[44] Abraham P, Avenell A, Park CM, Watson WA, Bevan JS. A systematic review of drug therapy for Graves' hyperthyroidism. Eur J Endocrinol. 2005 Oct;153(4):489-98.

[45] Razvi S, Vaidya B, Perros P, Pearce SHS. What is the evidence behind the evidence-base? The premature death of block-replace antithyroid drug regimens for Graves' disease. Eur J Endocrinol. 2006 Jun 1;154(6):783-6.

[46] Ohye H, Minagawa A, Noh JY, Mukasa K, Kunii Y, Watanabe N, et al. Antithyroid Drug Treatment for Graves' Disease in Children: A Long-Term Retrospective Study at a Single Institution. Thyroid. 2013 Aug 8;24(2): 200-7.

[47] Léger J, Gelwane G, Kaguelidou F, Benmerad M, Alberti C, the French Childhood Graves' Disease Study Group. Positive Impact of Long-Term Antithyroid Drug Treatment on the Outcome of Children with Graves' Disease: National Long-Term Cohort Study. J Clin Endocrinol Metab. 2012 Jan 1;97(1):110-9.

[48] Glaser NS, Styne DM, Organization of Pediatric Endocrinologists of Northern California Collaborative Graves' Disease Study Group. Predicting the likelihood of remission in children with Graves' disease: a prospective, multicenter study. Pediatrics. 2008 Mar;121(3):e481-488.

[49] Kaguelidou F, Alberti C, Castanet M, Guitteny M-A, Czernichow P, Léger J. Predictors of Autoimmune Hyperthyroidism Relapse in Children after Discontinuation of Antithyroid Drug Treatment. J Clin Endocrinol Metab. 2008 Oct 1;93(10):3817-26.

[50] Smith J, Brown RS. Persistence of Thyrotropin (TSH) Receptor Antibodies in Children and Adolescents with Graves' Disease Treated Using Antithyroid Medication. Thyroid. 2007 Sep 6;17(11): 1103-7.

[51] Read CH Jr, Tansey MJ, Menda Y. A 36-Year Retrospective Analysis of the Efficacy and Safety of Radioactive Iodine in Treating Young Graves' Patients. J Clin Endocrinol Metab. 2004 Sep 1;89(9):4229-33.

[52] Yoshihara A, Noh J, Yamaguchi T, Ohye H, Sato S, Sekiya K, et al. Treatment of Graves' Disease with Antithyroid Drugs in the First Trimester of Pregnancy and the Prevalence of Congenital Malformation. J Clin Endocrinol Metab. 2012 Jul 1;97(7):2396-403.

[53] Andersen SL, Olsen J, Wu CS, Laurberg P. Birth Defects After Early Pregnancy Use of Antithyroid Drugs: A Danish Nationwide Study. J Clin Endocrinol Metab. 2013 Nov 1;98(11): 4373-81.

Chapter 16

Hyperthyroidism in Children

Artur Bossowski and Karolina Stożek

Abstract

Hyperthyroidism is the state of excessive synthesis and release of the thyroid hormones by thyrocytes. Graves' Disease is the most common cause of hyperthyroidism in children. The condition may occur at any age but the prevalence increases with age. According to the classical paradigm, coexistence of genetic susceptibility, environment triggers and immunological dysfunction are responsible for its development. Diagnosis of Graves' Disease is based on presence of characteristic clinical symptoms, TSH receptor antibodies and excess of thyroid hormones. The management in pediatric population involves mainly pharmacotherapy (thyrostatics, β-adrenolitics), in resistant cases radical radioiodine I^{131} therapy or surgical treatment is necessary.

Keywords: hyperthyroidism, Graves' Disease, children, autoantibodies, antithyroid drugs

1. Introduction

Hyperthyroidism (hyperthyreosis) is the condition that occurs due to excessive synthesis and release of the thyroid hormones T_3 (triiodothyronine) and/or T_4 (thyroxine) by thyrocytes and as a result of hyperstimulation of cells having receptors specific to these hormones.

A negative feedback blocks the secretion of thyrotropin (TSH) from the pituitary gland. Subclinical hyperthyroidism is characterized by normal levels of free thyroxine (fT_4) and free triiodothyronine (fT_3), with TSH below the reference range in the blood.

The term "thyrotoxicosis" refers to the clinical syndrome associated with the increased level of thyroid hormones caused by their enhanced production by the thyroid gland, their excessive release resulting from the gland destruction (e.g. the Hashitoxicosis phase in chronic thyroidits of Hashimoto's type), as well as due to the exogenous supply of thyroid hormone preparations in an abnormal, too large dose, and casual poisoning with thyroid hormone preparations (thyrotoxicosis factitia). Thus, thyreotoxicosis refers not only to the level of hormones in the blood, but is also associated with the level of sensitive cells that undergo activation, which leads to the manifestation of subjective and objective symptoms.

2. Causes of hyperthyroidism in children

The causes of hyperthyroidism in children include:

- Graves' Disease (toxic diffuse goiter, struma diffusa toxica) accounting for 95–99% of hyperthyroidism cases in children and approximately 60% in adults.

IntechOpen

- toxic nodular goiter (Plummer's disease) being much less common in children than in adults; most frequently occurring as a single nodule, especially in older children.

- the Marine-Lenhart's syndrome, in which an overactive thyroid nodule co-occurs with Graves' Disease in the same patient.

- thyroiditis.

- the initial stage of Hashimoto's disease.

- phase 1 subacute (viral) thyroiditis.

- poisoning with thyroid hormones – iatrogenic hyperthyroidism.

- Iodine Basedow Syndrome – hyperthyroidism develops due to the application of inorganic iodides, which act as triggering factors that induce hyperthyroidism on the grounds of autoimmunization.

- amiodarone-induced thyrotoxicosis (amiodarone has a chemical structure resembling that of thyroxine, one tablet contains approximately 75 mg of iodine!)

- hyperthyroidism in the course of follicular and papillary cancers.

- McCune-Albright syndrome is associated with the point mutation of the gene encoding the alpha subunit of the Gs protein, resulting in permanent activation of adenylyl cyclase; its main components are: fibrous dysplasia, café au lait spots, overactivity of many endocrine glands.

- the so called early effect of radioiodine I^{131} treatment for the thyroid.

- ovarian goiter (struma ovarii) - a substantial amount of thyroid tissue in ovarian tumour.

- thyrotropic pituitary adenomas – secondary hyperthyroidism (elevated values of TSH and thyroid hormones).

- pituitary thyroid hormone resistance – elevated levels of TSH and thyroid hormones.

- false hyperthyreosis in patients taking biotin preparations – in some cases even TSH receptor antibodies appear [1, 2].

3. Etiology and etiopathogenesis of Graves' Disease

The disease is named after an Irish physician, Robert Graves, who was the first to describe the symptoms of hyperthyrosis. In non-English speaking countries, the two-word term is commonly used as the name of a German doctor, Karl Adolph von Basedow, is added. This is an autoimmune disease, in which stimulating antibodies activate TSH receptor, leading to the thyroid growth as well as to unrestrained production and release of thyroid hormones.

Last decades have shown a constant increase in the incidence of autoimmune thyroid diseases (AITD). It is estimated that the problem affects approximately 5% of the world population. However, Graves' Disease is rarely diagnosed in the pediatric population. Its prevalence accounts for about 0.02% and children constitute less than 5% of all the patients. Nevertheless, it is Graves' Disease that remains the most common cause of hyperthyreosis in children, being responsible for 10–15% of all thyroid disorders in this group. Among pediatric patients, Graves' Disease may occur at any age but the morbidity rate increases with age, having its peak in adolescence. Its annual incidence among younger patients is 0.1 per 100,000 as compared to 3.0 per 100,000 at puberty. In the USA, Graves' Disease affects 0.2–0.4% of children and adolescents, i.e. 1 per 10,000, whereas in Hongkong it is diagnosed in 14 children per 100,000 a year. Sex distribution in the age group of up to 11 years is comparable, but in the older age group, girls are more frequently affected than boys (6–8,1).

It is estimated based on the research into monozygotic twins that the etiology of AITD has genetic causes in approximately 80% of cases, as compared to 20% due to environmental factors. Hashimoto thyroiditis and Graves' Disease share some of the genes.

Genes likely to be responsible for the development of AITD can be divided into two groups:

1. genes modulating the immune system, i.e. *HLA-DR*, *CD40*, CTLA-4, PTPN22, CD25, *FoxP3*.

2. genes specific to the thryroid gland: the gene for thyroglobulin (Tg) and the TSH receptor (TSHR) gene.

Additional genes may also play a role, being involved in the differentiation of AITD phenotypes, disease severity and response to the therapy.

Genes whose mutations may be responsible for the disease onset include:

- *GD-1* (chromosome 14q31).

- *GD-2* (chromosome 20q11.2).

- *GD-3* (chromosome Xq21).

- *HLA-DR3* gene described mainly as the main gene in the development of Graves' Disease. The presence of arginine at position 74 of the HLA-DRβ chain predisposes to AITD disclosure, whereas glutamine at the same position shows protective functions.

- *CD40* performs a key function in the interaction between antigen-presenting cells and T lymphocytes. CD40, found on B cells, ensures normal signal for proliferation, differentiation and production of IgG. Therefore, the CD40 gene predisposes to the development of Graves' Disease, which is to a large extent B-cell dependent.

- *CTLA-4* is present on the surface of T cells and inhibits their excessive response to the antigen. Moreover, it shows the expression on regulatory T cells, thus playing a major role in promoting their suppresive functions.

- CD25 gene polymorphism inhibits Treg functions, thus promoting autoimmunity. A latest study has described the level of mRNA expression for the genes encoding T-bet and GATA3, main regulators of Th1 and Th2 differentiation, respectively, and for the cytokines secreted by (IFNγ) and Th2 (IL4) in patients with Graves' Disease. The levels of the expression of mRNA T-bet and IFNγ are substantially elevated in patients, whereas those of GATA3 and IL4 remain decreased.

Also mutations of the gene encoding the expression of thyroglobulin, located on chromosome 8 and the autoimmune regulator gene located on chromosome 21 predispose to Graves' Disease. Moreover, vulnerability to develop ophthalmopathy in the course of Graves' Disease has been studied, with the involvement of CTLA-4 genes, tumor necrosis factor α (TNFα), adhesion molecule 1 (ICAM-1), interferon γ (IFN-γ), insulin-like growth factor 1 receptor (IGF-1R), protein inhibiting the pathway of signal 3 transduction (SOCS3), thyroid peroxidase (TPO) and calsequestrin 1 (CASQ1) [3–5].

The environmental factors that trigger the cascade leading to AITD include:

- infections, both viral and bacterial, may be responsible for the loss of tolerance and development of AITD; in the etiology of Graves' Disease *Yersinia enterocolitica* is the best known pathogen having specific bindings to TSH, recognized by antibodies against TSH receptor; *Y. enterocolitica* ompF (outer membrane porin F) produces antibodies and according to some sources is responsible for the process of molecular mimicry;

- stress -stress hormones (glycocorticosteroids, catecholamines) may induce the production of IL4, IL6, IL12 by dendritic cells, stimulate Th2, Th17 or Th1 cells and lead to Treg cell apoptosis, which promotes the pathogenesis of Graves' Disease;

- radiation -radioiodine treatment for toxic nodular goiter may contribute to the development of Graves' Disease or ophthalmopathy; the effect of radiotherapy on thyroid function depends on a number of factors, such as age, sex, the presence of antithyroid antibodies, iodine intake, etc.;

- exposure to tobacco smoke -according to the available data the proportion of smokers is elevated in patients with orbitopathy (64.2%) and Graves' Disease (47.9%) as compared to the control group (30%); smoking increases the risk of Graves' Disease twice and orbitopathy 3–4 times; moreover, the risk is associated with treatment failure and severity of ophthalmopathy;

- excessive iodine supply -iodine-induced hyperthyrosis, also called iodine-Basedow syndrome, refers particularly to patients with nodular goiter or to a population in which salt iodination program has been recently implemented;

- medications -interferon-α, alemtuzumab, highly active antiretroviral drugs capable of AITD induction; a classic example of the hyperthyreosis-inducing drug is amiodarone, a benzuforan derivative rich in iodine, whose structure resembles that of thyroid hormones; there are two types of amiodarone-induced thyrotoxicosis (AIT):

    - I -caused by enhanced production of thyroid hormones,

    - II - manifested by inflammation and destruction of thyrocytes.

- vitamin D_3 deficiency.
- contaminations [6–9].

However, Graves' Disease can be associated with the involvement of a combination of factors. The disease may even appear a long time after contact with a stimulus. Immunologically, the pathogenesis of Hashimoto thyroiditis is based on the predominance of cellular response, whereas the pathogenesis of Graves' Disease is associated with humoral response. This is, however, a gross simplification, as these processes overlap. Up to now, it has been thought that hyperstimulated $CD4^+$ T cells play a major role in the pathogenesis of Hashimoto thyroiditis. T helper 1 cells (Th1) produce interferon γ. Anti-TSHR antibodies against TSH receptor, whose differentiation is induced by Th1 cells, belong mainly to the IgG1 subgroup. Th1 cells can also stimulate the production of antibodies by IL10 secretion, which in turn stimulates B cells. Helper T2 cells (Th2) secrete interleukin 4 (IL4) and lead to the stimulation and production of B cells and plasmatic cells, which produce IgG4 antibodies against thyroid-attacking antigens (**Figure 1**).

Th17 cells originate from Th under the effect of various factors, i.e. TGFB, IL6, IL21, IL23 or STAT3. They produce interleukin 17 (IL17), involved in the promotion of inflammatory processes. Th17 cells show the expression of CCR6, IL23R, IL12Rβ2 and CD161. Their large population has been found in patients with AITD. In turn, Tregs make up an opposite population of lymphocytes that are mainly involved in the inhibition of immune hyperreaction; hence, their function is impaired or their number is decreased in various autoimmune diseases, including AITD. The analysis of the Th17/Treg proportion in children showed a reduced number of phenotypes characteristic of Treg cells: $CD4^+IL17^+/CD4^+CD25^+CD127^-$ and $CD4^+IL17^+/CD4^+CD25^+CD127^-FoxP3^+$ in patients with Graves' Disease as compared to the control group.

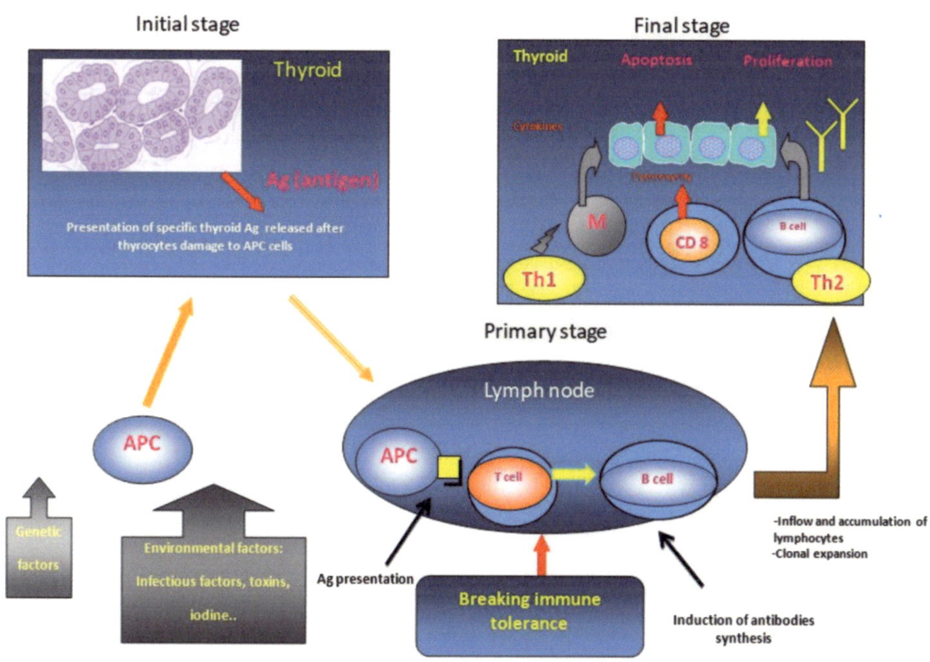

Figure 1.
Model of Graves' Diseases etiopathogenesis; APC – antigen presenting cell; M – macrophages, CD8 – cytotoxic cells; cells – Th1, th2.

Inflammation is an orderly process that should result in the elimination of a pathogenic factor and recovery of physiological condition, thus reflecting an effective immune response. One of the major traits of inflammatory condition is its self-limiting nature. The impaired suppresive function of lymphocytes leads ultimately to uncontrolled tissue injury and chronic inflammation. In the last few years, the maintenance of immunological tolerance has been ascribed to the subpopulation of B cells called B regulatory cells (Bregs). Their role has been emphasized in many autoimmune diseases which show both abnormal count and disturbed functionality of Bregs. Throughout the decades the knowledge of Bregs was based mainly on the research conducted on mice. The breakthrough was a study by Janeway et al., who in mice deprived of B cells observed a failure to recover after previous experimental autoimmune encephalomyelitis (EAE). Moreover, interleukin 10 (IL10) was found to be responsible for regulatory properties. Immature and mature B cells and plasmoblasts are thought to have a potential to differentiate towards Bregs producing IL10 both in mice and people. There is a strong potentiation of the function between Bregs and Tregs. On the other hand, Bregs inhibit differentiation of Th1 and Th17 cells by suppressing the production of proinflammatory cytokines as well as proliferation of dendritic cells (**Figure 2**).

Apart from IL10 secretion, Bregs are characterized by the production of other factors, i.e. transforming growth factor β (TGFβ) and interleukin 35 (IL35) (**Figure 3**). Through the production of TGF-β, Bregs activated by lipopolysaccharide (LPS) are able to induce the apoptosis of effector $CD4^+$ T cells and inactivity of $CD8^+$ T cells. Another mechanism inhibiting the immune response is due to the effect of IL35 which may inhibit the effector function of T cells; it also induces Bregs, promotes differentiation of B cells to Bregs secreting not only IL35, but also IL10.

Authors still pose a question whether Bregs constitute a separate cell line, in which a specific factor controls the expression of the genes responsible for their suppresive function or appear in response to the action of specific factors that stimulate B cells in a suitable environment. Immature and mature B cells and plasmoblasts and plasmatic cells may act as Bregs. Also B10 cells may differentiate into cells producing antibodies following termination of IL-10 production. In response to the inflammatory process, the level of Bregs increases and they gain the ability to regulate immunity. Thanks to the combination of antigen with B cell receptor (BCR), Bregs detect the inflammatory signal and induce regulatory effects [10–14].

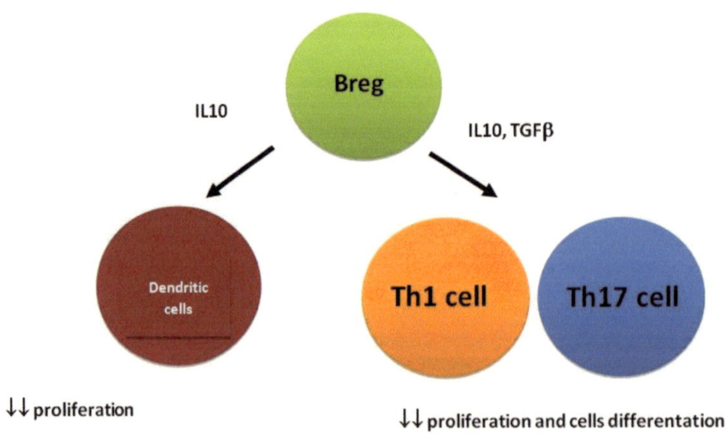

Figure 2.
Role of B regulatory cells in inhibiting differentiation of lymphocytes Th1 and Th17 and dendritic cells proliferation.

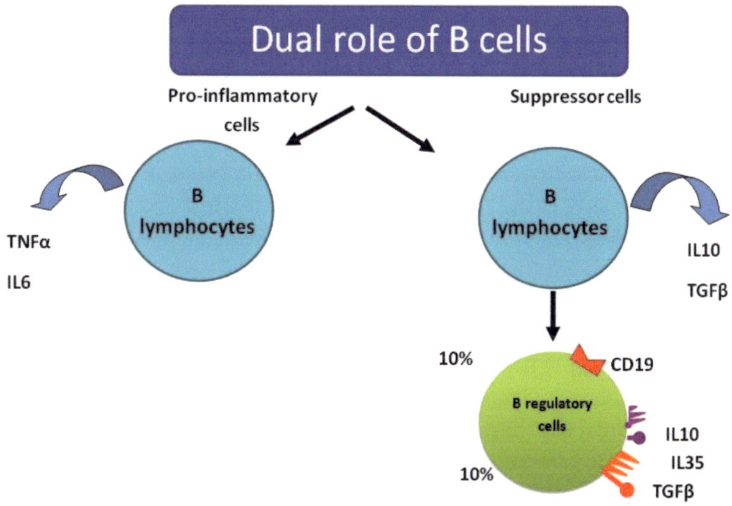

Figure 3.
Dual role of B lymphocytes. 10% of them release IL10, transforming growth factor beta (TGFβ) and interleukin 35 (IL35).

3.1 Autoantibodies

The major markers of Graves' Disease include TSHR-directed autoantibodies (TRAb). TSHR belongs to the family of glycoprotein hormone receptors and stimulates adenyl cyclase (cAMP) through G protein. The cAMP activates all the functions of thyroid cells, e.g. thyroglobulin synthesis, functioning of iodine pump, activity of thyroid peroxidase and release of hormones. Thyrotropin is a physiological agonist for the receptor.

Three types of TSH receptor antibodies can be distinguished:

- stimulating - thyroid stimulating immunoglobulins (TSI), which imitate the receptor ligand and increase the level of adenyl cyclase (cAMP), thus promoting the production of thyroid hormones and the growth of the gland.

- blocking - thyroid blocking immunoglobulins (TBI), inhibiting the activity of TSH and thus leading to hypothyreosis.

- neutral, whose effect on TSH receptor has not been yet examined.

In rare cases, both TSI and TBI are present or they are changed, one into the other, due to treatment. In clinical studies, the level of TRAb can be assessed using methods based on receptor binding (the so called binding assays), used to detect antibodies in the blood that compete with TSH for binding to its receptor (TSH binding inhibitory immunoglobulins, TBII or TRAb). However, in this way it is impossible to differentiate between their biological, stimulating or blocking activity.

The newest method, the so called bioassay (biological tests), is not routinely applied due to high costs. It can be used to determine the level of cAMP production after TSI binding to TSH receptor. The method is also used to monitor thyroid opthalmopathy and in the case of doubtful diagnosis of Graves' Disease due to borderline or negative TRAb values. Currently, no system is available to measure the activity of neutral antibodies. In our patients, TSI and TBI were determined with a biological test using Chinese hamster ovary cells with an embedded gene encoding the TSH receptor and with the luciferase system. TSI from a sample obtained from a patient binds to the receptor and via cAMP triggers the production of luciferase, thereby initiating a light reaction. The emission is measured with a luminometer. The measured values are compared to the reference values and in this way the presence of antibodies is confirmed or denied. The cut-off point in the analysis using a Thyretain TSI bioassay is the sample-to-reference ratio of more than 140% for the stimulating antibodies, and the degree of inhibition over 40% for the blocking antibodies.

Patients with hyperthyroidism and concomitant Graves' opthalmopathy showed significantly higher values of TSI/TSAb before and during treatment as compared to hyperthyroid patients without opthalmopathy (**Figure 4**). Patients in the prepubertal age had higher levels of TSI/TSAb than those in the pubertal age. Girls had significantly higher values than boys ($p < 0.02$) (**Figures 5** and **6**).

Moreover, the comparison of the proportion of positive values of TSI/TSAb vs. TBII in the whole group of patients with untreated Graves' Disease and

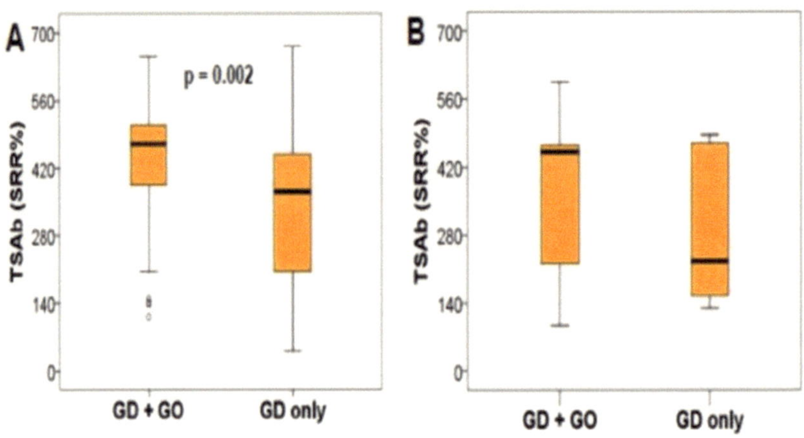

Figure 4.
Levels of thyroid stimulating immunoglobulins (TSAb): (A) untreated children; (B) children treated with Graves' Disease and with or without ophthalmopathy.

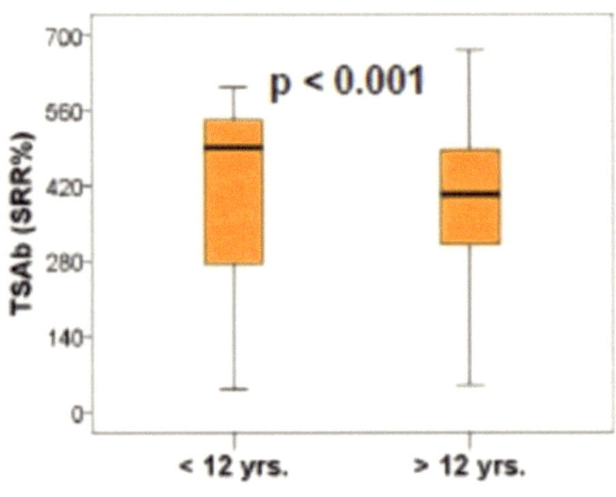

Figure 5.
Levels of thyroid stimulating immunoglobulins (TSAb) in children with Graves' Disease before and during adolescence.

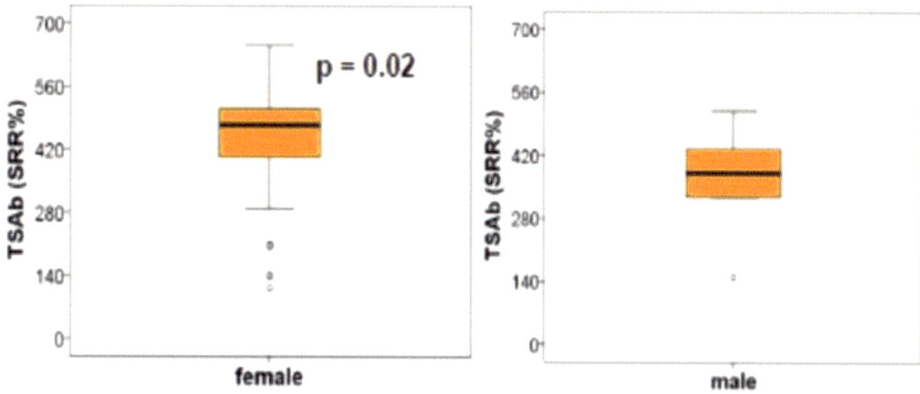

Figure 6.
Levels of thyroid stimulating immunoglobulins (TSAb) in females and males with Graves' Disease.

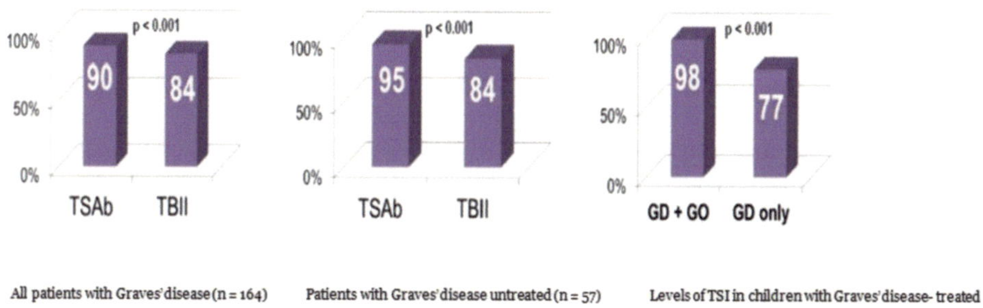

Figure 7.
Comparison of positive values of TSI/TSAb to TBII levels in all patients with Graves' Disease – untreated and with Graves' Disease and ophthalmopathy.

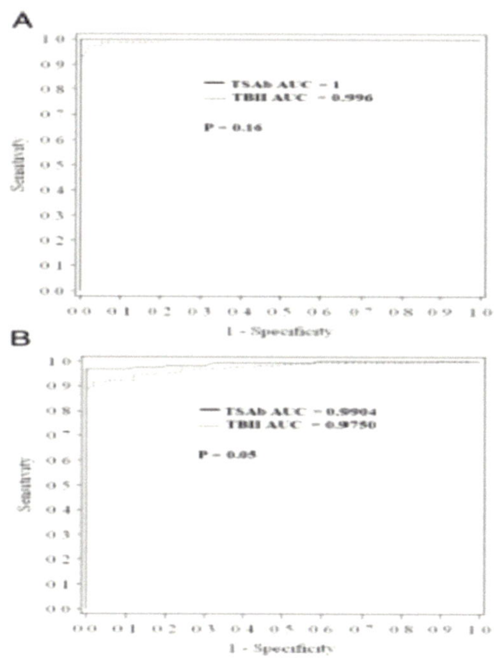

Figure 8.
ROC curves for TSI and TBII levels in patients with Graves' Disease; (A) untreated; (B) treated.

Graves' Disease with concomitant opthalmopathy revealed significantly higher values for TSAb than TBII in each group (**Figure** 7). The ROC curves for TSI and TBII in the above mentioned group of patients with Graves' Disease are presented in **Figure 8**.

Graves' Disease is also characterized by the presence of autoantibodies directed against various components of the thyroid, i.e. antibodies against thyroid peroxidase (anti-TPO), thyroglobulin (anti-TG). However, they are not highly specific and sensitive in the detection of this disease [15–17].

4. Clinical symptoms

Graves' Disease is a chronic disorder characterized by periods of exacerbations and remissions, with a differentiated clinical picture, slightly different in children as compared to adults. In the pediatric population, the CNS shows higher sensitivity to the excess of thyroid hormones and lower to the circulatory system. On the physical examination, the patient presents with restless behaviour and body mass deficiency despite good appetite. The child's skin becomes smooth, warm and moist, and the goiter is the most constant symptom. The thyroid goiter is usually evenly enlarged, with parenchymal density, smooth and painless. On palpation, throbbing and tremour of the gland can be felt, caused by enhanced blood flow, well heard (when auscultated above the thyroid) as a vascular murmur, mainly in the upper poles of the gland. The heart action is markedly accelerated and does not slow down at rest. In hyperthyroidism observed in the prepubertal group the growth rate and bone age advancement are accelerated due to increased release of growth hormone. The excess of thyroid hormones in early childhood is manifested by physical overreaction and concentration disorders. This effect is associated with the particular sensitivity of the CNS to the thyroid hormones, which affect α- and β-adrenergic postsynaptic receptors and increase serotonin release. In the prepubertal Graves' group neuropsychiatric symptoms have been observed including hyperirritability, locomotor anxiety, sleep and concentration disorders, which are manifested as worse academic performance and emotional lability. Ophthalmopathy in children with Graves' Disease is generally mild in nature and ocular lesions subside along with normalization of thyroid hormone secretion. Infiltrative-hydropic exophthalmos is rare. Pretibial edema in the pediatric group has a location similar to that in adults but is different in nature: it is soft and not well separated. **Table 1** presents the effect of hyperthyroidism on the respective systems.

Graves' Disease occurs in children with other autoimmune diseases, such as type 1 diabetes, Addison's disease, albinism, systemic lupus erythematosus, miastenia gravis, juvenile idiopathic arthritis, autoimmune thrombocytopenia, Addison-Biermer anemia. The risk of the disease is increased in children with trisomy 21, Turner syndrome and DiGeorge syndrome. In diabetic children metabolic balance is difficult to achieve. The course of the disease in these patients with concomitant hyperthyroidism is labile and it is difficult to compensate for glycemia. Demand for insulin increases, mainly as a result of developing insulin resistance and fast tissue insulin metabolism. At the same time intestinal glucose absorption is increased, gluconeogenesis is enhanced and glycogen synthesis is decreased. Moreover, in the states of thyrotoxicosis the secretion of growth hormone, which is also responsible for glycemia increase is elevated. In consequence, ketone acidosis frequently develops [1, 2].

Organs	Symptoms
Nervous system	Nervousness, irritability, emotional lability, sleep disturbance, headaches, learning difficulties, trembling of fingers, toes, tongue- fine tremor; motor incoherence, muscle weakness, excessive fatigue, especially of proximal muscles of limbs; reduction of tendon reflexes' duration;
Skin	Smooth, soft, satin skin; increased sweating and moistness; intensified warmth of the skin; vivid dermographism; delicate and breakable hair;
Eyes	Von Graefe's, Kocher's, Stellwag's, Popow's, Dalrynple's, Joffroy's signs- mild symptoms caused by stimulation of the sympathetic nevous system; Moebius' sign- lack of convergence; exophthalmos- bulging of the eye anteriorly out of the orbit;
Bones	Acceleration of growth rate and maturation of bone age in children; final height lower than expected due to early overgrowth of epiphyseal cartilages; intensive decay; limbs' pain; osteoporosis- typical for adults;
Circulatory system	Constant tachycardia; increase of systolic BP, decrease of diastolic BP (high amplitude of blood pressure); heart arythmia- premature atrial contractions, atrial fibrillation (especially in newborns); systolic murmur caused by hyperkinetic circulation; in ECG: increase of QRS amplitude; disturbance of repolarization phase; echocardiography: signs of hyperkinetic circulation;
Digestive system	Increased appetite combined with weight loss; accelerated intestinal passage and increased number of defecations; fatty diarrheas caused by inadequate secretion of pancreatic enzymes due to accelerated gastric emptying and increased intestinal peristalsis; absorption disorders;
Urinary tract	Increased thirst and polyuria due to increased index of glomerular filtration; hypercalcaemia, as the most frequent electrolyte disturbance in hyperthyroidism, impairs antidiuretic hormone activity, disturbs urine concentration and induces renal diabetes insipidus;
Reproductive system	Menstrual disorders; secondary lack of menstruation; decreased libido;

Table 1.
Impact of hyperthyroidism on different systems.

5. Diagnosis

5.1 Medical history and clinical examination

A detailed medical history and thorough clinical examination are indispensable for proper diagnosis. Clinical diagnosis of primary hyperthyroidism is confirmed by elevated levels of circulating thyroid hormones and TSH suppression to the values close to zero. In rare cases of hyperthyroidism, such as thyreotropinoma, ectopic TSH secretion and pituitary resistance to thyroid hormones, serum TSH level is usually elevated or inadequately normal, whereas the levels of thyroid hormones (fT_4 i/lub fT_3) are increased. With autoimmunization in Graves' Disease, the level of anti-TSHR antibodies is elevated. High titer of these antibodies allows for the exclusion of the toxic phase of Hashimoto thyroidits (hashitoxicosis) and subacute thyroiditis. Other antithyroid antibodies (a-TPO and a-ATG) are of minor importance. Very seldom, the co-occurrence of Graves' Disease and hashitoxicosis determines a positive titer of anti-TSHR antibodies.

5.2 Imaging investigations

Imaging investigations- thyroid ultrasound - is a subsequent stage in the diagnosis of hyperthyroidism; however, it is not indispensable for the diagnosis of Graves' Disease. In autoimmune hyperactivity, the thyroid is usually enlarged, with reduced echogenicity and markedly increased blood flow in color Doppler ultrasound (CDUS) and in power Doppler examination, with moderately increased flow in non-autoimmune hyperactivity caused by active mutation in TSH-R (**Figures 9** and **10**). Currently, due to high access to anti-TSHR antibody titer assays, gland scintigraphy with I^{123} or Tc^{99} is seldom performed. It used to be widely applied to differentiate between Graves' Disease, thyrotoxic phase of chronic lymphocytic thyroiditis, subacute thyroiditis and a hormonally active nodule.

5.3 Other examinations

If nodular lesions coexist, fine-needle aspiration biopsy (FNAB) of the thyroid should be performed. Elastography remains a complementary method to differentiate nodules [18].

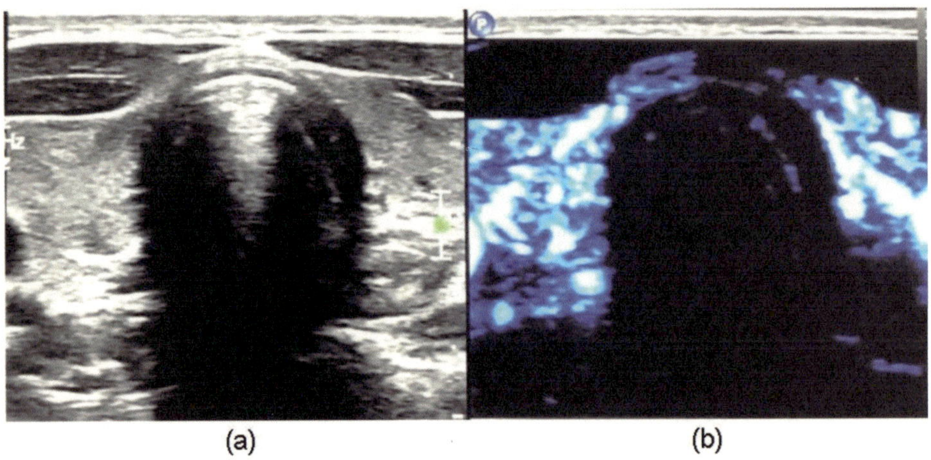

Figure 9.
Ultrasound image of hyperthyroidism in the course of active mutation in TSH receptor: (a) thyroid gland slightly enlarged bilaterally, inhomogeneous, hypoechogenic; (b) moderately increased vascular flow in Doppler ultrasonography.

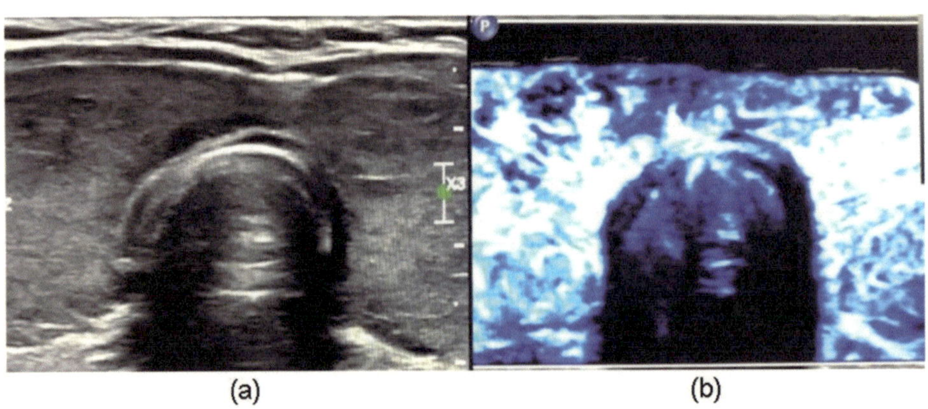

Figure 10.
Ultrasound image of hyperthyroidism in the course of Graves' Disease: (a) thyroid gland enlarged bilaterally, inhomogeneous, hypoechogenic; (b) increased, regular vascular flow in Doppler ultrasongraphy.

6. Treatment of hyperthyroidism

In most common type of hyperthyroidism in children with Graves' Disease causal treatment is unknown. The management involves pharmacotherapy (thyrostatics, β-adrenolitics), although sometimes radical radioiodine I^{131} therapy or surgical treatment is necessary. Some world literature reports indicate the application of immunotherapy in Graves ophtalmopathy in adults using rituximab (monoclonal anti-CD20 antibodies) to delete B cells. Thorough knowledge of the structure of human antibodies stimulating (M22) and blocking (Ki-70) TSHR has given great hope for their immunotherapeutic use in humans, including possible administration of blocking antibodies (TBI) to treat severe thyroid ophthalmopathy in the course of Graves' Disease. In children, conservative treatment with thyrostatics is most frequently used.

In clinical practice, two basic methods are used:

- the so called combined method ("block and replace" regimen), consisting in the inhibition of the production of thyroid hormones with a thyrostatic and administration of levothyroxin at a replacement dose (less recommended currently).

- adaptive method (titration regimen), based on monotherapy with a thyrostatic; smaller doses of the drug are used depending on the levels of thyroid hormones.

6.1 Thyrostatics

It is assumed that treatment with thyrostatics until eutyreosis is obtained usually lasts a few weeks (2–6 weeks), and complete treatment with gradually decreasing doses should be conducted for 24–36 months (**Figure 11A**). When Graves' Disease occurs in the prepubertal period the time of therapy prolons to 3–6 years (**Figure 11B**). In children thiamazoles are administered, namely imidazole, thiamazole (administered in one or two doses; 0.3–0.6 mg/kg/24 h, max. 30 mg/24 h), carbimazole (two or three doses daily; 0.4–0.8 mg/kg/24 h.

Propylothiouracyl, which 12–15 years ago used to be the most commonly administered medicine in the USA in the therapy of Graves' Disease, currently is not recommended and even contraindicated due to increased risk of severe liver damage. FDA reports have indicated that 1:2000 children may develop severe liver failure that will require transplantation as a consequence of propylothiouracyl administration. In 1:200 children reversible propylothiouracyl-dependent liver damage will occur. The only way to avoid liver injury is to withdraw this drug, limiting its use only to patients who are allergic to thiamazole and who have to be prepared to surgery or in children sensitive to thiamazole whose parents do not give their consent to radical treatment, as well as in the first trimester of pregnancy.

A -adrenolitic drug (athenolol 1–2 mg/kg in one dose or propranolol 1–2 mg/kg in 2–3 doses) is also administered for the first 2–4 weeks until euthyreosis is achieved to monitor hyperactivation of the cardiovascular system. Serum levels of fT_3 and fT_4 get normalized after 2–6 weeks, whereas TSH can be inhibited for a few months (3–6 on average). Therefore, in the initial phase of the treatment peripheral hormones should be monitored. Thyroid hormones usually need to be measured after 2 weeks, one month and then every month until TSH normalization. When f T_3 and f T_4 become normal the thyrostatic dose is

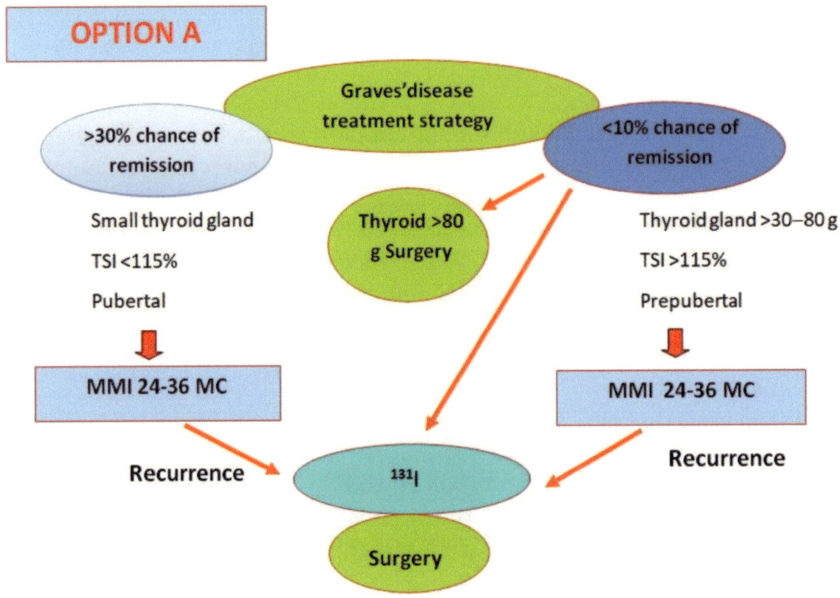

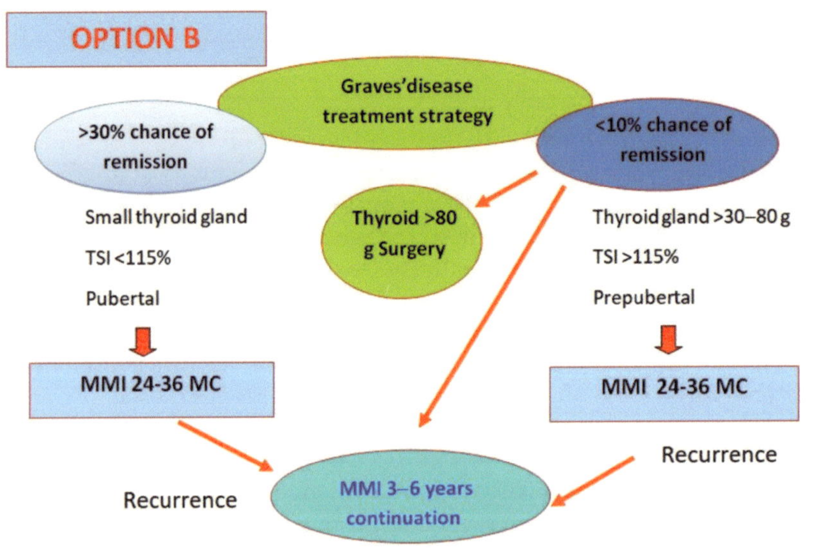

Figure 11.
*(A) Schemes of Graves' Disease treatment strategies: A option (**Figure 11A**) and B option (**Figure 11B**).*
*(B) Schemes of Graves' Disease treatment strategies: A option (**Figure 11A**) and B option (**Figure 11b**). Based on: Léger et al. [1].*

decreased by 30–50%, and then after the subsequent 3–6 weeks depending on the level of the hormones to the maintenance dose of 5–15/24 h. The persistence of antireceptor antibodies and difficulty in obtaining euthyrosis indicate high risk of relapse. Thus, remission is strictly related to the titer of TSI antibodies. When the titer is high, the chance of remission is 15%, and with a low titer approximately 50% of patients enter remission. Therefore, already at the start of the therapy, determination of TSI antibodies may help predict which patients are likely to achieve long-term remission of the disease.

The incidence of side-effects depends on the thyrostatic dose. All antithyroid drugs may cause goiter. Other undesirable effects include skin disorders, such as pruritus, urticarial or erythematosus exanthema, dyspepsia, arthralgia or transitory granulocytopenia (<1500 granulocytes/mm^3).

Agranulocytosis is rare (approximately 0.2% of cases). It should be remembered that as hyperthyreosis may lead to moderately increased neutropenia, complete blood cell count should be done prior to treatment and in any case of fever or strep throat. When the level of neutrophils is <1000/mm^3, the treatment should be discontinued or the dose decreased; at <500/mm^3 – further treatment is contraindicated.

In turn, the level of transaminases should be assessed prior to treatment implementation and possibly when a thyrostatic is introduced. Regular control of liver function is not justified. If symptoms of jaundice, gastrointestinal dysfunction or pruritis appear, measurements should include liver enzymes (ASPAT, ALT), total and bound bilirubin and ALP. Cholestatic jaundice, hepatitis or lupus-like syndrome are rare.

Other side-effects after propylothiouracyl administration include hepato-, neuro- and myelotoxic effects (with thrombocytopenia and agranulocytosis <250 granulocytes/mm^3) and vasculitis with the presence of ANCA antibodies. Thus, in the light of the current knowledge, children should not be treated with propylothiouracyl, and the recommended therapy should be based on thiamazole, radioactive iodine or surgery [19–22].

6.2 Radioiodine therapy

Radioiodine therapy is usually restricted to patients who are resistant to pharmacological treatment and who do not enter remission, or when they develop toxic reaction to a drug or have not complied with doctor's recommendations. The aim of the therapy is total destruction of the thyroid parenchyma by applying an ablative dose and in consequence obtaining permanent hypothyroidism. The advantages include easy application, lack of long-term side-effects and high efficacy of the first dose (approximately 95%). In the relapse of hyperthyroidism the subsequent dose of radioiodine can be administered 6 months after the first dose.

Young age (>5 years) is not a contraindication for this therapy, although much caution is required in children younger than 10. The risk of thyroid cancer in children exposed to I^{131} is the highest in those younger than 5 years due to increased vulnerability of the thyroid tissue to proliferative effects of ionizing radiation and gradually decreases in older age groups. Thus, children receive higher doses of radioiodine, i.e. a constant dose of 15 mCi, or doses dependent on the gland mass and its iodine uptake potential (150–200 μCi/g of thyroid tissue; 5.5–7.4 Mq/g; 12 000–16 000 cGy/g), so that to minimize the risk of secondary neoplasms. The radioiodine therapy should be followed by thyroxin substitution to manage hypothyroidim and avoid TSH increase. There is also no evidence that in the offspring of patients treated with I^{131} due to hyperthyreosis or thyroid cancer the risk of genetic defects is elevated (it is comparable to the risk noted in the general population).

Iodine (I^{131}) is usually administered after a break of 5–7 days in the application of the thyrostatic. Some suggest that antithyroid therapy should not be disrupted and the I^{131} dose needs to be increased by 20% to avoid the risk of an overactive thyroid storm. Otherwise, the use of -adrenolites and antiinflammatory non-steroids should be recommended to attenuate the symptoms of postradiation thyroiditis. Moreover, less common are nausea, pruritis of the neck skin, hypoparathyroidism or exacerbation of Graves ophthalmopathy. In this latter case, even though enhanced opthalmopathy in children is not frequent, protective treatment with glycocorticosteroids for 6–8 weeks should be considered (some recommend 3 months after radioiodine administration). Prolonged steroid therapy may have an effect on growth cartilage and body mass, and shows immunosuppresive action. Contraindications to radioiodine therapy are at the same time indications for surgery: large goiter >80 g, pressure symptoms, severe thyrotoxicosis with accompanying neurological symptoms, lack of iodine uptake of the thyroid, suspicion of a neopastic lesion, severe ophthalmopathy, age < 5 years, pregnancy and lactation, and also lack of consent to I^{131} treatment.

6.3 Surgical treatment

Surgical treatment of Graves' Disease is the oldest therapeutic method and total thyroidectomy which prevents relapse of hyperthyroidism is currently recommended. However, it is burdened with the risk of retrograde laryngeal nerve injury, hypoparathyroidism and more seldom hypothyroidism relapse (referring to 1–5% of children after total thyroidectomy vs. approximately 10–20% after partial or subtotal thyroidectomy). Sporadically, infection or keloid is observed at the site of the postoperative scar. The risk of complications depends to a large extent on the skills and experience of a surgeon. Importantly, prior to surgery a patient has to be treated with a thyrostatic drug and be in euthyreosis, receive iodide preparations (e.g. Lugol's solution or potassium iodide) 7–10 days before, 3–7 drops, each dose twice daily to reduce thyroid gland vascularity.

6.4 Excision of thyroid tissue

In rare cases of hyperthyroidism in children that is caused by the presence of autonomic tissue, radical treatment with thyroid removal or administration of ablation doses of radioiodine is recommended. In the state of thyroid hormone poisoning, the hormones need to be withdrawn and a -adrenolitic drug, e.g. propranolol, should be administered.

The therapy should be individually tailored and discussed both with the patient and the family [23–26].

7. Conclusions

- The diagnosis of Graves' Disease in children is based mainly on the determination of TSH suppresion and the presence of anti-TSHR antibodies.

- Thyroid ultrasound is not indispensable for the diagnosis; however, it allows for the assessment of the gland size and homogeneity.

- Scintigraphy is not required to diagnose Graves' Disease.

- The measurement of T_4 and T_3 is not obligatory in the diagnosis of Graves' Disease in children, but it is useful for treatment monitoring and to assess the prognosis of the disease relapse.

- Lack of anti-TSHR antibodies may suggest genetically inherited hyperthyroidism.

- The first-line treatment of Graves' Disease in children involves pharmacotherapy with imidazole, carbimazole, thiamazole at the initial dose of 0.4–0.8 mg/kg/24 h (0.3–0.6 mg/kg/24 h for thiamazole) depending on the disease severity to the maximum dose of 30 mg.

- Propylothiouracyl is contraindicated for children.
- Depending on patient's age, disease severity and the presence of anti-TSHR antibodies the initial therapy should last 3–6 years.
- Prior to the treatment implementation, peripheral blood cell count measurement should be performed to assess the grade of neutropenia caused by hyperthyroidism. Regular determination of blood count during check-ups is not necessary.
- Blood count should be performed if the patient is feverish or has strep throat. Neutrophil count $<1000/mm^3$ is an indication for treatment discontinuation or dose reduction; $<500/mm^3$ - further treatment is absolutely contraindicated!
- The level of transaminases should be determined prior to treatment. Regular control of liver function is not justified.
- When jaundice, gastrointestinal tract dysfunction or pruritis appear, liver enzymes (ASPAT, ALAT), total and bound bilirubin and ALP should be determined..
- Patients and their parents should be informed about possible side-effects of thyrostatics.
- Patients and their families should be informed about prognosis (50% of patients obtain remission after a few years of treatment) and possibilities of radical treatment.
- Female patients with Graves' Disease (both in the course of remission and after radical treatment) require endocrinology care prior to and during planned pregnancy.
- Indications for radical treatment include contraindications to pharmacology, poor results of pharmacotherapy, repeated prolongation of therapy, parents' and child's request.
- Thyroidectomy is a radical method applied in children before the age of 5 years or in the case of large goiter, nodular goiter or goiter pressing the organs.
- The experience of a surgeon performing thyroidectomy in children is the major factor responsible for postoperative complications.
- Radioiodine therapy is recommended after the age of 5 years if the goiter is not too large (more frequently in puberty).
- Education of patients and parents is important to ensure the best possible response to treatment.

Conflict of interest

The authors declare no conflict of interest.

Author details

Artur Bossowski* and Karolina Stożek
Department of Pediatrics, Endocrinology, Diabetology with Cardiology Unit, Medical University of Bialystok, Poland

*Address all correspondence to: abossowski@hotmail.com

References

[1] Léger J, Oliver I, Rodrigue D, et al. Graves' disease in children. Ann Endocrinol (Paris) 2018;79(6):647-55.

[2] Léger J. Graves' disease in children. Endocr Dev 2014;26:171-82.

[3] Bossowski A, Borysewicz-Sańczyk H, Wawrusiewicz-Kurylonek N, et al. Analysis of chosen polymorphisms in FoxP3 gene in children and adolescents with autoimmune thyroid diseases. Autoimmunity 2014;47(6):395-400.

[4] Lombardi A, Menconi F, Greenberg D, et al. Dissecting the Genetic Susceptibility to Graves' Disease in a Cohort of Patients of Italian Origin. Front Endocrinol (Lausanne) 2016;7:21.

[5] Rydzewska M, Góralczyk A, Gościk J, et al. Analysis of chosen polymorphisms rs2476601 a/G - PTPN22, rs1990760 C/T - IFIH1, rs179247 a/G - TSHR in pathogenesis of autoimmune thyroid diseases in children. Autoimmunity 2018;51(4):183-90.

[6] Ferrari SM, Fallahi P, Antonelli A, et al. Environmental Issues in Thyroid Diseases. Front Endocrinol (Lausanne) 2017;8:50.

[7] Katagiri R, Yuan X, Kobayashi S, et al. Effect of excess iodine intake on thyroid diseases in different populations: A systematic review and meta-analyses including observational studies. PLoS One 2017;12(3): e0173722.

[8] Wang B, Shao X, Song R, et al. The Emerging Role of Epigenetics in Autoimmune Thyroid Diseases. Front Immunol 2017; 8:396.

[9] Wiersinga WM. Clinical Relevance of Environmental Factors in the Pathogenesis of Autoimmune Thyroid Disease. Endocrinol Metab (Seoul) 2016;31(2):213-22.

[10] Bossowski A, Moniuszko M, Dąbrowska M, et al. Lower proportions of $CD4+CD25^{high}$ and CD4+FoxP3, but not $CD4+CD25+CD127^{low}$ $FoxP3^{+}$T cell levels in children with autoimmune thyroid diseases. Autoimmunity 2013;46(3):222-30.

[11] Bossowski A, Moniuszko M, Idźkowska E, et al. Decreased proportions of CD4 + IL17+/CD4 + CD25 + CD127– and CD4 + IL17+/CD4 + CD25 + CD127 – FoxP3+ T cells in children with autoimmune thyroid diseases. Autoimmunity 2016;49(5):320-8.

[12] Pyzik A, Grywalska E, Matyjaszek-Matuszek B, et al. Immune disorders in Hashimoto's thyroiditis: what do we know so far? J Immunol Res 2015; 2015:979167.

[13] Rydzewska M, Jaromin M, Stożek K, et al. Role of the T and B lymphocytes in pathogenesis of autoimmune thyroid diseases. Thyroid Res 2018;11:2.

[14] Stożek K, Grubczak K, Marolda V, et al. Lower proportion of CD19+IL-10+ and CD19+CD24+CD27+ but not CD1d+CD5+CD19+CD24+CD27+ IL-10+ B cells in children with autoimmune thyroid diseases. Autoimmunity 2020 Feb;53(1):46-55.

[15] Bano A, Gan E, Addison C, et al. Age may influence the impact of TRAbs on thyroid function and relapse-risk in patients with Graves' disease. J Clin Endocrinol Metab 2019;104:1378– 85.

[16] Diana T, Brown RS, Bossowski A, et al.Clinical relevance of thyroid-stimulating autoantibodies in pediatric graves' disease-a multicenter study. J Clin Endocrinol Metab 2014;99(5):1648-55.

[17] Stożek K, Bossowski A, Ziora K, et al. Functional TSH receptor

antibodies in children with autoimmune thyroid diseases. Autoimmunity 2018;51(2):62-8.

[18] Léger J, Carel JC. Diagnosis and management of hyperthyroidism from prenatal life to adolescence. Best Pract Res Clin Endocrinol Metab 2018;32:373– 86.

[19] John M, Sundrarajan R, Gomadam SS. Anti-thyroid drugs in pediatric Graves' disease. Indian J Endocrinol Metab 2015;19:340-6.

[20] Kahaly GJ, Bartalena L, Hegedüs L, et al. 2018 European Thyroid Association Guideline for the Management of Graves' Hyperthyroidism. Eur Thyroid J 2018;7(4):167-86.

[21] Léger J, Carel JC. Management of endocrine disease: Arguments for the prolonged use of antithyroid drugs in children with Graves' disease. Eur J Endocrinol 2017;177:R59–R67.

[22] Wang SY, Wang CT, Tien KJ, et al. Thyroid-stimulating hormone receptor antibodies during follow-up as remission markers in childhood-onset Graves' disease treated with antithyroid drugs. Kaohsiung J Med Sci 2019. doi: 10.1002/kjm2.12167.

[23] Committee on Pharmaceutical Affairs, Japanese Society for Pediatric Endocrinology, and the Pediatric Thyroid Disease Committee, Japan Thyroid Association (Taskforce for the Revision of the Guidelines for the Treatment of Childhood-Onset Graves' Disease), Minamitani K, Sato H, Ohye H, Harada S, Arisaka O. Guidelines for the treatment of childhood-onset Graves' disease in Japan, 2016. Clin Pediatr Endocrinol 2017;26(2):29-62.

[24] Rabon S, Burton AM, White PC. Graves' disease in children: long-term outcomes of medical therapy. Clin Endocrinol (Oxf) 2016;85(4):632-5.

[25] Rivkees SA. Controversies in the management of Graves' disease in children. J Endocrinol Invest 2016;39(11):1247-57.

[26] Ross DS, Burch HB, Cooper DS, et al. 2016 American thyroid association guidelines for diagnosis and management of hyperthyroidism and other causes of thyrotoxicosis. Thyroid 2016; 26:1343-421.

Chapter 17

Unusual Presentation and Rare Comorbidity of Graves-Basedow's Disease in Children

Agota Muzsnai

Abstract

Graves'-Basedow's disease (GD) is a well-defined hyperthyroid disorder caused by circulating antibodies that results the overproduction of thyroid hormones. All but a few children present with some degree of thyroid gland enlargement and most have two or more signs of excessive thyroid activity, such as tremor, irritability/nervousness, tachycardia etc. Fully developed clinical picture is easy to recognize while often the onset is insidious. Thyroid hormones affect many body systems, so signs and symptoms of Graves' Disease can be wide ranging. A survey on PubMed literature was conducted to gather all published pediatric Graves-Basedow's cases with unusual presentation at the time of diagnosis. We found all together 70 manuscripts with relevant information from 1978 to 2020 but mainly adult cases. One third of them were found to meet the criteria we focused on and were included in this paper, though in some situation the unusual findings do not consist part of hyperthyroidism, the rare manifestation is only a coexistence, or the serious disease even precedes the GD. Dermatopathy, hepatic dysfunction, impaired fluid balance, concomitant disorders in thyrotoxicosis, tricky laboratory findings, a phenomenon of metamorphic thyroid autoimmunity, peculiarities of thyroid dysfunction in children with Down syndrome, apparent associations, and reconstitution GD are highlighted in this chapter. Awareness about the relation of these remote findings to GD, or frequent coexistence with GD is important for early diagnosis. Finally, a reasonable suspicion for Graves' Disease may ultimately help to prevent unnecessary investigations and treatment.

Keywords: hyperthyroidism, thyrotoxicosis, thyroid autoimmunity, antibodies, rare disorder, Hashimoto thyroiditis, Turner syndrome, Down syndrome, reconstitution GD, children

1. Introduction

In pediatric age group the Grave's-Basedow disease (GD) is by far the most common cause of hyperthyroidism, accounting for greater than 95% of cases. The underlying process is an autoimmune reaction with cell proliferation and excess function (overproduction of thyroid hormone) caused by anti-thyrotropin receptor antibody (TRAb). When using term thyrotoxicosis, it depicts the clinical and biochemical manifestations of excess thyroid hormones. The annual incidence of thyrotoxicosis was less than 1 per 100,000 children <15 years of age in the last century and rised slowly above 1.5 per 100,000 by 2012 with the pubertal dominance up to 80%. In spite of the GD is a rare disorder in children, physicians should consider Graves' Disease in any child with clinical manifestations of hyperthyroidism, regardless of the age.

All but a few GD children present with some degree of thyroid gland enlargement and most have two or more signs of excessive thyroid activity. The clinical manifestations of hyperthyroidism during fetal life are tachycardia, cardiac arrhythmia, intrauterine growth retardation and may be associated with nonimmune fetal hydrops, craniosynostosis. Features of this condition in the neonate include irritability, tachycardia, hypertension, cardiac failure and arrhythmias, diarrhea, poor weight gain, vomiting, jaundice, hepatosplenomegaly, ophthalmopathy, craniosynostosis and thyroid enlargement. In childhood hyperkinesis, tachycardia, tremor, frequent stools, nervousness are the signs of hyperthyroidism but in young children these are less characteristic, often unrecognized. In school-age hyperthyroidism neuropsychiatric symptoms such as hyperactivity and poor school performance are common features. Adolescents usually present with classic signs including weight loss despite of good appetite, diarrhea, nervousness, and heat intolerance. Fully developed clinical picture is easy to recognize while often the onset is insidious. Thyroid hormones affect many body systems, so signs and symptoms of Graves' Disease can be wide ranging.

This chapter is aimed to draw attention to less common or less distinctive signs and symptoms which can be in relation to GD at the time of diagnosis. A survey was conducted on PubMed literature to gather all published pediatric Graves-Basedow's cases with unusual presentation at the time of diagnosis. We found all together 70 publications with relevant information from 1978 to 2020 but mainly adult cases. Half of them (36) were found to meet the criteria we focused on and were included in this paper, though in some situation the unusual findings do not consist part of hyperthyroidism, the rare manifestation is only a coexistence, or the serious disease even precedes the GD. Awareness about the relation of these rare manifestations or disorders to GD is essential to avoid wrong diagnosis, unnecessary investigations, or fatal outcome due to delay of diagnosis.

2. Unusual signs and symptoms

2.1 Dermopathy and acropachy

Thyroid dermopathy (TD), also called pretibial myxedema and thyroid acropachy (TA) together with Graves' orbitopathy (GO) are extrathyroidal manifestations of GD. Graves' ophthalmopathy in children not as common as in adults and less severe than in later age. Dermatological symptoms are rare and in general develop sequentially: Dermopathy is usually present if the patient is also affected with GO. The very rare acropachy occurs only in patients who also have dermopathy [1]. Or in other words, acropachy is an indicator of severity of ophthalmopathy and dermopathy. All have an autoimmune origin, the immune reaction is targeted to TSH receptor and, likely, the IGF-I receptor. Typical presentation of dermopathy is nonpitting edema or plaque-like lesions on the pretibial region, while thyroid acropachy presents as digital clubbing, swelling of digits and toes, and periosteal reaction of extremity bones. Awareness about the relation of TA to GD is important as clubbing usually is not a patient complaint and is noted only by clinical observers. Recently Kraus CN and al. reported a case of acropachy in a child as well as reviewed the literature of pediatric thyroid dermopathy [2].

2.2 Cholestasis

Hepatic dysfunction is commonly observed in patients with thyroid disease, it can be categorized mainly into group with either hepatocellular damage (transaminases elevations), or intrahepatic cholestasis (bilirubin elevation). In newborn, the hypothyroidism is the most typical thyroid disorder associated with cholestasis. Jaundice due to intrahepatic cholestasis may be a salient symptom in GD patients, and very occasionally, it is the presenting manifestation of thyrotoxicosis. The mechanism of liver injury in pure hyperthyroid states is not well understood, and no correlation was documented between abnormal liver biochemical tests and thyroid hormone levels. A contributing factor appears to be relative hypoxia in the perivenular regions, due to an increase in hepatic oxygen demand without an appropriate increase in hepatic blood flow [3], the other might be the thyroid hormones themselves with a direct toxic effect on hepatic tissue in hypermetabolic state [4]. If other possible causes of cholestasis are excluded, recovery occurs parallelly with restoration of euthyroidism. In the absence of another evidence of liver disease, and when jaundice is purely due to the hyperthyroidism, thionamide drugs may be used with monitoring of serum bilirubin and liver function tests [5]. Newborns and adolescent patient were reported with jaundice/hyperbilirubinemia as manifestation of GD hyperthyroidism [6–8].

2.3 Polydipsia, nocturnal enuresis

Disturbance of water homeostasis can lead to polyuria-polydipsia syndrome, which is a diagnostic challenge. Polydipsia is a nonspecific symptom in various diseases, often accompanied by polyuria. Increased thirst and/or nocturnal enuresis can be the main complains, and a careful case history usually reveals the primary reason (disturbed input or output). Polydipsia has been described as a presenting symptom of hyperthyroidism in adults. A few years back a serendipitous identification of GD in identical twin girls with polydipsia was published [9]. Though etiology of nocturnal enuresis is not fully understood, evidence is growing that enuresis may have a central origin: bedwetting children have lower brainstem reflex control (impaired prepulse inhibition) than normal controls [10]. A case of a 9-year-old boy has been reported by the same team who suffered from hyperthyroidism and a new appearance of enuresis. Bedwetting ceased and prepulse inhibition – measured as a parameter of central control – increased during on course of anti-thyroid therapy [11]. In our praxis we experienced two GD cases where nighttime incontinence was the presenting feature of recurrent hyperthyroidism.

3. Rare concomitant disorders

3.1 Thyrotoxic periodic paralysis

Thyrotoxic periodic paralysis (TPP) is a rare disease of the muscles secondary to hyperthyroidism presenting sudden attacks of short-term muscle weakness, stiffness, or paralysis. The underlying mechanism is malfunctions in the ion channels in skeletal muscle cell membranes: An increased influx of potassium into skeletal muscle cells leads to profound hypokalemia and paralysis. Hypokalemia in thyrotoxic hypokalemic periodic paralysis (THPP) results from an intracellular shift of potassium and not total body depletion. The symptoms may be mild or severe, and they may last for minutes or days, involving the whole body or just one or both limbs. The severity of the disease does not correlate with the hormone levels, and muscle paralysis simply resolves by achieving the euthyroid state. TPP most frequently seen in Asian men and also reported in Hispanic adolescent males [12, 13]. Fatal outcome of a 10-years-old girl with delayed diagnosis of hyperthyroidism should draw attention to the awareness about this rare but potentially lethal disorder [14].

3.2 Encephalopathy

Presenting feature of encephalopathy in GD and Hashimoto's thyroiditis would be similar (seizures, stroke-like episodes, cognitive decline, neuropsychiatric symptoms etc.) but characteristics of thyroid derangement is reversed. Thyroid function is not an issue in Hashimoto's encephalopathy which is renamed now as 'steroid responsive encephalopathy associated with autoimmune thyroiditis (SREAT)', while brain dysfunction is associated to hyperthyroid state in GD. Hecht T and coworkers reported on a 7-year-old girl with generalized seizures, somnolence, fever, and respiratory distress. The increase of sinus tachycardia with good hydration, sufficient analgesia, and hyperthermia led to the determination of thyroid hormones, and therefore finally to the diagnosis of a thyrotoxic crisis in Graves' Disease. Symptoms were disappeared by thyrostatic therapy [15]. They concluded that thyrotoxic crisis should be considered a differential diagnosis in case of resistant unexplained sinus tachycardia, seizures, and encephalopathy.

4. TSHR-blocking autoantibody (TBAb)

In Graves-Basedow's patients TRAb stimulates thyroid hormone synthesis by activating the TSH receptor (stimulating TRAb /TSAb/, TSHR agonist). TSHR antibodies that lack agonistic activity but are competitive inhibitors of TSH binding can cause hypothyroidism (blocking TRAb/TBAb/, TSHR antagonist). There is a wide variety of TSHR antibody assays employed in the past and nowadays. Depending on the underlying method, two types of assays are important for determination of circulating autoantibodies: Competition for ligand binding or measuring bio-response. A rare history of monozygotic 10-year-old twins was published who presented with hyper- and hypothyroidism, respectively [16]. Both girls had antibodies against thyrotropin receptors as measured by a radioreceptor assay. Analyzing further the sera in a functional bioassay, the TSH receptor antibodies of the hyperthyroid twin displayed stimulatory activity typical of Graves' Disease, while the antibodies of the hypothyroid twin acted as pure antagonists at the TSH receptor level. This is a proven pediatric case with hypothyroidism due to thyroid (or TSH)-blocking antibodies, where the pathogenesis was similar to GD. In the following 30 years an extensive work of research groups has led to significant improvements that has enabled bioassays to be employed routinely in clinical laboratories: 1, Two human monoclonal antibodies (MAbs) with TSHR agonist activity (M22 and K1-18), one human MAb with TSHR antagonist activity (K1-70) and one human MAb (5C9) with both TSHR antagonist and TSHR inverse agonist activity have been isolated [17]. 2, Currently available highly sensitive and specific assays to measure TRAbs use the human TSHR monoclonal antibody (Mab) M22 instead of the TSH [18]. Based on a research-use only service offered by RSR Limited, an adult case of woman with fluctuating hypo- and hyperthyroidism was published providing proof that a patient can produce a mixture of blocking and stimulating TSHR autoantibodies at the same time [19].

5. Metamorphic thyroid autoimmunity

Here we overview the phenomenon of metamorphic thyroid autoimmunity anticipating, that more investigational studies are needed to reveal the underlying mechanism, and larger epidemiological studies are needed to confirm that this finding is not unusual but is rather under-recognized in pediatric population. The term metamorphic thyroid autoimmunity was introduced by Ludgate M. and Emerson H. commenting cases with a conversion from Hashimoto thyroiditis (HT) to GD or vice versa [20–22]. A few years later Wasniewska M et al. aimed to ascertain HT in the history of GD children order to assess the relative frequency of this phenomenon [23]. Based on retrospective data of a cohort of 109 GB children and adolescents without coexistent chromosome abnormalities they calculated the frequency between 3 and 4%. Reporting results they confirmed the existence of a possible continuum between HT and GD within the spectrum of autoimmune thyroid diseases. In search of switching process from HT to GB in patient with either Turner syndrome (TS) or Down syndrome (DS) the same team found that antecedents of HT were significantly more common in chromosomopathy group (9/35 = 25.7%) compared to age-matched GD patients (4/109 = 3.7%) [24]. Guessing the clue of this immunological paradigm it should take into high consideration that attribute of HE is a cell-mediated destruction of thyroid tissue with hypo- or euthyroidism while GB is a TRAB-mediated gland activation presented in hyperthyroidism. In general, thyroid autoimmunity involves loss of tolerance to thyroid proteins in genetically susceptible individuals in association with environmental factors, no single mechanism explains the altered immune-reaction. Further immunological and genetic investigations can add explanatory information to this unusual pendulum swinging thyroid autoimmunity.

6. Peculiarities in Down syndrome

6.1 Asymptomatic vs. cumulative presentation

Thyroid derangement is the most frequently encountered endocrinopathy in Down syndrome (DS) affecting almost half of the patients (7 - 66%). Based on this fact the life-long monitoring of the thyroid function is recommended for all DS patients. Thyroid abnormalities encompass mainly any kind of hypothyroidism (congenital, primary, subclinical, or overt hypothyroidism), isolated hyperthyrotropinemia, Hashimoto thyroiditis or very rarely GD. Autoimmune thyroid disease is uncommon in young children with Down's syndrome but is common after 8 years of age [25]. A Spanish group [26] reported on three DS children with GD: Two of them were asymptomatic for thyroid hyperfunction (a 14-year-old girl and an 8-year-old boy), while the third child (a 12-year-old girl) presented goiter, nervousness, weight loss and tachycardia. In addition to the typical features of hyperthyroidism, the patient showed right-side heart failure and elevated transaminases, which disappeared with antithyroid treatment. Though annual biochemical screening for early detection of thyroid hypofunction is reasonable, regular auxological and clinical assessment in syndromic patients is also important.

6.2 Metamorphic thyroid autoimmunity

HT and GB are two different disease entities in the spectrum of thyroid autoimmunity presenting dominantly with hypothyroidism (HT) or with hyperthyroidism

(GB). A metamorphosis of both clinical and biochemical phenotype from HT to GD or vice versa has been discussed for more than 10 years [22] based on sporadic cases. A tapered Italian team conducted several retrospective studies to shed light on this phenomenon in pediatric population. In 2015 they published a research paper reconstructing the conversion process from HT to GD and the subsequent evolution of GD in a series of 12 children (7 girls/5 boys) with DS [27]. All patients fulfilled the criteria for diagnosis of HT and GD taking laboratory measurements and ultrasonography scan. Time interval between HT diagnosis and GB presentation ranged from 0.7 to 6.5 years, and Graves' Disease showed a milder clinical and biochemical course in this cohort. Summing up they conclude that „1, DS children might be incline to manifest over time a phenotypic metamorphosis from HT to GH and to subsequently fluctuate from hyperthyroidism to hypothyroidism; 2) in DS GD may have a mild biochemical and clinical course" [27].

6.3 Unusual scenario

A DS case with an unusual thyroid constellation were published by Nebesio TD and Eugster EA. „ A 10-year-old girl with Down syndrome was diagnosed with congenital hypothyroidism in the newborn period due to left thyroid hemiagenesis. Unexpectedly, her hypothyroidism resolved at the age of 3 years. After being off thyroid hormone replacement for 7 years and having normal thyroid function, she developed Graves' Disease with typical signs and symptoms of hyperthyroidism including diarrhea, inattention, and hyperactivity" [28]. This case highlights also the unpredictable course of thyroid disease which may occur in children with Down syndrome.

7. Coincidence in polyendocrinopathy APS3

The autoimmune polyglandular syndromes (APS1-4) encompass a wide clinical spectrum of disease with different (monogenic/complex) genetic etiologies and heterogeneous presentation. APS2 is defined by presence of primary adrenocortical insufficiency with either autoimmune thyroid disease or type 1 diabetes mellitus in the same patient. The clinical diagnosis of APS3 requires the presence of an autoimmune thyroid disease and an additional autoimmune illness other than Addison's disease; a frequent combination is pernicious anemia, vitiligo, alopecia, myasthenia gravis and Sjögren sy. Thyroid disease purports a variety of thyroid disorders. Hypothyroidism is more common than Graves' Disease, and GD tends to manifest at a younger age. Recently Klenczar K and coworkers reported on a 11-year-old female patient, who presented coincidence of T1DM with other autoimmune diseases, such as Graves-Basedow's disease, myasthenia gravis, vitiligo, and IgA deficiency [29]. The clinical picture of this case fulfilled the criteria of autoimmune polyglandular syndrome type 3.

8. Unexpected coexistence

Stickler syndrome is a rare genetically heterogeneous disorder of the connective tissue, caused by abnormal synthesis of type II, XI, or IX collagen. It is characterized by a distinctive facial appearance, eye abnormalities, hearing loss and joint problems. Ocular involvements are early onset cataract, myopia, abnormal vitreous humor, retinal detachment, and most of the patients exhibit short stature. Onesimo R et al. reported on a 5-year-old girl affected by Stickler syndrome who was diagnosed with GD in preclinical state, during health supervision and evaluation by pediatric endocrinologist for short stature [30]. None of her family member suffered from autoimmune thyroid disorder and her medical history was negative for autoimmune disease. Association between Stickler's syndrome and GD in this case seems to be an incidental coexistence.

9. Reconstitution Graves' Disease

Reviewing the manuscripts on Graves' Disease and rare comorbidity, a new issue has been raised. Growing numbers of publication on the association between biological treatment for life-threatening and/or medication-refractory disorders, and the development of autoimmune hyperthyroidism in adults, call the attention to secondary GD [31, 32]. The use of different modality targeting the immune system as a curative therapy (e.g. hematopoietic stem cell transplantation /HSCT/, antithymocite globulin/ATG/, antiretroviral therapy/ART/etc.), has had a profound impact on clinical outcomes. A subset of patients may experience immune restoration disease (IRD)/immune reconstitution inflammatory syndrome (IRIS) affecting the thyroid gland in two form, such as Hashimoto thyroiditis or Graves' hyperthyroidism. Although both are more common in children because of early thymic damage, it has received little attention in pediatric literature [33]. Sporadic cases were reported on challenging autoimmune processes: Defective T-cell function take place during the pathogenesis both of aplastic anemia (AA) and GD. Antithyroid drugs used for the management of GD may induce AA and GD may occur following treatment of severe aplastic anemia (SAA). The latter occurred in a 11-year-old girl who had been treated with allogenic HSCT at age of 8 years as having severe acquired AA [34]. A case of another child was published earlier with chronic relapsing severe aplastic anemia and GD [35]. Authors supposed a close relation in manifestation of hypertyroidism due to withdrawal of immunosuppressants. In adult patients the secondary GD may exhibit a fluctuating course, with alternating phases of hyper- and hypothyroidism, due to the coexistence of TRAb with stimulating and blocking function [36]. Clinicians need to remain vigilant when initiating immune reconstitution therapy, and a careful management and follow-up for thyroid function after these treatments are essential.

10. Discussion

In this chapter we presented a spectrum of unusual clinical findings, signs of Graves-Basedow's disease in childhood, but atypical laboratory results. Less common and less distinctive features detailed above are well documented in adults, which suggests that these are neither age-dependent nor characteristic to pediatric GD. Though the mechanism remains uncertain in majority of unusual manifestations, the recovery that occurs parallelly with restoration of euthyroidism, gives the evidence of their relation to GB hyperthyroidism. Metamorphic thyroid autoimmunity, a phenomenon of conversion from Hashimoto thyroiditis to Graves' Disease is also summarized without guessing the clue of this immunological paradigm. Existence of a continuum between HT and GD within the spectrum of thyroid autoimmunity is confirmed in pediatric population without coexistent chromosome abnormalities, also in children with Turner or Down syndrome. Beside this peculiar event sequence, GD in DS patient can be insidious by presenting delayed clinical symptoms even with multiple organ derangements. In some rare syndromic disorder regular clinical assessment and biochemical screening supports to reveal the occurrence of Graves' hyperthyroidism. Finally, a very vulnerable population with malignancy, immune deficiency syndromes, hemoglobinopathies and other disorders attract attention with a possible secondary GB following immune reconstitution therapy. Awareness about the relation of these remote findings to GD, or frequent coexistence with GD is important for early diagnosis, and a reasonable suspicion for Graves' Disease may ultimately help to prevent unnecessary investigations and treatment.

Author details

Agota Muzsnai
North-Buda Center, New St John's Hospital and Outpatient Clinic, Department of Pediatric Endocrinology, Budapest, Hungary

*Address all correspondence to: muzsnaia@freemail.hu

References

[1] Bartalena L, Fatourechi V: Extrathyroidal manifestations of Graves' disease: a 2014 update. J Endocrinol Invest. 2014 Aug;37(8):691-700. doi: 10.1007/s40618-014-0097-2. Epub 2014 Jun 10.

[2] Kraus CN, Sodha P, Vaidyanathan P, Kirkorian AY: Thyroid dermopathy and acropachy in pediatric patients. Pediatr Dermatol. 2018 Nov;35(6):e371-e374. doi: 10.1111/pde.13670. Epub 2018 Sep 6. PMID: 30187962

[3] Malik R and Hodgson H: The relationship between the thyroid gland and the liver. QJM, vol. 95, no. 9, pp. 559-569, 2002

[4] Owen PJ, Baghomian A, Lazarus JH, Godkin AJ: An unusual cause of jaundice. British Medical Journal, vol. 335, no. 7623, pp. 773-774, 2007.

[5] Hegazi MO, Ahmed S: Atypical clinical manifestations of Graves' disease: An analysis in depth. J Thyroid Res. 2012; 2012: 768019. Published online 2011 Nov 1. doi: 10.1155/2012/768019 PMCID: PMC3206356

[6] Beroukhim RS, Moon TD, Felner EI: Neonatal thyrotoxicosis and conjugated hyperbilirubinemia. J Matern Fetal Neonatal Med. 2003;13(6):426-428.

[7] Loomba-Albrecht LA, Bremer AA, Wong A, Philippset AF: Neonatal cholestasis due to hyperthyroidism: an unusual case and clinical implications. J Pediatr Gastroenterol Nutr 2012;54:433-434

[8] Regelmann MO, Miloh T, Arnon R, Morotti R, Kerkar N, Rapaport R: Graves' disease presenting with severe cholestasis. Thyroid. 2012 Apr;22(4):437-439. doi: 10.1089/thy.2011.0267

[9] Goldyn AK, Eugster EA, Nebesio TD: Serendipitous identification of Graves' disease in identical twins with polydipsia. J Pediatr Endocrinol Metab. 2010 Dec;23(12):1335-7. doi: 10.1515/jpem.2010.208. PMID: 21714468; PMCID: PMC4096950.

[10] Meir J, Eggert P: Prepulse inhibition of the startle reflex for differentiation of enuresis in children. Pediatr Nephrol. 2011 Jun;26(6):939-943. doi: 10.1007/s00467-011-1817-x. Epub 2011 Mar 5. PMID: 21373778

[11] Meir J, Roessner D, Eggert P: Enuresis in hyperthyroidism: a temporary lack of central control mechanism leads to nocturnal enuresis. Acta Paediatr. 2009; 99:145-146. PubMed: 19811458

[12] Al-Zubeidi H, Demeterco C, Jones KL: Thyrotoxic, hypokalemic periodic paralysis (THPP) in adolescents. J Pediatr Endocrinol Metab. 2015 Jan;28(1-2):157-161. doi: 10.1515/jpem-2014-0016. PMID: 25153560.

[13] Doležel Z, Novotná D, Schneiderová H, Papež J, Jouza M: Thyrotoxic periodic paralysis. Pediatr. praxi 2016; 17(6): 379-382 | DOI: 10.36290/ped.2016.083

[14] Satam N, More V, Shanbag P, Kalgutkar A: Fatal thyrotoxic periodic paralysis with normokalemia. Indian J Pediatr. 2007 Nov;74(11):1041-1043. doi: 10.1007/s12098-007-0194-8. PMID: 18057690

[15] Hecht T, Brand J, Vlaho S: Encephalopathy and sinustachycardia in childhood -- a possible differential diagnosis. J Pediatr Endocrinol Metab. 2012;25(1-2):149-151. doi: 10.1515/jpem-2011-0436. PMID: 22570965.

[16] Ilicki A, Marcus C, Karlsson FA: Hyperthyroidism and hypothyroidism

in monozygotic twins: detection of stimulating and blocking THS receptor antibodies using the FRTL5-cell line. J Endocrinol Invest. 1990 Apr;13(4):327-331. doi: 10.1007/BF03349571. PMID: 2164548

[17] Sanders J, Miguel RN, Furmaniak J, Smith BR: TSH receptor monoclonal antibodies with agonist, antagonist, and inverse agonist activities. Methods Enzymol. 2010;485:393-420. doi: 10.1016/B978-0-12-381296-4.00022-1. PMID: 21050929

[18] Furmaniak J, Sanders J, Sanders P, Miller-Gallacher J, Ryder MM, Smith BR: Practical applications of studies on the TSH receptor and TSH receptor autoantibodies. Endocrine. 2020 May;68(2):261-264. doi: 10.1007/s12020-019-02180-9. Epub 2020 May 29. PMID: 32472423

[19] Evans M, Sanders J, Tagami T, Sanders P, Young S, Roberts E, Wilmot J, Hu X, Kabelis K, Clark J, Holl S, Richards T, Collyer A, Furmaniak J, Smith BR: Monoclonal autoantibodies to the TSH receptor, one with stimulating activity and one with blocking activity, obtained from the same blood sample. Clin Endocrinol (Oxf) 2010;73:404-412

[20] Champion B, Gopinath B, Ma G, El-Kaissi S, Wall JR: Conversion to Graves' hyperthyroidism in a patient with hypothyroidism due to Hashimoto's thyroiditis documented by real-time thyroid ultrasonography. Thyroid. 2008;18:1135-1137. doi: 10.1089/thy.2008.0142.

[21] Hidaka Y, Tatsumi KI. Spontaneous transient Graves' thyrotoxicosis. Thyroid. 2008;18:1133-1134. doi: 10.1089/thy.2008.0159.

[22] Ludgate M, Emerson CH: Metamorphic thyroid autoimmunity. Thyroid. 2008 Oct; 18(10):1035-1037.

[23] Wasniewska M, Corrias A, Arrigo T, Lombardo F, Salerno M, Mussa A, Vigone MC, De Luca F: Frequency of Hashimoto's thyroiditis antecedents in the history of children and adolescents with Graves' disease. Horm Res Paediatr. 2010;73(6):473-476. doi: 10.1159/000313395. Epub 2010 Apr 15.

[24] Aversa T, Lombardo F, Corrias A, Salerno M, De Luca F, Wasniewska M: In young patients with Turner or Down syndrome, Graves' disease presentation is often preceded by Hashimoto's thyroiditis. Thyroid. 2014 Apr; 24(4):744-747.

[25] Karlsson B, Gustafsson J, Hedov G, Ivarsson SA, Anneren G. Thyroid dysfunction in Down's syndrome: relation to age and thyroid autoimmunity. Arch Dis Child. 1998;79:242-245.

[26] Soriano Guillén L, Muñoz Calvo MT, Pozo Román J, Martínez Pérez J, Baño Rodrigo A, Argente Oliver J.: [Graves' disease in patients with Down syndrome].An Pediatr (Barc). 2003 Jan;58(1):63-6. doi: 10.1016/s1695-4033(03)77994-6. PMID: 12628122

[27] Aversa T, Valenzise M, Salerno M, Corrias A, Iughetti L, Radetti G, De Luca F, Wasniewska M: Metamorphic thyroid autoimmunity in Down Syndrome: from Hashimoto's thyroiditis to Graves' disease and beyond. Ital J Pediatr. 2015 Nov 11;41:87. doi: 10.1186/s13052-015-0197-4. PMID: 26558364

[28] Nebesio TD, Eugster EA: Unusual thyroid constellation in Down syndrome: Congenital hypothyroidism, Graves' disease, and hemiagenesis in the same child. J Pediatr Endocrinol Metab. Author manuscript; available in PMC 2014 Jul 17.Published in final edited form as: J Pediatr Endocrinol Metab. 2009 Mar; 22(3): 263-268. PMCID: PMC4102130

[29] Klenczar K, Deja G, Kalina-Faska B, Jarosz-Chobot P: [Myasthenia gravis, Graves-Basedow disease and other autoimmune diseases in patient with diabetes type 1 - APS-3 case report, therapeutic complications]. Pediatr Endocrinol Diabetes Metab. 2017;23(3):159-164. Polish. doi: 10.18544/PEDM-23.03.0088. PMID: 29253037.

[30] Onesimo R, Cristina De Rose, Cipolla C, Silvia Della Casa, Leoni C, Salerni A, Ricci D, Zampino G: Basedow-Graves' disease in a pediatric patient with Stickler syndrome, a new endocrine finding to improve personalized treatment. Ital J Pediatr. 2020; 46: 178. Published online 2020 Dec 1. doi: 10.1186/s13052-020-00945-x PMCID: PMC7706036 PMID: 33256801

[31] Daikeler T, Labopin M, Di Gioia M, et al: Secondary autoimmune diseases occurring after HSCT for an autoimmune disease: a retrospective study of the EBMT Autoimmune Disease Working Party. Blood. 2011 Aug 11;118(6):1693-1698. doi: 10.1182/blood-2011-02-336156. Epub 2011 May 19. PMID: 21596847

[32] Daikeler T, Labopin M, Ruggeri A, et al: New autoimmune diseases after cord blood transplantation: a retrospective study of EUROCORD and the Autoimmune Disease Working Party of the European Group for Blood and Marrow Transplantation. Blood. 2013 Feb 7;121(6):1059-1064. doi: 10.1182/blood-2012-07-445965. Epub 2012 Dec 17.

[33] Sinha A, Abinun M, Gennery AR, Barge D, Slatter M, Cheetham T: Graves' immune reconstitution inflammatory syndrome in childhood. Thyroid. (2013) 23:1010-1014. 10.1089/thy.2012.0618

[34] Paketçi A, Demir K, Tüfekçi Ö, Acar S, Abacı A, Yılmaz Ş, Böber E: Graves' disease following allogenic hematopoietic stem cell transplantation for severe aplastic anemia: case report and literature review.J Pediatr Endocrinol Metab. 2018 Apr 25;31(5):589-593. doi: 10.1515/jpem-2017-0358. PMID: 29708883

[35] Kumar M, Goldman J: Severe aplastic anaemia and Grave's disease in a paediatric patient. Br J Haematol. 2002 Jul;118(1):327-329. doi: 10.1046/j.1365-2141.2002.03581.x. PMID: 12100169.

[36] Muller I, Moran C, Lecumberri B, Decallonne B, Robertson N, Jones J, Dayan CM: 2019 European Thyroid Association Guidelines on the Management of Thyroid Dysfunction following Immune Reconstitution Therapy. Eur Thyroid J. 2019 Jul;8(4):173-185. doi: 10.1159/000500881. Epub 2019 Jul 4. PMID: 31602359 PMCID: PMC6738237 DOI: 10.1159/000500881